CW00363152

The Mechanism of Acupuncture Therapy and Clinical Case Studies

The Mechanism of Acupuncture Therapy and Clinical Case Studies

Lily Cheung

Peng Li

and

Cheng Wong

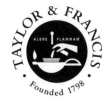

London and New York

First published 2001 by Taylor & Francis
11 New Fetter Lane, London EC4P 4EE

Simultaneously published in the USA and Canada
by Taylor & Francis Inc,
29 West 35th Street, New York, NY 10001

Taylor & Francis is an imprint of the Taylor & Francis Group

© 2001 Taylor & Francis

Typeset by EXPO
Printed and bound in Great Britain by MPG Books Ltd, Bodmin

Every effort has been made to ensure that the advice and information in this
book is true and accurate at the time of going to press. However, neither the
publisher nor the authors can accept any legal responsibility or liability for
any errors or omissions that may be made. In the case of drug
administration, any medical procedure or the use of technical equipment
mentioned within this book, you are strongly advised to consult the
manufacturer's guidelines.

British Library Cataloguing in Publication Data
A catalogue record for this book is available from the British Library

Library of Congress Cataloging in Publication Data
A catalog record has been requested

ISBN 0-415-27254-8

Contents

Foreword

Acupuncture has been practiced in China for well over two thousand years. However, it was not until President Richard Nixon's trip to China that acupuncture began to be accepted in Western countries, such as the United States and Europe. At this time, immigrants began flowing from China to these countries and the demand for acupuncture has increased steadily. Today, acupuncture is in its rightful place alongside Western therapies and payment for these services consumes a significant portion of our healthcare expenditures. Because of the increased demand for acupuncture and other alternative therapies, it is important for scientists and physicians to have a clear understanding of the mechanisms by which acupuncture can exert its beneficial effects.

In 1979 the World Health Organization held an interregional seminar in which it defined a number of diseases for which acupuncture could be considered to be potentially helpful. These include the treatment of acute infections and inflammation, dysfunction of the autonomic nervous system, pain, several cardiovascular diseases, asthma, tinnitus, drug abuse, mood and behavior disorders and various central and peripheral neurological diseases. Evidence for success in these disease states largely comes from reports in the literature confirming some evidence of efficacy. However, to date there have been no large-scale clinical trials. In November 1997, the National Institutes of Health published a consensus statement on acupuncture in which they examined a number of areas including public policy related to training and credentialing, adverse reactions, sham and the anatomy relating to meridians and acupoints. In addition, the National Institutes of Health indicated that there were a number of areas that should be devoted to future research in acupuncture. These include demographics, efficacy in various conditions, public policy and regulation and the biological basis underlying acupuncture's regulation of body organs.

As discussed in this monograph, pressure, heat and acupuncture needles have all been used in the form of therapy. Acupuncture needles either manipulated manually or stimulated with a low current and frequency have been best documented to induce beneficial effects. As discussed by Li, *et al.*, there appears to be a neurophysiological basis with many central neural pathways currently mapped. These pathways interact in a number of regions of the brain, many of which, either release or are affected by the release of endogenous opioids. This system appears to modify the activity of the autonomic system during physiological conditions such as exercise or other reflex inputs into the central nervous system or in pathologic disease states in which there is disordered neural and autonomic activity. Although many regions have been defined and their neurotransmitters identified, specific mechanisms underlying the regulation of activity of either reflex or descending neural control is poorly understood and requires further investigation.

The present work describes areas of our current knowledge and identifies gaps in our understanding. Hence, it provides a useful paradigm to educate both scientists and practitioners and to define areas of needed research for the future. The reader will find this monograph to be both informative and provocative since not only do the following chapters provide the status of our current knowledge but they also challenge scientists to better define acupuncture therapy.

John C. Longhurst, M.D., Ph.D.
Professor and Chair
Department of Medicine
University of California, Irvine
USA

Acknowledgements

Dr Lily Cheung has worked in clinical practice in London for many years. While working in the UK, I visited her, and was deeply impressed by her success in treating different kinds of disease. We talked often and exchanged ideas, and we finally decided to write a book which included all of Lily's clinical experience and the results of our research related to the mechanism of the effects of acupuncture.

Many results have been described in my monograph published in 1992[1]. This volume is an expanded and revised version of our work. It also includes the work of some of our colleagues from other universities, institutes and other countries. The monographs written by Huang KC[2] and Stux and Pomeranz[3] are very useful references. We are grateful to Professor Pomeranz for his good suggestions. We also appreciate Professor CY Chiang who helped us write Chapter 5. We should send many thanks to Professor FR Calaresu, HP Chen, JS Han, LF He, JS Tan, QZ Yin and J Yu, for sending us their important papers and information etc.

In editing this monograph, we wish to recall the warm and exciting experience of working with our colleagues over the past twenty years. Dr SX Lin is the first postgraduate student in our department who set up the chronic conscious animal model. I often recall the good days working with Professors T Yao, XQ Guo, QF Su, QL Gong, XY Sun and DN Zhu; and I miss my colleagues and students very much. They are Drs YF Xiao, Y Xia, DH Huangfu, Q Wang, SQ He, Q Lin, W Fan, W Wang, WH Wang, ZJ Sun, SY Sun and Z Zhang, etc. They worked very hard, had many clever ideas and made important contributions. I always remember my first wife, Professor RJ Lin, who died suddenly and untimely due to hard work over a long period and was exhausted at last. She was the first Chinese physiologist to set up a laboratory for intracellular recording of rostral ventrolateral medullary neurones *in vivo*. All my success, if any, was due to her help.

Our British friend, Dr TA Lovick, was the first foreign scientist to spend a period of time working with us in Shanghai. I learned much from her whilst working in Birmingham, and she has given us much help and has collaborated with us in the work which forms the basis of this volume. In recent years we have been pleased to collaborate with Professor JC Longhurst in California, USA, and have succeeded in setting up a feline model of reflex-induced myocardial ischemia, which can be inhibited by acupuncture. This work opened a new field of study, the mechanism of the inhibitory effect of acupuncture on myocardial ischemia, and will be very useful in cardiovascular medicine. We also wish to express our sincere thanks to Professors JH Coote, Y Hayashida, SM Hilton, XC Hu, A Sato, KM Spyer, JR Zhang, and Dr D Jorden for their very useful discussions, encouragement and help.

We wish to acknowledge that the projects related to the mechanism of acupuncture were supported by the National Natural Science Foundation of China, Science fund of the Chinese Ministry of Health, and National Educational Commission of China, as well as the IBRO Foundation for international collaboration and a NIH grant in the USA.

This monograph was written at the clinic of my son, Dr Jia Li, in Mississauga, Ontario, Canada. He supported me with the facilities for writing the monograph, and we often exchanged our ideas and had good discussions. He helped me to write Chapter 13 from his own work and experience. He also gave me the chance to have more clinical experience in treating chronic pain, cardiovascular disease and other diseases, difficult to treat by current western medicine. I would like to say many thanks to my present wife, Li-Ying Zhang, for taking care of me, helping me overcome difficulties and encouraging me to complete this monograph. I should also say many thanks to Mr J Fitzpatrick who helped me to correct my English writing.

This monograph is just a beginning to the scientific understanding of acupuncture and Traditional Chinese Medicine. It is to be hoped that more work will be done on this subject in the future.

Peng Li

References

1. Li, P. and Yao, T. ed. (1992) Mechanism of the modulatory effect of acupuncture on abnormal cardiovascular functions. Shanghai Med Univ Press, Shanghai.
2. Huang, K.C. (1996) Acupuncture the past and the present. Vantage Press, New York.
3. Pomeranz, B. and Paley, D. (1979) Electroacupuncture hyalgesia is medicated by afferent nerve impulses: an elctrophysiological study in mice. Exp Neurol, 66: 398–402.

SECTION 1
MECHANISM OF ACUPUNTURE THERAPY

Peng Li

In China, acupuncture has been used to treat patients with various kinds of diseases for more than two and a half thousand years. The Chinese ancients put forward the "meridian hypothesis" to explain the mechanism of acupuncture therapy. This was described in detail in the "Yellow Emperor's Classics of Internal Medicine." As physiologists, we realize that the so-called "meridian hypothesis" is merely our ancestor's understanding of the bodily regulatory systems and their functions, which existed long before the discovery and realization of the integrative function of the central nervous system and the humoral system. As the long history of clinical practice has proved acupuncture to have curative effects, it must have a physiological acupuncture and further clarify its mechanism.

My teacher, Professor Feng-Yen Hsu of the First Medical College of Shanghai, had a strong desire to investigate the mechanism of acupuncture in the late 1950s. He organized a research team, designed the projects, started the research work and experienced the sensation of acupuncture by being needled by us, his students. In the 1960s and 70s, most of the laboratories of physiology and the big hospitals in China were enthusiastic in studying the analgesic effect of acupuncture; we also worked in this area, and gained important data and experience. For example, we learned that using electric potential, resistance or impedance methods to detect the meridian line on the body is not viable. Although these methods were fashionable at one stage, and were introduced by the Japanese, they had many technical problems to do with basic physiological knowledge. The idea of searching for the meridian line on the body surface is also incorrect, so most physiologists and neuroscientists decided to stop such work.

From the late 1970s, we felt that too many people in our country were concentrating on one project, acupuncture analgesia. Even in studying the mechanism of acupuncture, there are many interesting and important topics which ought to be studied. So, we turned our attention to studying the effects of acupuncture on abnormal cardiovascular functions. In the first year we did a lot of experiments using different models and methods, but all failed. Finally we thought that this may be due to the aesthetics and surgery. It is already known that in their clinics, acupuncturists usually only perform acupuncture on conscious patients without anaesthetic. We recalled the work of Hu et al. in 1960, who reported a positive effect of acupuncture on experimental hypertension and hypotension in chronic conscious dogs (see chapter 4). We repeated that model and succeeded. We now knew that except in conscious animals, some anaesthetics could be used. Eventually, we also learned what kind of anaesthetic can be used, and what to do after surgical operations on animals.

Fortunately, over the past twenty years, our work has been going smoothly. We have been working together not only with Chinese colleagues, but also with colleagues of other countries. On the basis of our achievements, we published more than one hundred papers in Chinese and in international journals, and reported at many international congresses of physiology, neuroscience and acupuncture. Our research group won the first and second grade awards sponsored by the Chinese Ministry of Health and the Chinese National Education Commission eight times.

1 THE HISTORY AND DEVELOPMENT OF CHINESE MEDICINE

Cheng Wong

There is an ancient saying in China which echoes popular understanding that medicine and food have the same origin and it was through the search for food that medicinal qualities of plants and animals and insects were discovered. By the process of trial and error the identity and properties of various plants were recognised. Gradually the medicinal qualities of barks, leaves, roots, flowers, fruits, seeds were written up. Medicinal derivatives from animals and insects were also recorded.

Moxibustion was probably discovered from the use of fire. Use of warmth on parts of the body probably produced some relief of local pain. The initial use of heated stones and sand had been recorded and eventually the use of a plant like moxa (artemis vulgaris) developed for heat stimulation of definitive areas of the body.

Improvements in the use of tools led to the production of specialised tools for massage, draining of pus, bloodletting and the pricking of the skin. Various medical instruments such as these have been excavated in various parts of China. They probably indicate the beginning of acupuncture. The earliest instruments excavated were shaped from stone. These were known as Bian Stones—"bian" meaning the curing of diseases by pricking with a stone. Metal needles used in later times were believed to be developed from these primitive instruments.

As Chinese society began to recognise the existence of diseases, these were recorded in hieroglyphs inscribed on bones and tortoise shells according to the part of the body affected. These were the earliest records of their kind. As more diseases were recognised, these were recorded according to their characteristics. As the causes of diseases became clearer, superstitious beliefs began to fade into the background. They could see the link between diseases and food, climate, the environmental changes, mental factors and specific regional conditions. They also recognised that certain conditions could bring on an epidemic which could be contagious.

As usage and knowledge of medicinal substances expanded, these were taken in the form of medicated wine, compound prescriptions and decoctions and external applications. The practice of collecting herbs could be found reflected in folk songs before the 5th century BC. A good diet had been one of the requisites for healthy living. Uncontrolled eating was seen as one of the causes of diseases. To this day, avoidance of certain foods is used in preventing and treating disease. Food was seen as a way to combat pathogenic factors and for improving the energy resources of the body. Ge Hong wrote in the "Prescription for Emergencies" that he used seaweed to treat goitres and soy-beans for beri-beri. Since then the incorporation of herbs and many ordinary food substances into daily dietary recipes for treatment and health maintenance has become part of Chinese culture. During this period, there were also records of minerals being used as medicinal substances.

The theoretical system of Traditional Chinese Medicine (TCM), was believed to be formed during the second half of the 5th century BC to the middle of the 3rd century AD. The Huang Di Nei Jing (The Inner Canon of The Yellow Emperor) laid the theoretical foundation for TCM. This was believed to be compiled by many practitioners who collected and systemised various medical works between the 5th and the 3rd century BC. This was continuously studied and added to by others in later generations. One of the prominent physicians, Zhang Zhongjing, published "The Treatise on Cold Diseases and Miscellaneous Disorders" in the 2nd century. He laid down the principles for treatment according to the differentiation of the symptom-complex. Another well-known publication was "The Shen Nong's Classic of Herbalism", completed in the early part of the 1st century AD was a collection of experiences of many practising physicians. Although the original works had been lost, later versions were largely based on the knowledge from the original. It was in this Treatise that Zhang Zhongjing (150-219AD) laid down the principles of diagnosis namely, inspection; auscultation; olfaction; interrogation and palpation, and to differentiate these according to the 8 principles. He laid down 8 therapeutic methods, namely: diaphoresis, purgation, emesis, mediation, heat reduction, invigoration, tonification and resolution. These basic principles of treating each condition according to the overall symptoms continue to influence practice today. He was also the first to expound the idea that all diseases fall under one of 3 categories: 1) factors arising from inside the body; 2) factors arising outside the body; 3) factors from excesses in living and 4) those arising from trauma. The number of pharmaceutical forms recorded by Zhang includes decoction, boluses, powders, medicated wines, lotions for washing and bathing, fumigants, ear and nose drops, ointments and anal and vaginal suppositories.

Another eminent physician was Hua Tuo who lived in the 2nd century AD. He was also a skilled surgeon and believed to be the first to use anaesthesia. He actively promoted exercises as part of health care and developed a series emulating the movements of animals. His skills as an acupuncturist were well known. Some of his techniques are still used today. Around this time, some of the physicians were also involved in alchemy in order to attempt to supply the rulers at the time with life-prolonging elixirs. The search for immortality gradually lost favour after the 10th century but during that time there evolved an understanding of the chemical behaviour of some substances.

From the middle of the 3rd century AD. to the 14th century AD., medical practitioners began to study and systemise and add to the Huang Di Nei Jing and the Treatise on Cold Diseases & Miscellaneous Disorders. One of these physicians—Wang Shuhe wrote the "Classic of Sphygmology" in which he identified syndromes and determined treatment in line with the pulse conditions. He gave clear descriptions of methods used to differentiate pulse conditions and established the method for feeling the pulse at the "cunkou" position alone. In 1341, Dr. Du Ben published the "Ao's Golden Mirror of Cold Diseases" which concentrated on the appearance of the tongue and the pathological conditions related to the various types of tongue colour and coatings.

In 657 AD. the Tang government organised a revision of herbs and their use and issued the earliest official pharmacopoeia in the world. This work supplemented and revised the discrepancies and errors made earlier. The preparation and quality of herbs had always been closely linked with their therapeutic effects in clinical applications. From the time of the Shen Nong's Classic of Herbalism, it had already stated the importance of preparing herbs before use i.e., drying by sudden heat; times for collection and preparation; collection from cultivated and uncultivated land; genuine or fake; stale or fresh. In the 5th century, the first work in China dealing with herb preparation appeared and had been updated ever since. The different methods included steaming; baking; frying; boiling; roasting; infusing; water processing and a process known as calcining where the substance is heated in fire until red. The purpose of preparation was to enhance the therapeutic effects and in some cases to remove toxicity. Ready-made remedies also started to become popular and grinding was used to produce pills and powder. Baking and toasting were also methods used to preserve medicinal products.

The history of acupuncture and moxibustion can be traced back to antiquity. Archaeological findings of works on bamboo slips and silk revealed that over 3,000 years ago, physicians were already discussing meridians and moxibustion in their treatments. Well known physicians like Hua Tuo, Zhang Zhongjing and Bian Que were also skilled in acupuncture and moxibustion. The Huang Di Nei Jing and other publications had extensive discussions and theories relating to acupuncture, moxibustion, meridians, locations of points and manipulative techniques. In the 3rd century AD., Huangfu Mi published his theories and experiences exclusively on acupuncture and moxibustion. He determined the courses of the 12 regular meridians, the 8 extraordinary meridians and the major symptoms of related diseases. He specified the total number of acupuncture points and their locations. He determined the depth of needle insertions, the number of moxa cones for each treatment and the methods of manipulation according to diagnosis. At the same time, he described diseases according to their aetiology, pathogeneses, symptoms and the points to be used for treatment. Later works on acupuncture and moxibustion would be based on his work. Over the years, as records were lost and different interpretations were put on various works, there existed discrepancies and lack of agreement regarding meridians and point locations. Wang Weiyi (987–1067), a medical official in the Imperial Medical Bureau, made a careful study of past records and compiled a 3 volume summary which systemised the 12 regular meridians, the Du and the Ren meridians, and the locations of 354 points and their functions. This made it easier for physicians in the later generations to make sense of the theory and applications of acupuncture and moxibustion. One of Wang Weiyi's teaching tools was a 3 dimensional cast bronze model. This would be covered in a layer of wax and filled with water. When a student inserts the needle in the correct position, the water would leak. Around the same time, Wang Zhizhong established the unit for measuring and locating acupuncture points for each patient. During this period, some practitioners were also trying out methods for selecting points according to the time of day and to observe whether this would enhance the therapeutic effects.

Some physicians were also quite skilled in orthopaedics. In the 4th century, Ge Hong, recommended the use of bamboo splints for fractures. He recognised 3 major categories of traumatic injuries of bones and joints, namely: fractures; dislocations; open wounds. At the same time he classified the different types of fractures. In the 19th century, a taoist priest described methods of treatment for orthopaedic and traumatic disorders. These included methods of external fixation, suturing, external and oral medication for open fractures. From the 10th to the 14th century, wars were frequent in China. This helped to increase the skills of bone setting and treatment of knife and other traumatic injuries and the use of anaesthesia.

As communication and travel between countries became easier, there were cultural and medical exchanges between China, Rome, Japan and other South East Asian countries. Contacts with the Arab countries began in the 7th century AD. Herbs and medical expertise were exported to these countries as well as importing materials and local medical knowledge from these countries. From the 16th century onwards, western missionary doctors started to enter China. They brought with them, western medical knowledge. One of them, Michel Boym translated some of the chinese medical publications when he returned to Poland in 1656. These in turn were published in France, Italy and Germany and had a great influence on an English doctor, Sir John Floyer. Between the 12th and the 19th century, study and development of the various aspects of chinese medicine continued. During this period there was some improvement in the study of anatomy. The study of anatomy from cadavers only started from the 11th century. Even then, there remained a cultural stigma attached to such studies. Although there was to be a further improvement in this field, it was the import of western medicine that made the breakthrough in this field in China.

The use of acupuncture and moxibustion was encouraged after the 11th century, during the time of the Ming Dynasty. One of the more well known physician at the time, Yang Jizhou (1522–1620) wrote about his experiences of combining acupuncture and moxibustion and oral medication in his case histories. After the 18th century, the popularity of acupuncture and moxibustion went into decline as the ruler of the time concluded that "needling and burning" were not suitable for the nobles. In 1822, the Qing Dynasty government ordered the "Acupuncture and Moxibustion Department" in the Imperial Medical Academy to terminate its practice although it had remained popular with the common people. As a result there were not many important works published or written on the subject from that period.

In the meantime, acupuncture and moxibustion had been introduced into many of the European countries since the 17th century. Similarly, more missionary doctors came into China and translated western medical works into chinese. Western drugs began to be available in the country. European style hospitals were set up together with educational facilities. By the 19th century, western medicine was practised widely throughout China. An independent system of practice and education became established side by side with traditional chinese medicine. The study and use of western medicine gained in importance and influence after the opium war. Some of the local chinese became specialised in western medicine and others were even sent abroad to study. Missionary doctors became involved in treating the emperor in the imperial court. So western medicine gradually existed with traditional chinese medicine. As western influences expanded after the opium war, so did the education and use of western medicine. In such an atmosphere, extremes schools of thought were created. There was one group which rejected traditional chinese medicine and another which rejected western medicine. There were also others who could see the benefits of both systems and believed that integration would benefit everyone. One of the first to recognise this was Tang Zonghai (1862–1918). He believed the principles of both systems to be the same and integration would make better sense. Others who follow also believed that chinese herbal medicine can supplement western drugs and the differences in descriptions of causes and symptoms presents no barrier in the two systems working together to achieve the same outcome.

The regime prior to the People's Republic of China acted to discriminate against traditional chinese medicine both in practise and education. Publications and journals were also forbidden. When the communist party took over the country, doctors of traditional and western medicine were encouraged to co-operate and set up a health programme for the country.

After the founding of the People's Republic of China in 1949, three main areas of health were targeted—provision of health care to the masses; prevention; uniting the expertise of traditional and western doctors. Institutions for research were set up as part of medical colleges and universities. Doctors of TCM were invited to work in these institutions which in turn, provide them with further medical training. The teaching of TCM became part of the state programme for higher education. Research and systemisation of TCM became one of the priorities.

During this period, there were experiments in surgery using acupuncture analgesia which increased the understanding of the mechanism of acupuncture. New research methods began to be introduced to investigate the traditional theories of Yin and Yang, their deficiencies, concepts like the kidney essence and the therapeutic principle of strengthening the body's resistance and concepts like invigorating blood circulation to remove stagnation. At present there is a realisation that it is necessary to study and research chinese medical theory in the light of modern scientific theory. In the field of pharmacy, there is an urgent need to provide good quality herbs and to distinguish the genuine from the fake. Research continues to discover the active ingredients of herbal substances, their contra-indications, their side effects and the effect they have when taken with standard western drugs.

2 THE CONCEPTS IN TRADITIONAL CHINESE MEDICINE

Cheng Wong

Traditional Chinese Medicine considers the human body to be a part of nature. Thus, consideration of the human body is taken in its relation to its environment. The system that is in use now is developed from thousands of years of clinical practice and study. The basic principle is to apply treatment according to the differentiation of syndromes. This practice is influenced by the dialectical concepts of Yin and Yang and the 5 Elements (Wu Xing). These provide a guide to the course of the disease or dysfunction in the human body.

The basic theory was developed between 475 BC–24 AD. Through the chaos of the wars during this period and the various doctrines, the dialectical principals of Yin & Yang and the 5 Elements emerged. These principals were the results of the combined clinical experiences of practitioners over hundreds of years and who were also influenced by the philosophical thoughts at the time. The Huang Di Nei Jing was the first work to set down these theories systematically, followed by "The Classic of Questions" which cleared up some of the inadequacies of the former. From these, others developed the theory of meridians and Zang-fu organs; the influence of emotions, exogenous factors, climatic factors and other factors i.e. trauma and nutrition, as the causes of disease. Modern approaches stress the importance of research on conditions of for example, Yin deficiency (Xu); Yang Xu; the nature of cold and heat; the essence of the kidney, spleen and meridians and to understand them in terms of modern medical terminology.

According to TCM, the body is viewed as a system in which the Zang-fu organs are connected by meridians. This system can be influenced by the external environment. The 4 diagnostic methods and the "8 Principals" provide for the differentiation of syndromes (Bian Zheng). This is elaborated further by the "theory of Zang-fu organs". The aim of this differentiation is to describe the root cause of the patient's condition, taking into consideration the environmental condition and the patient's constitution. Each Zang-fu organ is always considered in relation to the whole. Harmonious function of the Zang-fu is necessary for homeostasis. This function is aided by the

12 meridians, qi, blood and body fluids. This integrity of the whole is expressed in terms of Yin & Yang and the 5 Elements. These theories provide the basis on which the stages of illness or "inequilibrium" are judged. Observation of the 5 sense organs, the constitution, complexion and pulse condition provide the basic clues for assessment.

"Differentiation of Syndromes" (Bian Zheng) allows for different syndromes to be found in the same disease and similarly the same syndrome to be found in different diseases. In summary, the practise of TCM encompasses a system of theories:

1   Yin & Yang and the 5 Elements
2   The Zang-fu organs
3   The concept of essence, qi, blood and body fluids
4   The meridian system
5   Aetiology and pathogenesis
6   Prevention and treatment

YIN & YANG

These concepts in materialism and dialectics helped the ancient Chinese to make sense of the opposing and at the same time, complementary forces in the material world. They helped to provide the language needed to explain similar changes going on in the body especially during ill health. Consequently, diagnosis and treatment can be systemised. Today, as a result of research and with a better knowledge of the pathological and physiological changes, doctors are able to see the limitations and inadequacies of the old system and be able to proceed with the essentials.

Originally, Yin was used to describe the shady slope of a mountain and Yang the sunny side. These terms were broadened to include all opposites. So when we are considering—a downward tendency, a movement towards the interior, a state of rest, the left in relation to the right—they will have a Yin quality and the opposites, a Yang quality. This abstract concept states that Yin and Yang is present in all things. It is their interdependence and their opposition that creates the duality and the changes we see in natural phenomena. It is applied when we are considering related objects or two aspects of one phenomena. Under certain conditions, Yin may tend towards Yang and Yang towards Yin. Every aspect can be divided infinitely into Yin and Yang. To apply Yin and Yang in Chinese Medicine is to be aware of the dynamic equilibrium created by opposition, interdependence and mutual transformation. A normal state of health in the body depends on the equilibrium created by the interaction of Yin and Yang in relation to its environment and in its reaction to external forces. Their interdependence reflects the relationship between the organs within the body. For example, qi pertains to yang and blood pertains to yin. Qi is responsible for the movement of blood but blood itself also provides the material basis for qi. Also in basic physiological functions, we see relative increases (yang) or decreases (yin) in activity. Their relative equilibrium helps to maintain homeostasis. In this state of relative equilibrium, one can dominate the other as yang dominates the day, and yin dominates the night. Any factors distorting this equilibrium will be represented by the recorded pathological manifestations of Yin and Yang. During the course of a disease, Yang may turn into Yin and vice versa. For example, persistent pyrexia associated with heat can turn into a yin syndrome when the body temperature drops presenting symptoms of pallor and a faint pulse and treatment will change accordingly.

When applying the Yin/Yang theory to the structure of the body, the external is considered yang, so is the dorsal part, the upper part, the lateral aspects etc. In terms of the internal organs,—the gallbladder; the stomach; large and small intestine; the urinary bladder are considered yang including the region referred to as the triple jiao. These are the Fu organs. The Zang organs are the liver; heart; spleen; lung and kidney. These are considered yin. The organs are also yang or yin in relation to each other. The tendons and bones correspond to yin and the skin, yang.

Normal physiological activity is seen as an expression of Yin and Yang. In terms of pathological changes, yang pathogenic factors damages yin and leads to yang syndromes. Yin pathogenic factors damages yang and gives rise to cold (yin) syndromes. Heat syndromes may appear when damaged yin is not controlling yang, giving rise to a false heat syndrome.

Generally speaking, cold syndromes are caused either by an excess of yin or a deficiency (Xu) of yang. Heat syndromes are caused by an excess of yang or a "xu of yin". When the deficiency of either reaches a critical stage, it brings about of "xu of yin and yang". Clinically, this will be observed in chronic conditions.

To use these manifestations accurately as a guide to diagnosis and treatment, the TCM practitioner must be skilled in using his own senses when considering the symptoms. When there is a simple excess of one or the other, treatment is directed to reducing the excess (Shi). When there is a relative excess as a result of a deficiency of the other, treatment will necessitate reinforcing the xu condition as well. If herbs are used for harmonising the yin & yang, it is important that the practitioner is familiar with the basic qualities of the herbs also in terms of yin and yang because this quality has a direct relationship to their actions.

THE 5 ELEMENTS

The ancient Chinese believe that there are 5 elements which are necessary for life. These are Wood; Fire; Earth; Metal and Water. They symbolise the relationship and actions occurring in nature and in our bodies. Various organs and their functions are attributed to the elements. These attributes provide a guide to the possible progress or regression of an illness and gives the doctor a clue to areas requiring treatment. For example, a preference for sour food and a taut pulse will indicate "liver" function problems (function here refers to the function of the liver according to the Zang-fu theory). In order to prevent this upset affecting the "spleen" function (according to the theory, when Wood-liver is in excess, Earth-spleen can be harmed), treatment will have to be given along the lines of "controlling Wood excess and tonifying Earth). Thus, even when the practitioner does not have a deep understanding of human physiology, he has a guide to dispense the right treatment, but only if his original assessment of the syndrome is correct.

THE ZANG-FU ORGANS

In Chinese medicine, the Zang-fu system, do not only refer to the organs themselves but also to the manifestations of their functions and the way their pathological changes are reflected on the surface of the body. Mental activities and emotions are also linked to the activities of the Zang-fu system, so one can influence the other.

The Zang organs for example, also share a common physiological function in producing and storing essence and qi. The Fu organs share containing, transporting, digesting and excreting. The other organs that do not fit into the above categories, e.g. the brain, uterus, blood vessels and bone—they share a function of storing essence and qi.

To extend the concept of integrity, each Zang organ is related to a Fu organ. For example, the kidney with the urinary bladder. Each Zang organ is also linked to a group of tissues and connected to the exterior via a sense organ. Pathology in organic function can be observed in the sense organ or manifested in the tissues. For example, the heart is linked to the blood vessels, circulation of the blood, mental activities and the tongue.

So problems with the heart function can manifest itself in symptoms of lassitude, poor memory, disturbed sleep, a pale puffy tongue and a pale complexion.

With this system, every aspect of the functions of the body comes under consideration. The TCM doctor, thus tends not to neglect other areas of the body when there is a problem with one part.

All these relationships stem from years of clinical observations linked to effective treatment. Concepts and ideas that do not work would be discarded in the process as is the situation in all forms of medicine.

ESSENCE, QI, BLOOD AND BODY FLUIDS

Essence (jing) is an essential part of the body that helps to maintain homeostasis. Qi is an abstract concept of the ancient philosophers which maintain that qi is the fundamental block of all living things and that their continued development depends on the proper functioning of qi. The concept of qi and its activities continue to be used to describe the changing activities of the body. Blood is another essential consideration in chinese medicine. Other then its obvious function and relationship to the heart, blood is closely related to the function of the liver, spleen and mental activities. Body fluids, another concept in chinese medicine, refers to all fluids normally secreted in the body i.e. saliva; gastric juices; etc. Their activities are controlled by the normal activities of the spleen, lung and kidney, helping to maintain the conditions of the joints, bone, brain, skin and all the muscles.

THE MERIDIANS

The development of the "meridians theory" is closely related to the practice of acupuncture. The meridians and collaterals (Jing-luo) forms a specific network to connect every part of the body and influence their activities. The system provides a guide particularly to clinical acupuncture. As they connect various parts of the body, they reflect disorders of particular organs or regions. Thus, for pain in the forehead, the Yang Ming meridian can be used for needle insertions. Through clinical observations, changes in the skin or tissues (presence of nodules for instance), can present itself according to the corresponding organic function. For example, with lung disease, tenderness or nodules may be palpated at point Feishu (UB 13—at level T3) or with appendicitis, at point Lanweixue (2 units inferior to point Zusanli) on the Stomach meridian. Through clinical observations, it was also recorded that certain herbs have an affinity for certain organs and their associated meridians. For example, Radix Angelicae Dahuricae is used for headaches associated with the Yang Ming meridian.

Thus, the meridian theory have always provided a guide to treatment after the correct syndrome had been diagnosed. Research into acupuncture this century has shown that the body's response to needle stimulation involves different types of endorphins, hormones and neurotransmitters in the body's effort to return the system back to a state of homeostasis. Only some of these substances have been identified and they have a direct relationship to the frequency and duration of stimulation and the correct combination and insertion of the needles.

AETIOLOGY

When the body is in good health, it is believed to be in equilibrium within itself and in relation to its environment. This equilibrium is not static. If conditions change either within or without the body, and the ability to adapt did not follow, the balance is lost and pathological symptoms will appear.

In Chinese medicine, the cause of disease is termed "pathogenic qi". The physiological functions that make up the ability to recover from a pathological process is termed "antipathogenic qi".

One group of "pathogenic qi" is the "Six Climatic Factors"—wind, cold, summer-heat, damp, dryness and fire. These are the normal seasonal changes in China. These changes are only harmful if they occur too abruptly or if the body is not adapting properly. Each seasonal factor has its own characteristics. Sometimes, disorders are caused by more than one factor e.g. wind, cold and damp can bring on a Bi-syndrome or damp and heat can affect the large intestine function. This concept also includes the idea of bacterial, viral infections and trauma from physical and chemical factors. If there are no obvious external influences, the 6 pathogenic factors are used to describe the endogenous factors. These are factors which appear to originate from within as a manifestation of organ dysfunction with resultant disturbances in qi, blood and body fluids. Thus disturbances can be described as endogenous wind or endogenous cold, etc.

Wind is a yang pathogen characterised by "upward, outward and dispersion". "Wind" will affect the yang part of the body first, i.e. the surface and upper part of the body. This can lead to sweating and headaches (as in flu). Wind is characterised by its unpredictability, so if wind is the cause, symptoms can be seen to spread throughout the system rapidly. One example is "wind-Bi" when one joint is affected after another. Another example is urticaria. In summary, the effects of "wind" are sudden and the resultant disturbances spread quickly. Wind usually combines with the other factors to disrupt the body.

Cold predominates obviously in winter. This can manifest as an exogenous attack, e.g. an obvious "cold" or an interior attack where the yang qi of the Zang-fu is affected as when cold symptoms are accompanied by diarrhoea and vomiting. Pathogenic cold usually produces pain due to qi and blood obstruction. Contractions may also occur. If the blood vessels are attacked, there will be symptoms of headaches, general aches and a tense pulse.

Summer-heat predominates in the summer especially at the end of the season. This will cause yang symptoms of high fever, restlessness, a flushed complexion and a bounding pulse. It can consume body fluids as in abnormal sweating causing dehydration with thirst and concentrated urine. In severe cases, it will lead to shortness of breath, lassitude and loss of consciousness. It can be accompanied by damp especially if it is a wet summer. This will present with additional symptoms of loose stools or nausea.

Damp is predominates towards the end of summer. This is usually the wettest part of the year in China. This can lead to spleen dysfunction with symptoms of water retention. It is a yin factor which will disrupt the normal flow of qi with symptoms of lung congestion, concentrated urine and disruption in bowel movements. If the yang qi is damaged, loose stools will result. Presence of discharges e.g. stickiness in eyes, or vaginal discharge, is representative of pathogenic damp. It usually attacks the lower parts of the body causing oedema.

Dryness predominates in the autumn when the humidity decreases during this period. This factor can be divided into a warm-dryness or a cool-dryness. Warm-dryness usually occurs in the early part of the season. Dryness will cause a parched throat, dry skin, lustreless hair, concentrated urine and constipation. It can impair lung function, which disturbs the normally descending lung qi and causes dry coughs and shortness of breath.

Fire and heat result from excessive yang. Heat can be wind-heat, summer- heat or damp-heat. Fire is usually seen to be produced internally as in heart- fire, hyperactivity of liver-fire and stomach-fire. Pathogenic fire tends to cause high fever, restlessness, thirst, perspiration and a bounding rapid pulse and further to insomnia, mania, anxiety delirium and finally coma. There may also be redness of the eyes, a red tip of the tongue, mouth ulcers, swelling and pain in the gums. Fire can also affect the liver and impair the tendons. This will stir up liver-wind with symptoms of high fever, coma, delirium, convulsions, neck rigidity and upward turn of the eyes. Haemorrhage may occur in one part or another of the body. Carbuncles, boils etc., are also examples of fire.

In addition to the climatic factors, the ancient chinese also believe that there are certain substances in the environment that are capable of causing diseases of epidemic proportions and transmitted via the mouth and nose. These were thought to arise from abnormal weather conditions, and pollution of the air, water or food.

The Chinese also classified emotions into 7 types. These were, joy, anger, melancholy, anxiety, grief, terror and fright. They believed that if emotions become too intense or extreme, functional disorders of related zang-fu organs result. Anger injures the liver and causes an upward surge of qi, excessive joy injures the heart and causes qi to scatter, anxiety injures the spleen and causes qi to stagnate, grief injures the lung and depresses qi and terror/fright injures the kidney and causes qi to descend. The upward surge of qi results in dyspnoea, a flushed complexion, red eyes even haematamesis and fainting. A scattering of qi produces an inability to concentrate or may lead to mental disorders. Depression of qi can cause lung dysfunction with dyspnoea and lassitude and low spirits. Terror can result in an abnormal downward flow of kidney qi represented by urinary incontinence, faecal incontinence, lumbago, nocturnal emissions and weakness in the lower limbs. To a lesser degree, fright results in mental restlessness and insecurity. Qi stagnation manifests itself in palpitations, amnesia, insomnia and dream disturbed sleep, poor appetite, abdominal distension, diarrhoea or loose stools. It is also believed that all emotions affect the heart first. Conversely, qi and blood disturbances resulting from other causes can lead to a manifestations of those emotions. Excessive emotions can also exacerbate existing conditions, e.g., anger can increase the pathological symptoms of a patient already suffering with hypertension. Generally speaking, excessive emotions affect the heart, liver or spleen either on their own or in combination.

Food is an essential part of life. According to ancient thought, it is the source of qi and blood. So, if food intake is inadequate, excess or improper, disruption of organ function will result. The immune system will be impaired. Excessive consumption of cold and raw foods can also damage the stomach and spleen. This results in cold-damp, with symptoms of abdominal pain and loose stools. Excess pungent or spicy food and alcohol cause phlegm and stagnation with symptoms of ulceration or haemorrhoids.

Physical exercise is also an important component of a healthy life. It helps to promote the proper functioning of the spleen and stomach qi. Adequate rest is also important to restore mental and physical energy. Excessive mental strain can damage the heart and spleen functions, leading to palpitations, poor memory, insomnia, dream-disturbed sleep, poor appetite, abdominal distension and loose stools. Excessive sexual activity reduces kidney qi and essence. This leads to general debility, soreness in the kidney region, dizziness, tinnitus, lassitude, diminished libido, nocturnal emissions, premature ejaculation and impotence.

Phlegm-fluid retention and blood stagnation are the results of organ dysfunction. Conversely, they can be viewed as causes for organ dysfunction. Phlegm or phlegm-fluid retention has broad manifestations in chinese medicine. They can refer to sputum or other forms of retained fluid or pathological manifestation of problems associated with fluid e.g., dizziness, nausea, vomiting, shortness of breath, palpitations or semi-consciousness. Phlegm can be cold, hot, dry, wind or damp. These conditions are usually caused by environmental conditions, bad eating habits or emotional distress. The organs usually affected are the lung, spleen, kidney and the qi of the triple jiao. The clinical manifestations are the results of the particular organ or organs affected. Phlegm blocking the lung will result in coughing, bronchial spasms and production of sputum. If it affects the heart, tightness of the chest or palpitations may result. If the heart meridian is obstructed, there may be a loss of consciousness or dementia may set in. If phlegm-fire affects the heart, mania occurs. When phlegm stagnates in the stomach, there is a feeling of fullness and there may be nausea and vomiting. Phlegm in the meridians may result in numbness of the limbs or hemiplegia. Dizziness is caused by phlegm affecting the head. Phlegm and qi stagnating in the throat produces the sensation of a lump affecting the throat. Fluids in the stomach produces gurgling sounds. If it stagnates in the costal region, there occurs a fullness in the chest and pain on coughing. If it stays in the diaphragm, there will be, coughing, dyspnoea especially in the recumbent position and puffiness. Oedema in the tissues and skin gives a feeling of heaviness in the body. Diagnosis is aided by observing the appearance of the tongue coating.

Blood stagnation is also a result of organ dysfunction. This may occur in the meridians, in the tissues or in the organs themselves. Impaired blood circulation results from stagnant qi, cold or heat in the blood. Stagnation in the heart produces palpitations, tightness in the chest, angina and a purplish colour of the lips and nails. Too much stagnant blood in the heart will eventually lead to mania. Blood stagnation in the lung, results in chest pain and haemoptasis. Stagnation in the stomach and the intestines causes haematemesis and constipation. Blood stagnation in the uterus results in lower abdominal pain, irregularities with menstruation with probably dark purplish menses and clots. In the liver, stagnation produces pain in the hypochondriac region. Gangrene in the extremities will be seen as stagnation in the limbs. Localised purplish or greenish skin colour in the skin represents stagnation blood on the body surface. Symptoms of obstruction in the blood vessels, haemorrhage or impaired blood circulation are believed to be caused by blood stagnation. If this occurs in the organs themselves, lumps or clots may be present. Common symptoms of blood stagnation will normally include stabbing, fixed pains aggravated by pressure and usually at night; localised purplish clots from external trauma or fixed tangible clots from internal disorders. These are usually accompanied by a dark complexion, dry scaly skin, cyanosed lips and nails, purplish tongue, petechia, ecchymosis, varicose veins under the tongue, and a thready and rough, deep and taut or intermittent pulse.

Pathogenesis

YIN AND YANG

The onset of disease or dysfunction, its development and outcome have a direct relationship to the body's constitution. Our resistance and ability to overcome disease (traditionally referred to as antipathogenic qi), creates the various pathological changes that can be described as disturbances or imbalances between yin and yang.

These changes are described as deficiency (xu) or excess (shi). Xu syndromes refers to a diminishing of "vital energy". Shi syndromes refers to the ascendant of the disease at the time—usually at the early or intermediate stages. Shi disturbances may be manifested as excessive phlegm production, indigestion, poor circulation, high fever, dysmenorrhoea, restlessness, lowering of the voice, abdominal pain, disruption to urinary and digestive system and a full and forceful pulse. Xu syndromes refers to the inadequacy of qi, blood, body fluids, the meridians and the zang-fu organs in resisting the progress of a disease at the time of examination. This is usually seen in a chronic condition and when the body's constitution is weak or in severe acute cases where the immune system has been rapidly compromised. The xu syndrome is usually associated with symptoms lassitude, pale and lustreless complexion, palpitations, shortness of breath, spontaneous sweating especially at night, feverish sensations in the palms, soles and chest, aversion to cold, cold limbs and a feeble pulse.

During the course of a disease or when complications set in both syndromes may be present.

Pathological changes described as imbalances between yin and yang can be classified into 5 categories:

1   Relative Excess of Yin or Yang
2   Relative Deficiency of Yin or Yang
3   The Deficiency of one affecting the other
4   The Excess of one affecting the other
5   The Exhaustion of Yin or Yang or both

QI & BLOOD

The deficiency and dysfunction of qi and blood is linked to the function of the zang-fu organs and meridians. Qi disturbances are represented by qi stagnation, adverse flow, sinking, blockage and collapse. Qi xu is represented by weakened resistance to a pathological process and manifested by lassitude, weakness, dizziness, spontaneous sweating and aversion to cold. The proper movement of qi ensures good health. Qi stagnation can arise from emotional upsets, indigestion, poor circulation, damp or phlegm. Stagnation of qi will interfere with the ascending function of the liver and spleen and the normally descending function of the stomach and lung or vice versa. Stagnation usually manifests as distension and pain, blood stasis and phlegm-fluid retention. Adverse flow refers to reversed movement of qi. For example, when the normal downward flow of the lung and stomach qi is reversed, it will be manifested by coughing, bronchial spasms and vomiting. The "sinking of qi" represents a type of qi xu characterised by the inability for proper upward flow of qi, with symptoms of distension and heaviness in the abdominal and lumbar region, frequent micturation, diarrhoea, shortness of breath, feeble voice and a weak pulse. "Qi blockage" and "qi collapse" is the extreme manifestation of qi disturbance, a good example of which is a comatose state. Qi xu and qi stagnation caused by blockage of the vessels by phlegm, cold or heat can lead to blood stasis which in turn leads to blockage of the meridians. This will result in symptoms of localised pain, lumps, dark complexion, dry scaly skin, cyanosed lips and a dark and purplish tongue.

Blood xu results from loss of blood and dysfunction of the spleen and stomach with symptoms of pallor, pale lips and tongue, dull nails, dizziness and giddiness, palpitations, lassitude, emaciation, numbness of limbs, stiff joints, dry eyes and blurred vision. Blood disturbances are usually linked to haemorrhage or prolonged illness. When the activities of the zang-fu organs are co-ordinated, the metabolism of the body fluids will run smoothly. Dry-heat and excessive emotions can disrupt the smooth flow of body fluids, resulting in insufficiency, represented by dryness the mouth, nose, skin, poor hair quality, cramps or vomiting and diarrhoea. Sometimes during fever, the distribution and excretion of body fluids are damaged and oedema results. This is usually associated with the function of the spleen, lung, liver and the triple jiao. This in turn can lead to qi stagnation. For example, in chronic bronchitis when there are symptoms of phlegm, coughing, orthopnea and tightness of the chest.

The dysfunction of qi, blood, body fluids and Zang-fu organs generally speaking, leads to the following pathological conditions:

1   The Stirring of Endogenous Wind
2   Endogenous Cold
3   Endogenous Damp
4   Endogenous Dryness from Fluid Consumption
5   Endogenous Fire/Heat

ENDOGENOUS WIND

This is closely related to the "Liver" with symptoms of dizziness, reeling, twitching and trembling. The manifestation of "wind" is caused by excessive yang or the failure of yin to control yang. The factors leading to this condition are usually:

- Emotional Frustration and Stress damaging the Liver and Kidney Yin
- Fever—the extreme heat consuming body fluids and affecting the tendons and blood vessels
- Insufficient Blood Production or Excessive Loss

ENDOGENOUS COLD

This represents Yang Xu with symptoms of pallor, aversion to cold, numbness or pain in the limbs or spasms. Cold is usually associated with the function of the spleen and the kidney, so there may be additional symptoms of oedema, diarrhoea or frequency of micturition.

ENDOGENOUS DAMP

This is related to a disturbance in the activity of the spleen leading to damp and phlegm. Obesity is a good example.

ENDOGENOUS DRYNESS

This is usually associated with prolonged illness when dehydration is present perhaps as a result of perspiration, diarrhoea, vomiting or haemorrhage in conditions affecting the lung, stomach and the large intestine.

ENDOGENOUS FIRE/HEAT

Excessive "fire" is usually due to environmental factors or extreme emotion. When it is due to yin xu, symptoms will be limited to specific parts of the body, as in toothaches, sore throats, dry mouth and lips and flushed cheeks.

THE MERIDIANS

The disturbances of qi and blood activities in the meridians are also seen to be causing organ dysfunction. A decrease in qi and blood for example will weaken the zang-fu organs. Muscular pain is believed to be due to a retardation of qi and blood flow. For example, if the flow in the Liver Meridian is affected, there may be symptoms of hypochondriac pain, goitres or lumps in the breasts. Disturbances of qi flow in the Yangming Meridians results in facial tics, delirium, rolling eyes; in the Shaoyang Meridians, deafness, weakness in the joints etc.

In TCM a thorough knowledge of the Meridian pathways coupled with observation of the physical signs will provide a good guide to the treatment plan.

THE ZANG-FU ORGANS

For an accurate assessment of syndromes, an understanding of the activities of the zang-fu according to traditional Chinese medicine, is important.

Each zang is said to be dependent on Kidney yin and Kidney yang. Conversely, any prolonged disturbance in the yin or yang of the zang will affect the Kidney.

The Heart—This opens into the tongue (problems with the heart can be detected in the tongue) and governs blood and control mental activities. Any symptoms relating to the circulation and emotional imbalance will be indicative of a disturbance in the "heart" function. Hyperactivity of the Ht.yang or Ht.qi will cause disturbances of the mind and produce a rapid pulse, red tongue, insomnia, palpitations, restlessness, dreaming, excitability or even hysteria. When the Ht.meridian is affected by excessive yang, there may be symptoms of ulceration in the mouth, dryness in the mouth or nose. When the disturbance affects its twin fu organ, the Small Intestine, symptoms of concentrated yellow urine and dysuria may appear. Chronic diseases usually causes Ht. Qi Xu, with impaired circulation and oedema. With Ht. Yang Qi Xu there are additional symptoms of lassitude, dullness, drowsiness and a general lack of interests. More extreme symptoms will include cold limbs, pallor, a purplish complexion, palpitations, angina, spontaneous sweating, a feeble and slow or a rapid and intermittent pulse. When the disturbance spreads to the Lung, breathlessness, coughing or bronchial spasms results. When the Kidney is affected, oedema is present. Ht. Yin Xu results from mental or emotional strain, prolonged illness. There are usually symptoms of feverish sensations in the palms and soles of the feet and chest, night sweats, insomnia, a thready pulse and a red tongue. A thready and weak pulse represents excessive consumption of Ht.blood, with symptoms of poor mental concentration, insomnia, excessive dreams, palpitation, fear, pallor and a pale tongue. Stagnation of Ht.blood causes a suffocating feeling in the chest. When this extends to the Heart Meridian there will be symptoms of palpitations, fright, chest pains, cold limbs, a feeble pulse and may even lead to coma.

The Lung—The main physiological function of the "Lung" is to control the respiration and to ensure the proper dispersal of qi throughout the body and the integrity of the water passageways. Disruption of this function will cause respiratory problems and retention of fluid, scanty urine and eventually obstruction of the Heart function. Disturbances of the Lung function are usually caused by external pathogenic factors with symptoms of stuffy nose, sneezing, sore or itchy throat, cough. When this occurs, the Lung qi is said to be deficient. When night sweats are present it is said that Lung Yin is insufficient. Normal Lung qi has a descending action in order to cleanse the respiratory tract. When this fails, sputum, dyspnoea and fullness of the chest with coughing results. Pathogenic Dry-Heat or emotional disturbances can cause a deficiency in the lung Yin leading to symptoms of a dry cough, production of sticky sputum, shortness of breath, afternoon fever, night sweats, flushed cheeks, feverish sensations in the palms, soles of feet and chest and possibly blood in sputum. Prolonged deficiency will lead to a deficiency in Kidney Yin.

The Spleen—The main function of the Spleen is transportation of nutrients, their distribution and maintenance of the integrity of the blood vessels. It is the yang component that controls these functions. Deficiency or injury of Yang Spleen Qi will cause disruption of these functions, eventually leading to Kidney Yang Qi Xu. Improper diet can cause Spleen Qi Xu. Symptoms of Qi Xu are, indigestion, may be a loss of taste, dizziness, abdominal distension, loose stools or diarrhoea, or prolapse of one of the internal organs. Haemorrhage can also cause Qi Xu. Diarrhoea with undigested food present or diarrhoea before dawn usually represents Spleen Yang Qi Xu. This condition can lead to damp, represented by fluid retention and disturbances in water metabolism. This can be complicated by exogenous damp. When jaundice appears, it indicates that the liver or gallbladder is involved. Spleen Yin Qi Xu will appear with the usual symptoms of spleen dysfunction but with a dry tongue and mouth or a red tongue with a little coating. Yin xu can lead to Stomach Yin Xu with symptoms of nausea and belching.

The Liver—This organ is believed to govern qi flow and the storing of blood. Clinical dysfunction is normally due to Qi & Yang Excess or Liver Yin & Blood Xu. The excess of Liver Yang is usually a consequence of Liver Yin Xu. Violent emotions causes stagnation of Liver qi with signs of distending pain especially in the hypochondriac region and swellings. When the stagnation extends into the Liver Meridian, it may lead to goitres, globus hystericus, distension, pain in the lower abdomen, dysmenorrhoea and anaemia. If it spreads to the stomach, it will cause belching, acid regurgitation or gastric pain. When Liver qi dysfunction spreads to the spleen, it causes abdominal pain and diarrhoea. When Liver qi is deficient and stagnant, Liver fire flares up. One of the causes of this is a sudden outburst of rage and other abnormal emotional activities. In this instance, Liver yang is in excess and produces a distending headache, red complexion, red eyes and may even cause ringing in the ears or deafness. When this excess yang spreads to the lung and stomach it produces symptoms of haemoptysis, epistaxis or syncope. A loss of blood, excessive pathogenic heat, prolonged illness or a weak spleen and stomach function can cause a deficiency of Liver blood. This type of deficiency can stir up endogenous wind with symptoms of muscle weakness, numbness in the limbs, joint problems or in the extreme, convulsions and coma. Other relating symptoms are dizziness, blurred vision, dry eyes and itchy skin. Emotional distress can also cause a deficiency of Liver yin which in turn causes Liver yang to become unrestrained. The pulse will probably be taut and rapid. In TCM, the Liver and the Kidney are observed to be sharing the same source. So a deficiency of Kidney yin will also lead to an uncontrolled Liver yang syndrome.

The Kidney—The major physiological function of the kidney is to store vital essence and regulate water circulation and metabolism. A disturbance of these functions result in growth impairment and problems with reproduction and water regulation with symptoms of scanty urine and oedema or polyuria. The Kidney's vital essence forms the foundation of the Yin and Yang of the whole body. "Vital essence" is composed of 2 parts—the kidney essence (shen jing—the yin aspect), and the kidney qi—the yang aspect. Deficiency of vital essence is commonly seen in the elderly when there are signs of senility or impotence. It is also used to explain congenital weaknesses or after prolonged illness or malnutrition. When this deficiency occurs in childhood, growth and development is impaired as seen in non-development of the sex glands during adolescence. A deficiency of "vital essence" can be brought on by the poor conservation of kidney qi as seen in excessive sexual activity. An overindulgence in sex is one of the chief reasons for a depletion in kidney qi. Symptoms relating to kidney qi depletion will be, premature ejaculation, incontinence of urine or faeces or incomplete emptying of the bladder or symptoms associated with the loss of control in the reproductive system and urinary system. A deficiency of Kidney yin is usually due to injury from a prolonged illness. Other causes are, fire arising from emotional upsets, from pathogenic heat and overuse of warm-natured tonics. This leads to uncontrolled Kidney yang resulting in a syndrome of Yin Xu & Fire Excess. When Kidney yang becomes deficient, it is said that the fire of the life gate is in decline. This is usually due to a deficiency of the Heart and Spleen Yang or and overindulgence in sex. This eventually leads to a Cold syndrome with a decline in reproductive ability and disturbances in water metabolism, the clinical manifestations of which are, impotence, sterility, oedema, diarrhoea with undigested food.

The Gallbladder—The main function of this organ is to store and excrete bile thus helping the Spleen and Stomach in their functions. The GB function is also closely associated with the Liver function. Emotional upsets and damp heat are the main causes of disturbances with resulting jaundice. When phlegm and heat affects the meridian, it can produce symptoms of irritability, insomnia and mental instability.

The Stomach—Its normal function is to digest food. Stomach qi is observed to have a descending tendency. So any disturbance will cause qi to ascend giving symptoms of dyspepsia, gastric pain, abdominal distension, belching or vomiting. Bad eating habits or prolonged illness can cause a deficiency of Stomach qi which will bring about indigestion and other symptoms of stomach dysfunction. An advanced stage of febrile or chronic disease can lead to a deficiency of Stomach yin with loss of appetite, dry red tongue with no coating or a mirror-like tongue. An excess of cold or raw foods or ingestion of drugs of a cold nature will cause a syndrome of "Cold in the Stomach". Stomach fire is a result of qi stagnation from pathogenic heat, alcoholism or excess of pungent, hot and greasy foods. Excess fire from the Liver and Gallbladder can also result Stomach fire. The symptoms of fire in the Stomach are usually digestive hyperactivity, hunger, bitter taste in the mouth, thirst and constipation. There may also be further symptoms of nausea, vomiting, painful and swollen gums, epistaxis or haematemasis.

The Small Intestine—The main function is digestion. Dysfunction results in abdominal pain after meals, diarrhoea, vomiting and abdominal distension. Dysfunction can have an effect on the urinary system with symptoms of dysuria and incontinence.

The Large Intestine—Its main function is the excretion of wastes. This can be disturbed by dysfunction of the Stomach and Lung with symptoms of constipation if qi is deficient, or loose stools from damp cold and damp heat. Kidney xu can also affect the Large Intestine with symptoms of frequency of urine, loose stools or even faecal incontinence or a rectal prolapse.

The Urinary Bladder—The principal function of this organ is to excrete urine. Dysfunction will be represented by frequent micturation, dysurea, turbid urine, retention or incontinence. This function is closely linked with the function of the Kidney.

THE EXTRAORDINARY FU ORGANS

TCM has a separate category for the brain, bones, blood vessels and the uterus. In addition to their known conventional organic function, traditional medicine ascribes various causes for their dysfunction in terms of the relating organs, qi and blood.

The Brain—Certain mental dysfunction as failing vision, hearing loss, reduced responses to stimuli, are believed to be the result of a deficiency in Kidney qi. Dysfunction of the Heart, Lung, Spleen and Liver, will also cause disturbances in Brain function.A deficiency of yang qi will also cause dizziness as well as ear and eye disorders.

Bones—In TCM the Marrow is closely allied to the Bones. Deficiency from malnutrition or consumption of yin from pathogenic heat or cold in the lower jiao or insufficient blood and essence will affect the bones and marrow.

Blood Vessels—These are thought to be passageways for blood as well as for qi. It is qi which controls the flow. Depletion of body fluids or an accumulation of phlegm and cold will result in stagnation qi and thus affect the smooth passage of blood flow. When the Spleen qi is weak, haemorrhage may occur.

The Uterus—Early menstruation, menorrhagia, prolonged menstruation or functional uterine bleeding are reflections of heat in the blood or a failure of the Liver to store blood or a failure of Spleen qi to control blood. Delayed menstruation, oligomenorrhoea, dysmenorrhoea, anaemia or lumps in the abdomen or pelvis occurs when there is "cold" in the Uterus arising from qi and blood stagnation or insufficiency of qi and blood or a deficiency of yang qi. The Uterus can also be influenced by cold-damp or heat-damp from the surrounding areas. Emotional strain or an overindulgence in sex are also possible causes of uterine dysfunction. Insufficiency of qi and blood in the Chong and Ren Meridian also causes uterine dysfunction as these two channels are observed to originate in the Uterus. The Chong and Ren are also closely connected to the Kidney and Liver Meridians. Inadequate qi and blood in the Kidney and Liver Meridians will in turn affect the Uterus. The Chong Meridian is also closely connected to the Stomach and Spleen Meridian whose function of transporting and transforming of nutrients is important for the healthy functioning of the Uterus.

Specific Points and their Applications

YUAN-SOURCE POINTS AND LUO-CONNECTING POINTS

There is one point on each of the 12 meridians where the original qi is said to be retained. This is the Yuan point of the meridian. This point is usually used in a Shi/Xu syndrome. Pairs of Yin/Yang meridians are connected by a Luo-Connecting point and is used when it is necessary to treat both meridians. The Yuan and Luo points can be used on their own or in combination.

Meridian	Yuan Point	Luo Point
Lung	Taiyuan (Lu. 9)	Pianli (LI. 6)
Large Intestine	Hegu (LI. 4)	Lieque (Lu. 7)
Stomach	Chongyang (St. 42)	Gongsun (Sp. 4)
Spleen	Taibai (Sp. 3)	Fenglong (St. 40)

Meridian	Yuan Point	Luo Point
Heart	Shenman (Ht. 7)	Zhizheng (SI. 7)
Small Intestine	Wangu (SI. 4)	Tongli (Ht. 5)
Urinary Bladder	Jinggu (UB. 64)	Dazhong (K. 4)
Kidney	Taixi (K. 3)	Feiyang (UB. 58)
Pericardium	Daling (P. 7)	Waiguan (SJ. 5)
Sanjiao	Yangchi (SJ. 4)	Neiguan (P. 6)
Gall Bladder	Qiuxu (GB. 40)	Ligou (Liv. 5)
Liver	Taichong (Liv. 3)	Guangming (GB. 37)

THE BACK SHU POINTS AND THE FRONT MU POINTS

These are points where the qi of their corresponding Zang-fu organs is said to be infused. Disturbances of the Zang-fu are reflected on these points as tenderness or hardness. The Back Shu are located on either side the vertebra and the Front Mu are on the chest and abdomen. They are used for treating their respective Zang-fu disturbances, e.g. the Lung Back Shu for bronchitis. The Back Shu are also useful for treating problems related to sense organ, e.g. the Kidney Back Shu for tinnitus. The two sets can be used on their own or in combination.

Zang-fu	Back Shu Points	Front Mu Points
Lung	Feishu (UB. 13)	Zhongfu (Lu. 1)
Pericardium	Jueyinshu (UB. 14)	Tanzhong (Ren. 17)
Heart	Xinshu (UB. 15)	Jujue (Ren. 14)
Liver	Ganshu (UB. 18)	Qimen (Liv. 14)
Gall Bladder	Danshu (UB. 19)	Riyue (GB. 24)
Spleen	Pishu (UB. 20)	Zhangmen (Liv. 13)
Stomach	Weishu (UB. 21)	Zhongwan (Ren. 12)
Sanjiao	Sanjiaoshu (UB. 22)	Shimen (Ren. 5)
Kidney	Shenshu (UB. 23)	Jingmen (GB. 25)
Large Intestine	Dachangshu (UB. 25)	Tianshu (St. 25)
Small Intestine	Xiaochangshu (UB. 27)	Guanyuan (Ren. 4)
Urinary Bladder	Pangguangshu (UB. 28)	Zhongji (Ren. 3)

THE FIVE SHU POINTS

On each of the 12 meridians, in the area distal to the elbows and knees, there are 5 points of specific qualities. These are the Shu Points. The flow of qi from the most distal to the 5th point is said to correspond to the source and flow of a river to the sea. Thus the first most distal Shu point is the Jing or Well , then follows the Ying-Spring, Shu-Stream, Jing-River and finally, the He- Sea. The latter point is where the qi is said to be most abundant. Jing-Well points are indicated for mental problems and tightness in the chest area. Ying- Spring points are used for febrile diseases. Shu-Stream points are for Bi Syndromes or painful joints caused by pathogenic wind and damp. Jing-River points are generally useful for coughs, throat disorders and asthma. He-Sea points are good for problems in the abdomen and pelvis.

Each of the Shu points also correspond to one of the Five Elements. In the Yin meridians, the first point corresponds with Wood. In the Yang meridians the first point corresponds with Metal. Thus, each meridian has a "Mother" and a "Son" point. For example, in the Lung meridian(Metal), the "Earth" point, Taiyuan (Lu 9), is the "Mother" point and the "Son" point will be Chize (Lu 5), a Water point. When this particular system is used for treatment, the rule is to "reinforce the Mother for xu syndromes and reduce the son for a shi syndrome". For example, when the patient is suffering with chronic cough, shortness of breath, a low voice and a weak thready pulse, it is probably better to needle at point Taiyuan.

Meridian Upper Limb	1 (Wood) Jing-Well	2 (Fire) Ying-Spring	3 (Earth) Shu-Stream	4 (Metal) Jing-River	5 (Water) He-Sea
Lung	Shaoshang (Lu. 11)	Yuji (Lu. 10)	Taiyuan (Lu. 9)	Jingqu (Lu. 8)	Chize (Lu. 5)
Pericardium	Zhongchong (P. 9)	Lagong (P. 8)	Daling (P. 7)	Jianshi (P. 5)	Quze (P. 3)
Heart	Shaochong (Ht. 9)	Shaofu (Ht. 8)	Shenmen (Ht. 7)	Lingdao (Ht. 4)	Shaohai (Ht. 3)
Lower Limb					
Spleen	Yinbai (Sp. 1)	Dadu (Sp. 2)	Taibai (Sp. 3)	Shangqui (Sp. 5)	Yinlingquan (Sp. 9)
Liver	Dadun (Liv. 1)	Xingjian (Liv. 2)	Taichong (Liv. 3)	Zhongfeng (Liv. 4)	Ququan (Liv. 8)
Kidney	Yongquan (K. 1)	Rangu (K. 2)	Taixi (K. 3)	Fuliu (K. 7)	Yingu (K. 10)

Meridian Upper Limb	1 (Metal) Jing-Well	2 (Water) Ying-Spring	3 (Wood) Shu-Stream	4 (Fire) Jing-River	5 (Earth) He-Sea
Large Intestine	Shangyang (LI. 1)	Erjian (LI. 2)	Sanjian (LI. 3)	Yangxi (LI. 5)	Quchi (LI. 11)
Sanjiao	Guanchong (SJ. 1)	Yemen (SJ. 2)	Zhongzhu (SJ. 3)	Zhiqou (SJ. 6)	Tianjing (SJ. 10)

Meridian Upper Limb	1 (Metal) Jing-Well	2 (Water) Ying-Spring	3 (Wood) Shu-Stream	4 (Fire) Jing-River	5 (Earth) He-Sea
Small Intestine	Shaoze (SI. 1)	Qiangu (SI. 2)	Houxi (SI. 3)	Yanggu (SI. 5)	Xiaohai (SI. 8)
Lower Limb					
Stomach	Lidui (St. 45)	Neiting (St. 44)	Xiangu (St. 43)	Jiexi (St. 41)	Zusanli (St. 36)
Gall Bladder	Qiaoyin (GB. 44)	Xiaxi (GB. 43)	Linqi (GB. 41)	Yangfu (GB. 38)	Yanglingquan (GB. 34)
Urinary Bladder	Zhiyin (UB. 67)	Tonggu (UB. 66)	Shugu (UB. 65)	Kunlun (UB. 60)	Weizhong (UB. 40)

Meridians	Mother Point (Reinforcing)	Son Point (Reducing)
Lung	Taiyuan (Lu. 9)	Chize (Lu. 5)
Large Intestine	Quchi (LI. 11)	Erjian (LI. 2)
Stomach	Jiexi (St. 41)	Lidui (St. 45)
Spleen	Dadu (Sp. 2)	Shangqiu (Sp. 5)
Heart	Shaochong (Ht. 9)	Shenmen (Ht. 7)
Small Intestine	Houxi (SI. 3)	Xiaohai (SI. 8)
Urinary Bladder	Zhiyin (UB. 67)	Shugu (UB. 65)
Kidney	Fuliu (K. 7)	Yongquan (K. 1)
Pericardium	Zhongchong (P. 9)	Daling (P. 7)
Sanjiao	Zhongzhu (SJ. 3)	Tianjing (SJ. 10)
Gall Bladder	Xiaxi (GB. 43)	Yangfu (GB. 38)
Liver	Ququan (Liv. 8)	Xingjian (Liv. 2)

XI-CLEFT POINTS

The Xi points are sites where the qi of each meridian converges. They are situated in the extremities in each of the 12 main meridians and in the 4 extra meridians (Yinwei, Yangwei, Yinqiao, Yangqiao). They are usually used for acute disorders in the related organs or in the areas supplied by the affected meridian.

	Meridian	Xi-Cleft Point
Yin Meridians of the Hand	Lung	Kongzui (Lu. 6)
	Pericardium	Ximen (P. 4)
	Heart	Yinxi (Ht. 6)
Yang Meridians of the Hand	Large Intestine	Wenliu (LI. 7)
	Sanjiao	Huizong (SJ. 7)
	Small Intestine	Yanglao (SI. 6)
Yang Meridians of the Foot	Stomach	Liangqiu (St. 34)
	Gall Bladder	Waiqiu (GB. 36)
	Urinary Bladder	Jinmen (UB. 63)
Yin Meridians of the Foot	Spleen	Diji (Sp. 8)
	Liver	Zhongdu (Liv. 6)
	Kidney	Shuiquan (K. 5)
Extra Meridians	Yangqiao	Fuyang (UB. 59)
	Yinqiao	Jiaoxin (K. 8)
	Yangwei	Yangjiao (GB. 35)
	Yinwei	Zhubin (K. 9)

THE LOWER HE-SEA POINTS OF THE SIX FU ORGANS

The Fu organs; stomach, large intestine, small intestine, gall bladder, urinary bladder and the sanjiao, are closely related to the Yang Meridians of the Foot. One point on each of the related meridian is particularly useful for treating disturbances of the related organ and this is termed the Lower He-Sea Point.

Meridians	Fu-Organ	Lower He-Sea Point
Foot Yangming	Stomach	Zusanli (St. 36)
	Large Intestine	Shangjuxu (St. 37)
	Small Intestine	Xiajuxu (St. 39)
Foot Shaoyang	Gall Bladder	Yanglingquan (GB. 34)
Foot Taiyang	Urinary Bladder	Weizhong (UB. 40)
	Sanjiao	Weiyang (UB. 39)

THE EIGHT INFLUENTIAL POINTS

According to traditional thought, the body can be classified into 8 "tissues". Acupuncture points had been discovered to have a particular effect on each of these and they were termed Influential Points.

Tissue	Influential Point
Zang organs	Zhangmen (Liv. 13)
Fu organs	Zhongwan (Ren 12)
Qi (the respiratory system & breathing)	Shanzhong (Ren 17)
Blood	Geshu (UB. 17)
Tendons	Yanglingquan (GB. 34)
Vessels and the Pulse	Taiyuan (Lu. 9)
Bones	Dazhu (UB. 11)
Marrow	Xuanzhong (GB. 39)

Zhangmen (liv. 13) will be effective for treating weaknesses of the "Spleen" function. For qi disturbances of the Fu organs i.e. vomiting and diarrhoea, Zhongwan will be a point of choice. Disturbances of the respiratory system, as in cough and asthma, pt. Shanzhong should be used as part of the prescription. Geshu is effective for conditions related to "blood" disturbances as in wasting diseases or haemetemasis. Yanglingquan is used in conditions causing muscle or joint weakness. Weaknesses relating to a deficiency of vital energy as reflected also in the pulse, then Taiyuan can be included. Dashu is found to be useful for painful joints and rheumatism. In conditions associated with the "Marrow" as in paralysis, then Xuanzhong can be chosen to increase effectiveness of treatment.

THE EIGHT CONFLUENT POINTS

There are four points in the upper limbs and four in the lower limbs which were said to connect the eight extra meridians to the 12 regular meridians. Thus, they are useful in treating conditions related to both.

Areas of Influence	Confluent Point	Regular Meridian	Extra Meridian
Heart, chest, stomach	Neiguan (P. 6)	Pericardium	Yinwei
	Gongsun (Sp. 4)	Spleen	Chong
Neck, shoulders, back, inner canthus	Houxi (SI. 3)	Small Intestine	Du
	Shenmai (UB. 62)	Urinary Bladder	Yangqiao
Retro-auricular region, cheek, outer canthus	Waiguan (SJ. 5)	Sanjiao	Yangwei
	Linqi (GB. 41)	Gall Bladder	Dai
Throat, chest, lung	Lieque (Lu. 7)	Lung	Ren
	Zhaohai (K. 6)	Kidney	Yinqiao

The point on the upper limb can be used together with the corresponding point on the lower limb, for example, Lieque can be used with Zhaohai for problems relating to the throat and lung.

3 THE ANATOMICAL AND PHYSIOLOGICAL RULE OF ACUPOINTS

Peng Li

For more than two thousand five hundred years, acupuncture has been used to treat different kinds of diseases by ancient Chinese doctors. According to their knowledge and clinical experience, they put forward the "meridian theory" to explain the mechanism of acupuncture therapy, which was described in detail in the "Yellow Emperor's Classics of Internal Medicine." Afterward, a great number of acupuncture points were added, which are considered extra-meridian points. Since clinical reports showed that acupuncture really could cure many diseases, many scientists have tried to find out what the mechanism of acupuncture is. There are several ways in which to approach it.

What are the Meridians on the Body?

Many researchers tried to find out the fourteen channels and acupoints on our body as suggested meridian theory. Early in by the 1950s, someone reported that the skin resistance or impedance over occupants is lower than that of surrounding skin. Nakatani[17] of Japan proposed that different areas of the body can have abnormally higher or lower conductivity, and that such abnormal conduction is very closely related to the meridian lines. He called "Rydoraku channels" them which in Japanese means "a good conduction line." According to his proposal, various kinds of instruments were designed and sold out. Many scientists including many Chinese doctors bought these machines and tried to find out the channels. When they could not find them, they tried to design new machines. They tried to use electric potential, resistance or impedance etc. to repeat what Nakatani reported, but no definite positive results could be found. The problem with these attempts was mostly attributed to pressure artefacts from electrodes. Another important problem was that they usually put the indifferent electrode on the palm. They did not know that the palm is the main source of skin galvanic reflex, which is related to the activity of sweat glands innervated by sympathetic cholinergic fibres, and is very sensitive to psychological change.[13] The change of potential or resistance underneath the indifferent electrode is much bigger than on other skin areas they locked at, and surely will cover all the difference between acupoints and non-acupoints. So how is it possible to get reliable results? A group at the Shanghai Institute of Physiology reported that in animals with a bone fracture of the leg, some low resistance points come out on the skin, e.g., ear, but no meridian lines could be found. Their result is reliable.

In the 1960s, a doctor in North Korea claimed that he had found the channels and acupoints on animals. He published a monograph with some beautiful pictures to show the structure and physiological evidence of the acupoints and channels. This was big news! Many Chinese scientists were sent to his lab, and were ordered to learn from him. Professor F.Y. Hsu. was in one of the first groups sent there, along with some other professors. After he came back, he report to the officer of the Chinese Ministry of Health and said that the Korean doctor's findings were false. Soon, it was proved that both the morphological and physiological evidence were mistakes due to technical error. This is a lesson for all of us.

In 1985, Vernejone[22] injected a radioactive isotope subcutaneously into humans and claimed that vertical lines of migration were seen only from acupoints and resembled meridian lines in their distribution. However, in this work, lymphatic and venous drainage has not been ruled out. The explanation for this isotope migration raised serious doubts.

In China, some research groups are continuously using different kinds of techniques to search for the unique morphological evidence of meridians on the body. They not only measured the electric potential, electrical resistance and impedance of the acupoints, but also used ultrasound, infrared, radioactive isotopes, electro microscopes etc. in order to find the channels on or underneath the skin. Some of them even tried to buy very expensive machines, e.g., computerised tomography (CT), magnetic resonance imaging (MRI) etc.; so that they could try to scan the body from head to foot to see where the channels were Unfortunately, although they continue to work hard, and often believed that they had found something, no one scientific has produced a reliable report.

It can be concluded that despite so many years and so many scientists and doctors trying to find out the unique morphological structure of meridians on the body all have failed. What is the problem? Are the techniques or the instruments they used not advanced enough? No, they used all the new techniques and instruments in the world. Then, is the "meridian theory" wrong? If it is wrong, why during acupuncture has the patient felt a dull aching numbness or itching a propagation sensation, which the Chinese acupuncturists called "De Qi" In about 10% of the population, needling causes a sensation to radiate along the meridian away from the needle.[2,3] How to explain the effect of acupuncture and "De Qi"? Why do we not try an other way of understanding the meridian hypothesis by modern physiology and neuroscience?

The Anatomical Structures Underneath Acupuncture Points

In 1973 researchers at the Shanghai First Medical College[6] reported the relationship of acupoints and their surrounding nerves. They showed that no unique structures have been found under acupuncture points (acupoints); if there is something, they are nerves and nerve endings. In 1996, Yu et al.[25] studied the three-dimensional structure of NeiGuan (Pe 6) and found that normal tissue, including receptors and nerve endings, contribute to this acupoint but that was nothing unusual Chiang et al. at the Shanghai Institute of Physiology[4] reported that in normal adults, vascular occlusion of the upper arm could not prevent the analgesic effect of acupuncture needling of a point on the hand (Hegu, LI 4). On the other hand, infiltration of procaine in the deep tissues around the point of acupuncture abolished entirely the analgesic effect, suggesting that a nerve rather than humours were responsible for the mediation of the effect.

In 1978 Kline et al.[10] reported that electrical stimulation (2 mA, 2 ms, 4 Hz) of the Zusanli (St36) acupoint elicited significant decreases in arterial blood pressure and heart rate, when the tip of the needle was close to branches of the peroneal nerve. Cutting the sciatic nerve or paralysing the animal with succinylcholine or gallamine abolished these responses, whereas direct stimulation of the intact peroneal nerve still elicited a decrease in arterial blood pressure and heart rate in paralysed animals. Their results suggested that the decrease of arterial blood pressure and heart rate induced by acupuncture was due to the activation of motor fibres resulting in muscle contraction and subsequent excitation of muscle and/or joint receptors, which elicited an inhibitory reflex. Their results also showed that there was no significant depressor effect if the acupuncture needle was inserted at rather than in a control point, close proximity to somatic nerves.

In 1984, Dung[7] listed the anatomical structures found in the vicinity of acupoints. They are large peripheral nerves, nerves emerging from a deep to a more superficial location, cutaneous nerves emerging from a deep fascia, nerves emerging from bone foramina, motor points, neuromuscular attachments, blood vessels in the vicinity of neuromuscular attachment, along a nerve composed of the fibres of varying diameters, bifurcation points of the peripheral nerve, ligaments rich in nerve endings and suture lines of the skull. So his data confirms that no particular structure dominates at acupuncture points. The major correlate is the presence of a nerve, either in large nerve bundles or nerve endings.

Heine[9] also revealed that 80% of acupoints correlate with perforations in the superficial fascia. Through these holes, a cutaneous nerve vessel bundle penetrates to the skin. More details about the structure underneath the acupoints were described in some anatomical atlases of acupoints.[20] These details can be summarised as follows:

(1) Acupoints on the face and forehead region are located along the terminals or cutaneous branches of the trigeminal nerve and facial nerve. They are either at the nerve trunk where it leaves the foramen or at the end of its terminal branch. Sometimes it is at the site of anastomosis of two different nerves or at the point at which a nerve branches bilaterally. On the posterior aspect of the head and neck, most acupoints are found along the occipital nerves. Acupoints in the front of the neck lie along the terminal branches of the cervical plexus.

In the external ear, many acupoints can be used to treat different kinds of diseases, and in this small area, both the medial and lateral auricle receive innervation from the vagus nerve, glossopharyngeus nerve and the combination branches of the facialis and occipitalis minor nerve. The medial ear also receives branches from auriculo-temporal nerve, auricular magnus nerve and occipital major nerve. This is the anatomical base on which acupuncture applied on the auricle could cure many splanchnic and somatic diseases.

(2) On the trunk, typical spinal nerves have six cutaneous branches that reach the skin of the body wall in the thorax and abdomen. Each of these branches corresponds to an acupoint. The effects of these acupoints are usually related to the splanchnic organs that are in the same or nearby spinal segments.

(3) On the forearm and hand, acupoints are mostly related to the ulnar nerve, median nerve and radial nerve, which are often used to treat diseases in the area those nerves innervate, and also to treat diseases on the head, face and in the chest. Those acupoints on the lower limbs

were related to a sciatic nerve, peroneal nerve, tibial nerve and femoral nerve etc. These acupoints are usually used to treat the disease on the lower limbs and in the abdomen or pelvis.

In histological examinations Croley(5) showed twice as many papillae within the area of acupuncture points as non-acupuncture points. There was a concentration of dermal papillae containing capillary loops with sympathetic wrappings with the contained nerve endings, within group of acupoints is innervated by superficial somatic nerves, and is mostly unmyelinated fibres. The innervation of some main acupoints used to treat cardiovascular diseases are listed in the following table.

Table 1   Innervation of Acupoints

Acupoints	Nerves beneath the acupoint	Spinal segment
Neiguan (Pe 6)	Median Nerve	C6-T1
Ximen (Pe4)	Median Nerve	C6-T1
Shenmen (He 7)	Ulnar Nerve	C8-T1
Quchi (LI 11)	Radial Nerve	C5-T1
Zusanli (St 36)	Deep Peroneal Nerve	L4-S3
Sanyinjiao (Sp 6)	Tibial Nerve	L4-S3
Jueyingshu (UB 14)	4th and 5th thoracic nerves	T2-4
Xinshu (UB 15)	5th and 6th thoracic nerves	T3-5
Renzhong (Du 26)	2nd branch of the trigeminal nerve and buccal branch of the facial nerve	
Chenjiang (Ren 24)	3rd branch of the trigeminal nerve	
Shixuan (Ex 30)	Cutaneous nerves	

How to Select Acupoints?

According to the results of recent research, many scientists and doctors now understand that commonly used acupoints can be classified into three kinds.

"AH SHI" POINTS

To treat pain on the patient's leg, arm, back or any part of the body, needles are usually placed very close to the site of pain. These points are called "Ah Shi" points, which in Chinese means "these acupoints are where the patient has pain": It seems peculiar, but is easy to manage and very effective. This is because these acupoints are near the site of pain, and they are afferent inputs which will converge to the neurons of the same or nearby segment of the spinal cord or even higher centres. The afferent inputs induced by needling will inhibit the afferent input from the pain site (see next chapter). Of course, the local effect of needles should also be considered. Nevertheless, "Ah Shi" points are not the only points we should choose, and if we only choose the "Ah Shi" points, the effect will not be very successful.

ACUPOINTS ON THE SAME OR NEARBY SPINAL SEGMENT

To treat some diseases, such as angina pectoris, Neiguan (Pe 6), Xinshu (UB 15) etc. are the loci of the acupuncture points. Han[8] showed that acupoints are endowed with more nerve fibres including pressure and stretch receptors, and have more myelinated group II fibres in their innervation, if compared with the non-acupoints. Lu[16] found that in the acupoint Zusanli (St 36) area, there are 1550 myelinated fibres and 577 non-myelinated fibres, their ratio is 2.7:1. In the non-acupoint area, there are only 640 myelinated fibres and 860 non-myelinated fibres, their ratio is 0.7:1. He also showed that the ratio of Aα, β, γ, to Aδ in Zusanli is 3.10:1, while in the nonacupoint the ratio is 1.61:1. So the myelinated fibres in the acupoints are much more than in the nonacupoints. Their physiological evidence will be discussed in the next chapter.

Some work[24] reported that the acupoints are motor points, at which the nerve enters the muscle, and it approximates but is not identical to the end plate zone of motor nerve endings. For example, some acupoints are just proximal to the Achilles tendon, or immediately proximal to the tendon insertion on a bony prominence. Some acupoints are at the arterial arch of hand or foot, e.g., Hegu (LI 4) on the back of the hand, and Taicho (Liv 3) on the back of the foot. Needling on these acupoints is very effective in influencing sympathetic activity.

What Kinds of Nerve Fibres are Activated by Acupuncture?

In 1973 Chiang et al.[4] showed that the essential correlate of analgesia by acupuncture was a "De Qi" sensation that is the feeling of numbness, fullness and sometimes soreness. If procaine was injected intramuscularly, all the feeling and the analgesic effect of acupuncture could be abolished. In the same year, the Shanghai Institute of Physiology[1] where Chiang was working further reported that electromyogram recordings showed that during "De Qi", there is pronounced muscle activation accompanied by the acupuncturist noting the grab of the needle.

In 1978 Toda and Ichioka[21] reported that type II afferent was sufficient for acupuncture analgesia in the rat. In 1979, Pomeranz and Paley[18] recorded the afferent of mice from Hegu (LI 4, located in the first dorsal interosseous muscle), and also found that type II afferent was enough to produce acupuncture analgesia.

In 1985, Wang et al.[23] did some observational experiments on humans with direct micro electrode recordings from single fibres in the median nerve, and performed acupuncture on the distal side. They saw that during "De Qi" numbness was related to the activation of type II muscle afferent fibres; heaviness, distension and aching were due to the activation of type III fibres, and soreness was related to the activation of type IV unmyelinated fibres. The acupuncturists have also noticed that when the patient got the "De Qi" sensation, the muscle grabbed the needle.

It should be mentioned that to treat different diseases the acupoints selected are different. The fibres activated during acupuncture to treat other kinds of disease may be not the same as acupuncture analgesia. For example, to treat cardiovascular diseases such as hypertension, coronary heart disease, angina pectoris, arrhythmia and cardiac insufficiency etc., acupuncturists prefer to use Neiguan (Pe 6), Shemen (He 7), Jueyingshu (UB 14), Xinshu (UB 15), Ximen (Pe 4), Zusanli (St 36), Sanyingjiao (Sp 6), Quchi (LI 11), Taichong (Liv 3) etc., and sometimes auricular acupoints are also used. Deep somatic nerves innervate all these acupoints, and more myelinated fibres are involved. On the other hand, to treat hypotension and shock, Renzhong (Du 26), Chenjiang (Ren 24) and Shixuan (tips of the fingers and toes) are usually used. This later chosen. For genitourinary diseases, we may choose Sanyinjiao (Sp 6). These acupoints, although sometimes located on the extremities and not at all near the organs, may be form on the area of referred pain. In meridian theory, Neiguan (Pe 6) is on the channels that go to the heart. In recent research work it was shown that Neiguan (Pe 6) has projections to the same or nearby spinal segment (C6–T1) and that the sympathetic preganglionic neurons innervate the myocardium and coronary artery (T1–5). Stimulation of these acupoints will send more afferent discharges to these neurones (directly at the spinal level, or activate the inhibitory system at the supra-spinal level), inhibit the sympathetic output, decrease the cardiac oxygen demand and inhibit the myocardial ischemia, and so release the angina (see chapter 8). Similarly, Sanyinjiao (Sp 6) is innervated by the tibial nerve and has projections to L4–S3, near the spinal centre of a micturition reflex, etc.

DISTAL ACUPOINTS

Sometimes acupoints on a distal site are used. Traditional Chinese doctors usually like to make differential diagnoses according to the syndrome, pulse, tongue etc., and then they will choose the acupoints according to the meridian theory, which will sometimes be far from the diseased organ, and have no projections on the same or nearby spinal segment. The effectiveness of these acupoints may be due to the convergent inputs of these somatic areas and the related organs in the brain, and the integrative function of the neurons of the brain. It is already known that neurons in the reticular formation of the brain stem received afferent inputs from different parts of the body. It has extensive interconnections with the sensory, motor, and integrative nuclei and pathways all along the brain stem. Lin et al.[15] used horseradish peroxide (HRP) to trace the afferent projections from the "stomach meridian of foot-Yangming". He saw that 3–4 days after injection of 30% HRP into Zusanli (St 36) or Jiaxi (St 41), the HRP labelled cells were found in the nuclei gracilis, cuneatus and spinal branch of the trigeminal nucleus. So they concluded that stimulation of Zhsanli (St 36) or Jiaxi (St 41) could excite the nucleus gracilis, and spread to nucleus cuneatus and the spinal branch of the trigeminal nucleus. This may be the mechanism that in some people stimulates the acupoints on the foot so that there is some feeling directed along the trunk to the face. Our experiments also showed that the neurons in the rostral ventrolateral medulla (RVLM) could receive inputs from different brain areas and different somatic nerves.[14] Recently we found that the cardiovascular neurons in RVLM also receive projections from the great splanchnic nerve, deep peroneal nerve etc. Stimulation of the deep peroneal nerve could inhibit the response induced by the splanchnic inputs.

The meridian theory only explained the spatial and functional relationship between the somatic part and the internal organs. To analyse the mechanism, surely we should use the knowledge and techniques of physiology and neuroscience etc. In addition physiology and neuroscience will open a new area when investigating the mechanism of acupuncture. Before scientists can solve all these problems, we will keep the meridian theory in mind. Maybe it is something we cannot understand with our present knowledge, and if we dismiss it, we may lose some very important information. So, to do acupuncture in the right way, doctors cannot work as a technician or physiotherapist. He or she should be qualified to perform both western and Chinese medicine. This means they should learn the basic sciences of medicine, not only western medicine, but also the principal points of traditional Chinese medicine.

References

1. Anonymous (Shanghai Institute of Physiology) (1973) Electromyographic activity produced locally by acupuncture manipulation. *Chin Med J*, **53**: 532–535 (in Chinese)
2. Bensoussan, A. (1994) Acupuncture. meridians—myth or reality? Part 1. *Comp Ther Med*, **2**: 21–26.
3. Bensoussan, A. (1994) Acupuncture meridians—myth or reality? Part II. *Comp Ther Med*, **2**: 80–85.
4. Chiang, C.Y., Chang, C.T., Chu, H.L. and Yan, L.F. (1973) Peripheral afferent pathway for acupuncture analgesia. *Sci Sin*, **16**: 210–217.
5. Croley, T.E. (1996) In Hung, K.C. ed. *Acupuncture the past and the present*. Chapter 4 *Acupuncture points-histological properties*. p.47 Vontage Press, New York.
6. Department of Anatomy, Shanghai First Medical College (1973) The relationship between channels, acupoints and their surrounded nerves. In *A selection of the theoretical study of acupuncture anaesthesia*. Shanghai Science and Technology Publisher. p.251–264 (in Chinese).
7. Dung, H.C. (1984) Anatomical features contributing to the formation of acupuncture points. *Am J. Acupunct*, **12**: 139–143.
8. Han, C.C. (1996) In Hung, K.C. ed. *Acupuncture the past and the present*. *Chapter 4 Acupuncture points-histological properties*. p.47 Vontage Press, New York.
9. Heine, H. (1988) Akupunkturtherapie-perforationen der oberflachlichen korperfaszie durch kutane GefaB-Nerverbulbet. *Therapentikon*, **4**: 230–244.
10. Kline, R.L., Yeung, K.Y. and Calaresu, F.R. (1978) Role of somatic nerves in the cardiovascular responses to stimulation of an acupuncture point in anaesthetized rabbits. *Exp Neurol*, **61**: 561–570.
11. Huang, K.C. (1996) *Acupuncture the past and the present*. Vantage Press, New York.
12. Li, P. and Yao, T. ed. (1992) *Mechanism of the modulatory effect of acupuncture on abnormal cardiovascular functions*. Shanghai Med Univ Press, Shanghai.
13. Li, P., Zheng, X.Z., Jin, W.Q. and Zhao, X.J. (1962) Studies on skin potential and skin galvanic reflex in human subjects. *Acta Physiol Sin*, **25**: 171–181 (in Chinese).
14. Lin, R.J., Gong, Q.L. and Li, P. (1991) Convergent inputs to neurones in the nucleus paragigantocellularis lateralis in the cat. *Neuroreport*, **2**: 281–284.
15. Lin, W.Z., Xu, M.H., Fan, L. and Guo, H.Y. (1994) The connecting function of the stomach meridian of foot-Yangming in the nerve network of spinal cord and brain stem. *Shanghai J. Acup Moxib*, **13**: 225.
16. Lu, G.W. (1983) Characteristics of afferent fibre innervation on acupuncture point Zusanli. *AM J. Physiol*, **245**: R606–612.

17. Nakatani, Y. and Yamashita (1977) *Ryodoraku acupuncture*. Ryodoraku Research Institute, Osaka.
18. Pomeranz, B. and Paley, D. (1979) Electroacupuncture hyalgesia is mediated by afferent nerve impulses: an electrophysiological study in mice. *Exp Neurol*, **66**: 398–402.
19. Stux, G. and Pomeranz, B. (1998) *Basics of acupuncture*, 4th ed. Springer, Berlin.
20. The cooperative group of Shandong Medical College and Shandong College of Traditional Chinese Medicine (1990) *Anatomical atlas of Chinese acupuncture points*. Shandong Science and Technology Press, Jinan, China.
21. Toda, K. and Ichioka, M. (1978) Electroacupuncture: relation between forelimb afferent impulses and suppression of jaw opening reflex in the rat. *Exp. Neurol.*, **61**: 464–470.
22. Verneijoul, P. de, Parras, J.C. et al. (1985) Etude des meridiens d'acupuncture par les traccurs radioactifs. *Bull Acad Natl Med (Paris)*, **169**: 1071–1075.
23. Wang, K., Yao, S., Xian, Y. and Hou, Z. (1985) A study on the receptive field of acupoints and the relationship between characteristics of needle sensation and groups of afferent fibres. *Sci Sin*, **28**: 963–971.
24. Wong, J. and Cheng, R. (1987) *The science of acupuncture therapy*, 2nd ed. p.35–36 Kola Mayland Co. (Hong Kong).
25. Yu, A.S., Zhao, Y.X., Li, X.L. and Nian, Z.G. (1996) Morphological research in Neiguan (Pe 6)'s three-dimensional structure. *Shanghai J. Acup Moxib*, **15**: 30–31.

4 THE ANALGESIC EFFECTS OF ACUPUNCTURE

Peng Li and C.Y. Chiang

Over the past few decades, knowledge the physiological basis of the control of pain has increased more than at any time in history. This growth has been mainly in studies of the neural and neurochemical basis of analgesia at various levels of the central nervous system such as the spinal cord, brainstem and higher subcortical centres. Under the impetus of a number of important discoveries not only has pain research experienced a unique progress but moreover the advances achieved have paved the way for the development of therapeutic approaches in the treatment of pain. One of these methods is acupuncture or electroacupuncture (EA). Although acupuncture was introduced in the Western world as early as the 16th century it remained largely unknown until in late 1950s when the first reports of operations under acupuncture analgesia were reported from China. Since then, acupuncture has achieved world fame and has become increasingly employed throughout the world. It is estimated that more than one million practitioners outside China administer acupuncture treatment for chronic pain, and of these, more than three hundred thousand are physicians.[35]

Clinical Studies

In China acupuncture has been used widely to stop pain and treat other diseases for more than four thousand years. In Western countries, in the early 1920s Goulden reported that Dr. Davis had introduced the use of acupuncture in the treatment of sciatica and that over two decades more than one hundred cases of sciatica and other forms of neuritis had been treated with acupuncture.[28]

In the 1960s some hospitals in Shanghai and Beijing, China started to perform operations of pulmonary lobectomy under the acupuncture anaesthesia. In the early stages, the procedure was quite complicated. Before surgery, every patient was given some pre-medication, e.g. a small dose of dolantine, etc. Then, in the operating theatre, about ten needles were punctured in each of the patient's limbs. During the operation the head acupuncturist issued his instructions through a signal board to four subordinate acupuncturists, who according to the instructions twisted the needles in the patient's limbs. It took 30 minutes of needle manipulation before the operation began. In a successful case, under the surgical lamp, while scissors, scalpel and haemostats moved busily over a long chest cut, the patient, calm, with eyes open, was chatting with nurses peacefully without any expression of suffering. At that time, no one could explain the mechanism. Soon after, this technique was much simplified. Electroacupuncture was applied, and its use spread to the whole country and was applied to nearly all operations, including thyroidectomy, neurosurgery, open-heart surgery with extracorporeal circulation, gastrointestinal surgery, caesarean section, and tubal ligation, etc. This method is cheap and does have benefits for the patients, being, safe, with far fewer side effects, and no postoperative complications. Normal physiological functions were restored promptly after operation. However, several years later, doctors had more experience and concluded that acupuncture anaesthesia should not be available to every patient or for all operations. It is more not suitable for the abdominal gastrointestinal surgery, because acupuncture cannot block the response of pulling the gastrointestinal tract.

Moreover, acupuncture anaesthesia is based on its analgesic effect, and so is not available for every patient. About one third of achieve a patients could not suitable analgesic effect by acupuncture or EA. Cao, et al.[2] reported that those people whose sympathetic activity could be inhibited by acupuncture would show a suitable analgesic effect with acupuncture. If their sympathetic activities are very high and cannot be inhibited by acupuncture, there is a mild or even no analgesic effect. So, some doctors are trying to use various chemicals or herbs to improve the efficiency of acupuncture analgesia. D-phenylalanine,[7] haloperidol and pimozide (dopamine receptor antagonists),[43] metoclopramide (antidopaminergic and anticholinesterase action),[28] etc. were believed to potentiate the analgesic effect of acupuncture. N_2O[26] or fentanyl[30] was also used with acupuncture to get a better analgesic effect.

For chronic pain, such as headache, migraine, back and lumbar pain, sciatica, neuralgia, etc. all could be relieved by acupuncture or EA. In most reports the effective rate is 60-80%. Cheng and Pomerenz[9] obtained a 90% success rate in the treatment of musculoskeletal pain with acupuncture. In Dr. LL Cheung's clinic and our acupuncture clinic in Mississauga, many patients experienced pain relief immediately after acupuncture, and if treated continuously every day or every other day, after a course (about 7–10 times) most patients will be symptom-free.

It is clear now that acupuncture analgesia or anaesthesia is not a placebo or psychological effect. Controlled clinical trials on chronic pain have proved that acupuncture helps from 55%–85% of patients, while placebo controls benefit only 30%–35% of cases. Moreover, the effect of acupuncture is long lasting, and repeated acupuncture treatments potentiate this effect, while the placebo is much more transient and repeated placebos become less and less effective each time.[38] The important duty for us is to explain its mechanism.

Mechanism of Acupuncture Analgesia

PERIPHERAL AFFERENT PATHWAY FOR ACUPUNCTURE ANALGESIA

Early in 1966, at the First National Conference on Acupuncture Anaesthesia in Shanghai Han, et al.[19] reported that 194 volunteering students were tested to see the effect of electroacupuncture (EA) on single acupoint Hegu (LI 4), when their pain threshold rose gradually within a period of 30 minutes. About two thirds of the subjects showed a 100% or more increase in pain threshold. For comparison, different acupoints, e.g. Hegu (LI 4), Zusanli (St 36) or Taichong (Liv 3) were punctured; the speed of recovery from pain thresholds once the needles were removed was remarkably similar. So it was postulated that there is a chemical basis for acupuncture analgesia.

In 1973 Chiang et al.[10] did experiments on 21 normal adults and demonstrated that the analgesic effect of acupuncture (with the needle twisting maneuver) is related to the De Qi sensation: the feeling of numbness, fullness, and sometimes soreness. Vascular occlusion of the upper arm could not prevent the analgesic effect of acupuncture needling of a point on the hand, Hegu (LI 4), from being mediated to other regions of the body as manifested by raising the thresholds of pain at those regions. However infiltration of procaine in the deep tissues around the point acupuncture entirely abolished the analgesic effect, while subcutaneous injection did not block the De Qi sensation and the analgesic effect of acupuncture either. So, it is suggested that nerves but not humours were responsible for the mediation of the effect. The analgesic effect from test points has been shown to be bilaterally distributed and widespread but somewhat segmental in nature. They also reported that when needles were inserted into the patient, acupuncturists would feel a grab of the needle by the muscle when proper De Qi was achieved. Shen and Wu et al.[1] recorded electromyogram around acupoints during De Qi and showed pronounced muscle activation accompanied by the acupuncturist's noting the grab of the needle.

In 1979 Pomeranz and Paley[36] stimulated Hegu (LI 4) in mice, and recorded the impulses from the nerves involved in producing acupuncture analgesia. They found that type II afferent was sufficient to produce acupuncture analgesia. In 1981 Lu, et al.[31] did experiments on cats and rabbits. They stimulated the peroneal nerve to induce pain response, and needled on Zusanli (St 36), and Quchi (LI 11) to get an analgesic effect; they also used a non- acupoint (1–1.5 cm lateral and lower than Zusanli) which had no analgesic effect as a control. The dorsal roots of L6–S1 were dissected and single fibre's recordings were made during stimulation of the Zusanli and non-acupoint. In this way they could record the neurogram and calculate the conduction velocity of the fibres activated during EA. Their results showed that type II and III afferent were important for acupuncture analgesia. Dilute procaine (0.1%) blocking type IV fibres had no effect on analgesia, while an anodal blockade or ischemic blockade of types II and III type fibres abolished acupuncture analgesia. They also found that underneath the effective acupoints there are more myelinated fibres; the ratio of myelinated fibres to non-myelinated fibres is 2.7:1, while underneath the non-acupoints there are fewer myelinated fibres; the ratio of myelinated fibres to non-myelinated fibres is 0.8:1. Therefore, morphological findings supported their electrophysiological results. Compare the analgesic effect of Quchi and Zusanli: the later is more effective than the former, maybe due to the similar segmental distribution of nerve fibres in the lower limb. However, Melzack et al.,[33] based on their measurement of muscle excitability points, proposed muscle nerve entry zones corresponding to traditional acupoints. This suggestion complies with findings that stimulation of muscle afferent is important for producing analgesia.

In 1984 Chung, et al.[14] did experiments on monkeys in which type I and II fibres of the tibial nerve were stimulated. This resulted in only a slight inhibition of the pain responses of the spinothalamic pain tract. When the stimulus strength was increased to a level that excited type III fibres, a powerful inhibition was observed. However, increasing the stimulus strength to excite type IV fibres is not necessary, as it induces stress analgesia and unbearable pain in conscious patients. Hou et al.[27] reported that the muscle potential recorded from the acupoints located in fleshy muscle is discharged by the intrafusal fibres of muscle spindles. They demonstrated that the afferent fibres conveying needling sensation impulses were mainly the fibres of groups III and IV. Tang et al.[39,40] showed that the type IV fibres are more effective for acupuncture analgesia. Nevertheless, most reports believed that activation of type IV fibres is not necessary. In contrast, activation of type II and III fibres are enough to induce analgesic effect. In 1985 Wang, et al.[41] made single fibres recordings on humans, and showed that Type II muscle afferents produced numbness, type III fibres gave sensations of heaviness, distension and aching, and type IV fibres caused soreness. As soreness is an uncommon aspect of De Qi, they concluded that the simulation of muscle afferent fibres (type II and III) produces De Qi sensation.

NEUROTRANSMITTERS INVOLVED IN THE ACUPUNCTURE ANALGESIA

Endogenous opioids

In 1976, Pomeranz and Chiu[35] used the mouse squeak latency paradigm and gave EA at Hegu (LI 4). They saw that naloxone iv could completely block the acupuncture analgesia and caused hyperalgesia. Sham EA produced no effect and naloxone alone produced very little hyperalgesia. They suggested that endorphin is implicated in the acupuncture analgesia. In 1977, Mayer et al.[32] studied acute laboratory-induced tooth pain in human volunteers. By manual twirling of needles in Hegu (LI 4), they increased the pain threshold of the volunteers. This effect was reversed by iv naloxone, while iv saline had no blocking effect. They also studied a control group of subjects receiving placebo injections. The placebo subjects were told to expect a strong analgesic effect, but none was observed. In 1978, Chiang, et al.[11] reported that in the summer of 1976, they did experiments and analysed data with signal detection theory on young medical volunteers. The changes of pain perception were detected by percutaneous electrical stimulation and radiant heat tests. Acupuncture applied on Hegu (LI 4) could have an analgesic effect, which was not found in either placebo-acupuncture or rest experiments. Intramuscular injection of naloxone (0.8 mg) could partially reverse the acupuncture analgesia, but naloxone itself had no marked influence on pain perception in normal subjects. They also found that the verbal report criterion of pain (a psychological factor) was also mildly changed.

Since these early reports there have been numerous studies in which systemically administered endorphin antagonists have been used to test the endorphin related acupuncture analgesia hypothesis. Most results provide support for this hypothesis, and more opioids were found: which could be grouped into three families: the enkephalin, the endorphin and the dynorphins.[3,4,5] By using the antibody microinjection technique Han, et al.[21] further showed that enkephalin seemed to be the mediator for acupuncture analgesia both in the brain and in the spinal cord, and β-endorphin to be effective only in the brain not in the spinal cord.

Dynorphin is analgesic at the spinal level, but not in the brain. Later by microinjection of type-specific antagonists of opioids receptors, antiserum and radioimmunoassay they concluded that low frequency (2 Hz) EA release endorphin and enkephalin, and high frequency (100 Hz) EA release dynorphins.[20] Gao, et al.[17] observed that after EA of Zusanli (St 36) for 50 minutes, them μ opioid receptor density was significantly increased in the following examined structures: the caudate nucleus, cingular gyrus, septal area, preoptic area, amygdaloid nucleus, periaqueductal grey, interpeduncular nucleus, dorsal raphe nucleus, raphe magnus nucleus, cervical and lumbar enlargement. Recently He, et al.[25] reported that after EA on Zusanli (St 36), the propiomelanocortin (POMC) mRNA level in the hypothalamic arcuate nucleus increased gradually and significantly for over four days. And successive EA on the fourth day could enhance the transcription to prevent the mRNA level from declining. Guo, et al.[18] found that EA in rats elevated precursors of the three endorphins, preproenkephalin, preprodynorphin and preproendorphin mRNA in the brain. It lasted 24–48 hours after 30 minutes of EA, indicating a prolonged increased rate of synthesis of these opioids. These results could explain the enduring effects of EA and the potentiation of repeated daily treatments.

Some sceptics are concerned that acupuncture may be a kind of stress induced analgesia, but many facts showed that this is not the case. For example: Sham EA on nearby non-acupuncture points induced no analgesia; acupuncture analgesia is naloxone reversible, but stress induced analgesia is only partly antagonised by large doses of naloxone. Plasma cAMP levels decrease during acupuncture analgesia but rise during stress induced analgesia. The periquaductal gray is essential for acupuncture analgesia but not for stress induced analgesia. A dorsolateral spinal cord lesion eliminates acupuncture analgesia but not stress induced analgesia, etc.[48]

In 1978 Han, et al.[21] noticed that if the analgesic effect of EA was assessed at 30 minute intervals for six sessions, a sustained decrease of the EA effect was demonstrated, leading to a complete abolishment of the EA analgesia at the end of six hours. This phenomenon is very similar to the development of tolerance after repeated administration of morphine, and called it was tolerance to acupuncture analgesia. They hypothesised that a prolonged and profound activation of the opioids system by EA might trigger an opposite mechanism that releases some endogenous antagonists to counteract the effect of opioids. Their later experiments confirmed this: icv or intrathecal injection of a picomole dose of cholecystokinin octapeptide (CCK-8) resulted in a complete abolishment of EA analgesia. On the other hand, acupuncture tolerance can be postponed or reversed by the icv or intrathecal injection of CCK antiserum, indicating the importance of endogenous CCK in producing acupuncture tolerance. This may explain the fact that when EA was used for anaesthetic purposes in surgical operations lasting for 6–8 hours, the effect of analgesia decreased with time and became unsatisfactory by the end of the operation. To avoid this outcome, EA may be administered intermittently rather than continuously during the course of the operation. In animal experiments it was also show that when rats were made tolerant to low frequency EA analgesia, they were still susceptible to high frequency EA, and vice versa. Therefore, alternative applications of low and high frequency EA may be used to avoid tolerance.

Serotonin
In 1975–1978, Han, et al.[19] showed that acupuncture analgesia was decreased dramatically when the brain of the rabbit was depleted of its 5-HT content by parachloro-phenylalanine (pCPA, 5-HT synthesis blocker), 5,6 dihydroxy tryptamine (DHT, chemical denervator), or the 5-HT receptor blocker cinanserin. The analgesic effect was potentiated markedly when the cerebral content of 5-HT was raised by the administration of 5-HTP, the 5-HT precursor. Flurospectrophotometric determination of the content of 5-HT in the central nervous system demonstrated a positive correlation between the effectiveness of acupuncture analgesia and the cerebral content of 5-HT. During acupuncture, both the synthesis and release of 5-HT increased. When the former prevailed over the latter, there was a net increase in the cerebral content of 5-HT. In clinical studies, it was also found that chlorimipramine, the tricyclic compound that selectively facilitated serotonergic transmission, was very effective in potentiating the effect of acupuncture analgesia. Numerous experiments showed that electrolytic or chemical lesions to Raphe Magnus and Dorsalis, which contains most of the serotonin cells and their descending and ascending axons, blocked acupuncture analgesia.[15,16] Using double labelling immunocytochemistry, He, at al.[23,24] showed the co-localisation of C-fos protein and serotonin in the nucleus raphe dorsalis, nucleus raphe centralis superior and rostral ventromedial medulla. It is interesting that the expression of c-fos in the serotoninergic neurons of the brain stem could only be found in animals after EA on Zusanli (St 36) for one hour, where as control animals had a very low level of Fos labelling and co-localisation with 5-HT was rarely seen. All the evidence from animal and clinical studies seemed to point to the conclusion that acupuncture activates the serotonergic system in the brain and the spinal cord, which is

essential for mediating the effect of acupuncture analgesia.[6,8] Nevertheless, local microinjection studies showed that the descending serotonin inhibitory system might not be as important as the raphe projections to the forebrain. Because intrathecal injection of serotonin antagonists over the spinal cord produced no blockade of acupuncture analgesia, lesions of the ascending raphe tracts caused a selective decrease of cerebral serotonin and a correlated decrease of acupuncture analgesia in rats. If spinal cord serotonin does not mediate acupuncture analgesia, why does a lesion of the descending system in the spinal cord block acupuncture analgesia? Indeed, the raphe magnus serotonergic descending neurons are activated by EA.[13] On the other hand, Mayer and Walkins suggested that there is a synergism between descending serotonin and norepinephrine.[38] The next paragraph will discuss this possibility.

Catecholamines

Han, et al.[21] reported that central catecholamines might play a role opposite to that of 5-HT. Facilitation of catecholamine transmission in the brain by IC injection of DOPA, the direct precursor for dopamine (DA) or dihydroxyphenylserine (DOPS), precursor for norepinephrine (NE) resulted in attenuation of the effect of acupuncture analgesia. In contrast, blockades of NE transmission by phentolamine, the α-adrenoceptor blocker, spiroperidol, the DA receptor blocker, or 6OHDA, the chemical neurotoxin for catecholaminergic nerve terminals, was accompanied by a marked potentiation of the effect of acupuncture analgesia. It was also shown that there was a decrease in the content of NE in the brain following EA stimulation. In contrast to these findings, a repeated icv injection of a-methyltyrosine (a-MT) to block the synthesis of NE resulted in a decrease in the content of NE and could not increase the efficacy of acupuncture analgesia. Further experiments showed that EA accelerated both the synthesis and release of NE in the central nervous system. Since the dramatic increase in release could not be compensated by the increase in the rate of synthesis, a partial depletion in the tissue content of NE ensued. Intrathecal injection of NE antagonists blocked acupuncture analgesia, which showed the importance of descending NE pathways.[19] Further evidence indicated that even in the brain the action of NE was different in different nuclei. An antagonistic effect on acupuncture analgesia could be demonstrated in the periaqueductal gray (PAG) and in habenula, but not in amygdala and nucleus accumbens. In the hypothalamus it may even facilitate the effect of EA. Therefore, compared with the role-played by 5-HT in acupuncture analgesia, the function of NE is much more complicated.

Other neurotransmitters

Some reports showed that during acupuncture analgesia the ACh content in the cerebral cortex, hypothalamus and caudate nucleus increased. By push-pull infusion, it was observed that the release of ACh in caudate nucleus increased during acupuncture analgesia. In clinical studies, during acupuncture applied to patients suffering from pain, ACh in the cerebrospinal fluid collated from lateral ventricles increased. In animal experiments microinjection of atropine or scopolamine to block the cholinergic receptor could attenuate the acupuncture analgesia. On the other hand, microinjection of physostigmine to inhibit cholinesterase and increase ACh could enhance the effect of acupuncture analgesia.[22,43]

Although there are some experiments to show that microinjection of haloperidol and pimozide to block the DA receptors in caudate nucleus could enhance the effect of acupuncture analgesia, while microinjection of apomorphine or L-DOPA will attenuate its effect, some other reports showed opposite results.[22] The influence of DA on acupuncture analgesia needs further study.

GABA is an inhibitory amino acid in the brain, but it was shown to attenuate the effect of acupuncture analgesia. Whenever GABA in the brain increased the effect of acupuncture analgesia decreased.[43] All this needs further investigation.

A CEREBRAL NEURONAL LOOP FOR ANALGESIA

Integration in the spinal cord

It is well known that an injury or nociceptive stimulation activates the sensory receptors of type III and IV fibres, which send impulses to the spinal cord and synapses onto the spinothalamic tract, and interns to the thalamus and cortex. Electrophysiological recordings (31) showed that these nociceptive inputs evoke continuos high frequency firing of the nociceptive neurons in the V layer of the dorsal horn. Many reports showed that acupuncture could activate type II and III (sometimes IV fibres also), send signals not only to the spinal cord sensory cells, but also pass through the anterolateral tract (ALT) and project to the midbrain and hypothalamic-pituitary complex. In the spinal level it activates some enkephalin or dynorphin cells. These reduce the release of the pain transmitters and attenuate pain. The analgesia effect will be better if the acupoints selected are on the same or nearby segments of the nociceptive inputs.

Supraspinal integration

When the signals from the acupoints are transmitted to the supraspinal centers via ATL, it may activate different neurons. In the 1970s and 1980s, many labs in China did a lot of work to make lesions on different nuclei, e.g. nuclei raphe, PAG, nucleus arcuatus, caudate nucleus, etc. Their purpose was to find out the pathway of the inputs induced by acupuncture. In 1976, Du and Chao[15] first showed that destroying the area of nucleus raphi abolished the analgesic effect of acupuncture. Han suggested that one of the signals from ATL projects and excites neurons in the PAG, which release enkephalin. Then it in turn activates the raphe nucleus, causing it to send impulses down through dorsal lateral tracts (DLT) to release 5-HT and NE onto the spinal "pain" cell to inhibit it.[21]

From the adjacent area of nucleus raphe, nucleus reticularis paragigantocelllularis may also be activated and send signals via DLT to the spinal cord, releasing NE to block pain transmission.[38]

Signals of acupuncture will also be transmitted to nucleus arcuateus (ARC), which is full of endorphin and is related to the analgesic effect of acupuncture, stress and morphine. Yin, et al.[45,46,47] did research to show that acupuncture could activate the endorphin neurones in ARC which have projections to periaqueductal gray (PAG), dorsal raphe nucleus (DR), and nucleus locus coeruleus. From there it sends projects via ascending projections to the parafascicular nucleus in the thalamus, and descending projections to the dorsal corn of the spinal cord, and inhibits the evoked response to noxious stimulation. This is the fast analgesic effect of acupuncture. From ARC there are also projections to the median eminence, terminated at the primary capillary plexus. So, β-endorphin may be released into CSF and plasma from the pituitary and induce the slow analgesic effect.[28,47]

Other nuclei including the nucleus anterior caudate, accumbens, amygdala, habenula and orbital cortex, etc.[37,43] are also reported to relate to the analgesic effect of acupuncture. He, et al.[22] did research to show that the caudate nucleus is an important central link in the expression of acupuncture analgesia, in which opioid peptides and ACh promote expression and dopamine antagonises it. They believe that in the pathway for pain modulation from the caudate nucleus, PAG is an important brain area in which the opioid peptidergic activity evokes descending and ascending controls over pain transmission at both the spinal and supraspinal level, resulting in analgesia. By using immunocytochemistry, He, et al.[23] further showed that in rats following EA of Zusanli (St 36) the expression of c-fos labelled cells were found in the lumbar spinal cord, mainly distributed ipsilaterally in the medial $\frac{2}{3}$ of laminae I-II, with a few scattering in laminae III–VII and X. Invariable labelling was also found in the medial thalamus. A few cells were also found in the ventral posterolateral nucleus, and dense labelling was seen in some limbic structures. This result suggested that EA activate a number of fine fibres, which in turn activate the relayed cells projecting to the thalamus via the ventrolateral funiculus. It is interesting to see that stimulation of some acupoionts could activate the neural firing of the above nucleuses; bilaterally microinjection of naloxone (1 μg) or lesions made in these nucleuses could block or attenuate the acupuncture analgesia. Interestingly, stimulating one of these nuclei also produces notable analgesic effect. It seems that all these nuclei are connected in a closed loop, and that breaking one link would result in a collapse of the whole system.

Experiments showed that there is a serotonergic pathway from PAG to the nucleus accumbens, and a descending pathway from the nucleus accumbens down to PAG, with a relay station at habenula. In habenula and PAG met-enkephalin was released as a transmitter. From PAG neural pathways are sent upward to the thalamus and downward to the spinal cord to suppress transmission of signals of pain. Han called this loop as a "meso-limbic loop of analgesia," which can be activated both by morphine and EA. Amygdala and arcuate nucleuses of the hypothalamus are also included in this loop.[21]

Recently, Tang, et al.[42,49,50,51,52] did a series of work to show that the thalamic nucleus submedius (Sm) is not only a centre to accept noxious input, but also an important thalamic centre to modulate pain feeling. The Sm- ventrolateral orbital cortex (VLO)-PAG may contribute a pain modulatory pathway, activating the brainstem descending inhibitory to system to modulate the noxious reception at the spinal level. Acupuncture analgesia may be due to the activation of this system.

Therefore, acupuncture analgesia includes different integration levels: the spinal cord, PAG, hypothalamus-pituitary and the VLO-Sm-PAG pathway.

Clinical Application

Although the mechanisms of acupuncture analgesia are quite complicated and need further study, some of the results are useful for clinical application.

SELECTION OF PATIENT

Since about one third of patients gain no or mild analgesic effect by acupuncture, it is necessary to choose the patient before an operation using acupuncture anaesthesia. If the patient's sympathetic activities are high and cannot be inhibited by acupuncture, EA is not available. However, some kinds of chemicals or herbs that can increase the analgesia effect of EA will be helpful.

SELECTION OF ACUPOINTS

Either for acupuncture anaesthesia or for analgesic effect on chronic pain, three kinds of acupoints can be chosen. The local points, which are close to the site of pain (Ah Shi Point), could induce a segmental release of endorphins in the spinal cord corresponding to the area of stimulation. They can also activate the PAG, hypothalamus-pituitary and VLO-Sm-PAG pathway. Since the enkephalinergic neurons are closely associated with pain perception neurons they inhibit noxious input very quickly, while pain relief is almost immediate and usually gives more intensive analgesia than distal nonsegmental needling.

Regional acupoints are acupoints in the same or nearby segmental area of the spinal cord, such as Quanliao (SI 18) for surgery of the frontal area of the head, Neiguan (Pe 6) to release the pectoris angina, etc. They are effective because they are found in the same or nearby spinal segment, and also may activate PAG, hypothalamus-pituitary and the VLO-Sm-PAG pathway.

Distal acupoints are far away from the painful region, but can still activate the midbrain PAG, hypothalamus-pituitary and VLO-Sm-PAG pathway, and achieve analgesic effect. Some Traditional Chinese doctors choose; these distal points according to the meridian hypothesis.

To induce EA anesthesia or treat chronic pain, not only local points are chosen, some regional and distal acupoints will also be used to achieve better effect.

CHOOSE OF THE STIMULATION PARAMETERS

Usually low current and low frequency (2–4 Hz) stimulation is chosen to treat chronic pain or induce anaesthesia. This releases enkephaline in the spinal cord and enkephaline and endorphin in the supraspinal center.[21] It produces analgesia of a slower onset and longer duration, outlasting the

20 minutes stimulation session by 30 minutes and up to many hours. Its effects are cumulative, becoming increasingly better after several treatments. On the other hand, low current and high frequency (50–200 Hz) stimulation induced analgesia has a rapid onset but of very short duration, with no cumulative effects. It may result from the release of dynorphin in the spinal cord.[20] Maybe other transmitters, e.g., GABA are involved.[43] High intensity should not be used to avoid stress as it may hurt the patient.

Since low frequency stimulations produce a cumulative effect, repeated treatments produce more and more benefits for the patient. However, repeated treatment of EA will cause tolerance. To avoid this problem, EA usually need only be given twice a week. Another way is to give the low frequency and high frequency stimulation alternatively. It may delay the tolerance because the transmitters they release are different.[21] For getting a good effect of acupuncture anaesthesia some pre-medication may need to be applied to the patient before surgery.

References

1. Anonymous (Shanghai Inst Physiol) (1973) Electromyographic activity produced locally by acupuncture manipulation. *Chin Med J*, **53**: 532–535 (in Chinese).
2. Cao, X.D., et al. (1990) Acupuncture analgesia. In Xu CF, et al. edited: *Neurobiology*, p 287, Shanghai Med Univ Press, Shanghai, China.
3. Chen, X.H. and Han, J.S. (1992) All three types of opioid receptors in the spinal cord are important for 2/15 Hz electroacupuncture analgesia. *Eur J. Pharmacol*, **211**: 203–210.
4. Chen, X.H. and Han, J.S. (1992) Analgesia induced by electroacupuncture of different frequencies is mediated by different types of opioid receptors: another cross-tolerance study. *Behav Brain Res*, **47**: 143–149.
5. Chen, X.H., Geller, E.B., et al. (1996) Electrical stimulation at traditional acupuncture sites in periphery produces brain opioid-receptor-mediated antinociception in rats. *J. Pharm Exper Ther*, **277**: 654–660.
6. Cheng, R. and Pomeranz, B. (1980) Electroacupuncture analgesia could be mediated by at least two pain-relieving mechanisms: endorphin and non-endorphin systems. *Life Sci*, **25**: 1957–1962.
7. Cheng, R. and Pomeranz, B. (1980) A combined treatment with D-amino acids and electroacupuncture produces a greater anesthesia than either treatment alone: naloxone reverses these effects. *Pain*, **8**: 231–236.
8. Cheng, R. and Pomeranz, B. (1981) Monoaminergic mechanisms of electroacupuncture analgesia. *Brain Res*, **215**: 77–92.

9. Cheng, R. and Pomeranz, B. (1987) Electrotherapy of chronic musculoskeletal pain: comparison of electroacupuncture-like TENS. *Clin J. Pain*, 2:
   143–149.
10. Chiang, C.Y., Chang, C.T., Chu, H.L. and Yang, L.F. (1973) Peripheral
    afferent pathway for acupuncture analgesia. *Sci Sin*, 16: 210–217.
11. Chiang, C.Y., Ye, Q., Shen, Y.T. and Zhu, F.X. (1978) Effects of naloxone
    on experimental acupuncture analgesia evaluated by sensory decision theory.
    Acta Zool Sin, 24: 1–10.
12. Chiang, C.Y., Du, H.J., Chao, Y.F., Pai, Y.H., Ku, H.K., Cheng, J.K., Shan,
    H.Y. and Yang, F.Y. (1979). Effects of electrolytic lesions or intracerebral
    injections of 5.6-dihydroxytryptamine in raphe nuclei on acupuncture
    analgesia in rats. *Chin Med J*, 92: 129–136.
13. Chiang, C.Y. and Huang, G.F. (1990). Raphe-spinal serotonergic neurons
    activated by electro-acupuncture in rats. In Yamada T Edited: *Pregr. Orient.
    Med.*, ICOM Press, Tokyo, P.123–128.
14. Chung, J.M., Willis, W.D., et al. (1984) Factors influencing peripheral nerve
    stimulation produced inhibition of primate spinothalamic tract cells. *Pain*,
    19: 277–293
15. Du, H.J. and Chao, Y.F. (1976). Localization of central structures involved
    in descending inhibitory effect of acupuncture viscero-somatic reflex
    discharge. *Scientia Sinica*, 19: 137–148.
16. Du, H.J., Zimmerman, M., et al. (1984) Inhibition of nociceptive neuronal
    responses in the cat's spinal dorsal horn by electrical stimulation and
    morphine microinjection in nucleus raphe magnus. *Pain*, 19: 249–257.
17. Gao, M., Li, K.Y. and He, L.F. (1997) Changes of mu opioid receptor
    binding sites in rat brain following electroacupuncture. *Acupunc &
    Electrotherap Res*, 22: 161–166.
18. Guo, H.F., Tian, J., et al. (1996) Brain substrates activated by electro-
    acupuncture (EA) of different frequencies (II): Role of Fos/Jun proteins in
    EA-induced transcription of preproenkephalin and preprodynorphin genes.
    Brain Res Molecular Brain Res, 43: 167–173.
19. Han, J.S., Terenius, L. (1982) Neurochemical basis of acupuncture
    analgesia. *Annu Rev Pharmacol Toxicol*, 22: 193–220.
20. Han, J.S., Xie, G.X. (1984) Dynorphin: important mediator for electro-
    acupuncture analgesia in the spinal cord of the rabbit. *Pain*, 18: 367–377.
21. Han, J.S., ed. (1987) *The neurochemical basis of pain relief by acupuncture.*
    China Medical and Pharmaceutical Science and Technical Press, Beijing,
    China
22. He, L.F. (1992) Caudate nucleus and pain modulation. *News in Physiol Sci*,
    7: 203–207.
23. He, L.F., Zhou, J.X., Gao, M., Du, J.H. and Da, C.D. (1992) Expression of
    c-fos protein in the rat central nervous system in response to electro-
    acupuncture. *Chin J. Physiol Sci*, 8: 359–363.

24. He, L.F., Wang, M.Z., Gao, M. and Zhou, J.X. (1992) Expression of c-fos protein in serotonergic neurons of rat brainstem following electro-acupuncture. *Acupunc Electrotherap Res. Int J.*, **17**: 243–248.
25. He, L.F., Yu, Y.H. and Gao, M. (1995) Temporal alterations of proopiomelanocortin mRNA level in rat hypothalamic arcuate nucleus following electroacupuncture. *World J. Acu-Mox*, **5**: 36–41.
26. Herget, H.F., LAllemand, H., et al. (1976) Combined acupuncture analgesia and controlled respiration. A new modified method of anesthesia in open heart surgery. *Anaesthesist*, **25**: 223–230.
27. Hou, Z.L. (1989) The receptors of needling sensation at the acupuncture points and the afferent fibres conveying needling sensation impulses. *Acupunct Res*, **14**: 127–131.
28. Huang, K.C., ed. (1996) *Acupuncture. The past and the present.* Vantage Press, New York
29. Kaada, B., Jorum, E. and Sagvolden, T. (1979) Analgesia induced by trigeminal nerve stimulation (electroacupuncture) abolished by nuclei raphe lesions in rats. *Acupunct Electrother Res*, **4**: 221–234.
30. Kho, H.G., Eijk, R.J., et al. (1991) Acupuncture and transcutaneous stimulation analgesia in comparison with moderate-dose fentanyl anesthesia in major surgery. Clinical efficacy and influence on recovery and morbidity. *Anesthesia*, **46**: 129–135.
31. Lu, G.W. (1983) Characteristics of afferent fibre innervation on acupuncture point zusanli. *Am J. Physiol*, **245**: R606–612.
32. Mayer, D.J., Price, D.D. and Raffi, A. (1977) Antagonism of acupuncture analgesia in man by the narcotic antagonist naloxone. *Brain Res*, **121**: 368–372.
33. Melzek, R., Stillwell, D.M. and Fox, E.J. (1977) Trigger points and acupuncture points for pain: correlations and implications. *Pain*, **3**: 3–23.
34. Peets, J. and Pomeranz, B. (1985) Acupuncture-like transcutaneous electrical nerve stimulation analgesia is influenced by spinal cord endorphins but not serotonin: an intrathecal pharmacological study. In: Fields, H., et al. (eds) *Advances in pain research and tehrapy*. Raven, New York, p519–525.
35. Pomeranz, B. and Chiu, D. (1976) Naloxone blocks acupuncture analgesia and cause hyperalgesia: endorphin is implicated. *Life Sci*, **19**: 1757–1762.
36. Pomeranz, B. and Paley, D. (1979) Electroacupuncture hyalgesia is mediated by afferent nerve impulses: an electrophysiological study in mice. *Exp Neurol*, **66**: 398–402.
37. Shen, E., Ma, W.H. and Lan, C. (1978) Involment of descending inhibition in the effect of acupuncture on the splanchnically evoked potentials in the orbital cortex of cat. *Sci Sin*, **21**: 677–685.
38. Stux, G. and Pomenraz, B. (1998) Basics of Acupuncture 4th ed Springer, Berlin
39. Tang, J.S., Chen, L.S., Wang, K.M. and He, Z.L. (1981) Influence of blocking the nerve fibers by DC current on the acupuncture analgesia. *Chin Med J*, **61**: 267–269.

40. Tang, J.S. and Yuan, B. (1989) A study on the afferent fibers responsible for the acupuncture analgesia. *Acupun. Res.*, **14**: 135–136.
41. Wang, K., Yao, S., Xian, Y. and Hou, Z. (1985) A study on the receptive field of acupoints and the relationship between characteristics of needle sensation and groups of afferent fibres. *Sci Sin*, **28**: 963–971.
42. Wang, Y.X., Yuan, B. and Tang, J.S. (1997) Role of thalamic nucleus submedius in the inhibitory effect of acupuncture on the transmission of noxious reception in the spinal dorsal horn. *Acupun Res*, **22**: 24–26.
43. Xu, C.F., et al. (eds) (1990) *Neurobiology*. Shanghai Med Univ Press, Shanghai China (in Chinese)
44. Xu, Z.B., Pan, Y.Y., Xu, Z.F., Mo, W.Y., Cao, X.D. and He, L.F. (1983) Synergism between metoclopramide and electroacupuncture analgesia. Acupunc & Electrotherap Res. *Int J*, **8**: 283–288.
45. Yin, Q.Z., Duanmu, Z.X., Guo, S.Y., Yu, X.M. and Zhang, Y.J. (1984) Role of hypothalamic arcuate nucleus in acupuncture analgesia A review of behavioral and electrophysiological studies. *J. Trad. Chin Med*, **4**: 103–110.
46. Yin, Q.Z. (1986) Hypothalamic arcuate nucleus and analgesia. Fudan lectures in neurobiology. II–5, 33–46.
47. Yin, Q.Z. (1996) Hypothalamic arcuate nucleus and the modulation of pain. Symposium of the 70th Annual Congress of Chin Physiol Sci. *CAPS news communication*, **15**: suppl 198–201.
48. Zhang, A.Z. ((1980) Endorphin and analgesia research in the People's Republic of China (1975–1979). *Acupunct Electrother Res Int J*, **5**: 131–146
49. Zhang, Y.Q., Tang, J.S., Yuan, B., Jia, H. (1995) Inhibitory effects of electrical stimulation of thalamic nucleus submedius on the ra6t tail flick reflex. *Brain Res*, **696**: 205–212.
50. Zhang, Y.Q., Tang, J.S., Yuan, B. and Jia, H. (1997) Inhibitory effects of electricallly evoked activation of ventrolateral orbital coartex on the tail-flick reflex are medaited by periaqueductal gray in rats. *Pain*, **72**: 127–135.
51. Zhang, Y.Q., Tang, J.S. and Yuan, B. (1996) Inhibitory effect of electrical stimulation of thalamic nucleus subgmedius on the nociceptive responses of neurons in the spinal dorsal horn in the rat. *Brain Res*, **737**: 16–24.
52. Zhang, S., Tang, J.S., Yuan, B. and Jia, H. (1998) Inhibitory effects of glutamate-induced activation of thalamic nucleus submedius are mediated by ventrolateral orbital cortex and periaqueductal gray in rats. *European J. Pain*, **2**: 153–163.

5 THE DEPRESSOR EFFECT OF ACUPUNCTURE ON HYPERTENSION

Peng Li

Clinical Studies

In 1956 Zhang[24] found that application of acupuncture to proper acupoints could produce a depressor effect on some types of hypertension. The Acupuncture Research Group of An Hui Medical College (1961)[1] also reported an observation on the acupuncture therapy of hypertension. They showed that in stages 1 and 2, especially for neural hypertension, acupuncture was highly effective, but for stage 3, acupuncture was less effective. In 1994 Qi[13] reviewed the research work of therapeutic effect of acupuncture on hypertension in China. She mentioned that most doctors used Quchi (LI 11), Renying (St 9), Zusanli (St 36), Sanyinjiao (Sp 6), Hegu (LI 4) and Taichong (Liv 3) etc. They kept the needles in the body for 20–40 minutes, did it every day and all got very good results. Their effectiveness ranged from 75%–90%. Someone also claimed that acupuncture could improve the microcirculation and blood viscosity in hypertensive patients. So there is clinical evidence that acupuncture can lower blood pressure in patients with different types of hypertension. It is important to elucidate its mechanism. During the past few years we did a series of experiments on hypertensive models, and showed that somatic afferent inputs produced by acupuncture or direct stimulation of somatic nerves cause changes in the activities of the central nervous system, leading to a reduction of the sympathetic outflow, which in turn results in a decrease in high blood pressure.

The Depressor Effect of Electroacupuncture (EA) on Noradrenaline (NA) Infusion Induced Hypertension in Dogs

In 1960 Hu et al.[4] reported an experimental hypertensive model in dogs by intravenous infusion of NA at a constant rate. They showed that EA had a significant depressor effect. In 1979 our department tried to set up other hypertensive animals in acute experiments under anesthesia, but all failed. Then in 1980, Professor Hsu asked his student Dr. Lin SX and me[9] to learn from Hu et al., and use a similar model and design to analyse its mechanism.

Experiments were performed on conscious dogs, which were trained to lie on the table calmly for 2–4 hours and be familiar with all the experimental procedures. Their carotid artery was implanted into a skin bridge on the neck beforehand. During experiments, their carotid or brachial systolic blood pressure (SPB) was measured indirectly by a special by designed cuff and manometer. The value of this was nearly the same as that measured directly on a polygraph. Heart rate was derived from the electrocardiogram (ECG), and in some dogs, the mesenteric blood flow was also measured. EA was administered to the dog's Zusanli (St 36) or Neiguan (Pe 6). A current of 2–4 volts, 0.5 ms in pulse duration, 1–2 Hz was applied for 20 minutes after the control data of SPB, HR and MBF were obtained.

EFFECT OF EA ON NORMAL DOGS AND HYPERTENSIVE DOGS INDUCED BY INTRAVENOUS INFUSION OF NA

The mean + SE of SBP in normal dogs was 132 ± 13 mmHg, and their HR was 93 + 6 beats/min. EA applied to Zusanli (St 36) with a current of 2–4 V, 1–100 Hz had no significant effect. This is consistent with the observations in healthy human beings.

In 7 conscious dogs, when NA was infused intravenously at a constant rate (0.25 mg/ml, 0.22–0.44 ml/min), the SBP was raised to 178 ± 20 mmHg (that is 40–60 mmHg higher than normal level), and could be maintained for more than one hour. HR decreased markedly at the beginning of NA infusion, and then returned to the control level within 10–20 minutes. When EA was applied to Zusanli (St 36) or Neiguan (Pe 6) for several minutes, the SBP dropped 20–30 mmHg, which is statistically significant in comparison to before EA and the control group ($n = 10$, $P < 0.01$). It was maintained at a low level during EA for 20–30 minutes, and returned to a high level slowly (about 30–40 min) when EA was stopped. The change of HR after EA had no statistical significance. Since in this model the depressor effect of EA is significant, we would like to analyse whether it is due to the decrease of cardiac output or the dilatation of some splanchnic vessels.

CHANGES OF CARDIAC FUNCTION AND MESENTERIC BLOOD FLOW (MBF) DURING DEPRESSOR EFFECT OF EA

To detect the change of cardiac function during the depressor effect of EA, the carotid pulse, phonocardiogram and ECG were used to measure the systolic time intervals. The value of preinjection period/left ventricular ejection time (PEP/LVET) is inversely proportional to the cardiac output.[4] When the NA induced hypertension was depressed by EA, there was no significant change in HR and PEP/LVET, and this depressor effect could not be blocked by intravenous injection (iv) of atropine. Therefore it is believed that the depressor effect of EA on this NA induced hypertension is not due to the decrease of cardiac output, HR, or vagus activity.

Nevertheless, the MBF measured by an implanted magnetic flow probe decreased about 50–60 ml/min when NA was infused intravenously, and increased markedly (over 40 ml/min) during the depressor period by EA. This finding indicated that the vasoconstriction of mesenteric vessels induced by NA infusion could be inhibited by EA. It is suggested that in this experiment, the vasoconstriction induced by NA infusion is partly caused by its direct action in vascular smooth muscle and partly due to the increase of sympathetic vasoconstrictor tone (see next paragraph). The depressor effect of EA is mainly due to vasodilatation of the mesenteric vessels, and this was due to centrally mediated inhibition of the sympathetic vasoconstriction tone. This suggestion is supported by the fact that the depressor effect of EA could not be found when the dogs were anaesthetised by pentobarbital or urethane-chloralose.

IS THE BARORECEPTOR REFLEX ESSENTIAL IN THE DEPRESSOR EFFECT OF EA?

It was found in these experiments that during intravenous infusion of NA in conscious dogs, not only was the BP kept at a high level, but also the respiratory rate was often markedly increased. It was thought that the baroceptor and chemoreceptor reflexes might be activated and were important in the depressor effect of EA.

To examine this proposal, another series of experiments[5] were carried out (n = 8), in which the dog's sino-aortic nerves were cut chronically. The BP was elevated to a very high level; the SBP may go up to more than 200 mmHg, but 5–7 days after surgery the dog's BP recovered to its normal range. In these animals, intravenous infusion of NA could raise the SBP up to 185 + 12 mmHg, and HR increased rather than decreased.

In such cases, EA could no longer produce a significant depressor effect. Therefore it seems likely that the depressor effect of EA depends on the existence of baroreceptive or chemoreceptive reflex, or both.

To examine the importance of the baroreceptor reflex, $\alpha_{1 \, agonist}$ phenylephrine (0.5 mg/ml, 0.11–0.22 ml/min) was infused intravenously in six intact dogs. The SBP could be raised to 155 ± 8 mmHg, and HR decreased from 112 ± 5 to 83 ± 9 beats/min. While there is no marked change of respiration, PO_2 in arterial blood did not decline. In such a hypertensive status, EA had no significant depressor effect, although the baroreceptor was strongly stimulated. This means that the depressor effect of EA is not mainly due to the activation of baroreceptor reflex.

THE ROLE OF CHEMORECEPTOR REFLEX IN THE DEPRESSOR EFFECT OF EA

On the other hand, when we measured the CO_2 concentration in the expired air of the dogs with NA infusion, it increased from $3.7 \pm 0.1\%$ to $4.7 \pm 0.3\%$. In the arterial blood the PCO_2 increased from normal level to 44 mmHg, and PO_2 of which decreased from 98 ± 6 to 75 ± 10 mmHg. Intravenous injection of propranolol (0.5 mg/kg) could prevent the decline of PO_2 and the excitation of respiration, while the SBP could still be kept at a high level (170 ± 5 mmHg). These results suggested that NA could increase the tissue metabolism and markedly increase the oxygen consumption and CO_2 production via activation of β receptor. So the chemoreceptors were excited. The pressor effect of NA infusion was partly due to a chemoreceptive pressor reflex besides its direct vasoconstrictor effect on the vascular smooth muscles. The depressor effect of EA on hypertension induced by intravenous infusion of NA might be due to the inhibition of chemoreceptor reflex. The following experiments supported this suggestion.

In four conscious dogs, when lobeline was infused intravenously at a constant rate (0.6–1.2 mg/ml, 0.22–0.44 ml/min), the SBP could be raised and maintained at a level 20–40 mmHg higher than the control. This pressor effect of lobeline is due to the excitation of arterial chemoreceptors, since lobeline produces no pressor effect in sino-aortic denervated dogs. In such cases, EA could decrease SBP to its control level. After cessation of EA, the SBP increased to a high level again.

In another series of supplementary experiments,[11] rabbits were anaesthetised by urethane-chloralose (700 mg/kg and 35 mg/kg iv respectively). It was shown in these rabbits that the carotid-occlusion pressor reflex, the renal sympathetic nerve excitation and pressor reflex induced by hypoxia could be inhibited by deep peroneal nerve stimulation. This nerve is located just underneath the acupoint Zusanli (St 36).

Based on these results, it is believed that the depressor effect of EA on the NA infusion induced hypertension is due to the inhibition of the chemoreceptive pressor reflex.

ENDOGENOUS OPIOIDS INVOLVED IN THE DEPRESSOR EFFECT OF EA

It was known that during EA endogenous opioids increased in blood and cerebrospinal fluid.[12,18,and 25] We tried to examine whether the endogenous opioids were also involved in the depressor effect of EA.

In the hypertensive dogs induced by intravenous infusion of NA, an intravenous injection (iv) of morphine (0.1 mg/kg) caused a significant depressor effect for about 15 minutes, while the depressor effect of EA could be blocked by iv naloxone (0.2 mg/kg). Moreover, in experiments performed either on conscious dogs or anaesthetised rabbits, the inhibitory effect of EA on chemoreceptor pressor reflex could be blocked by iv naloxone. All these results showed that opioid receptors might be excited in the depressor effect of EA.

To examine whether the opioid receptors in the brain were activated during the depressor effect of EA, a second series of experiments was carried out.[10] In conscious dogs, when BP was raised by NA infusion and maintained at a high level, morphine (4 μg in 2 μl) was microinjected into the midbrain periaqueductal grey (PAG), the hypothalamic supramammillary area (HSM) or the dorsal area of hippocampus (dHPC). The location of the microinjection was identified according to the atlas of Lim, et al.[7]. It caused an obvious depressor effect for about 15 minutes, with no significant change in HR. When naloxone (4μg in 2 μl) was microinjected into these areas, the depressor effect of EA was blocked. Micorinjection of normal saline into these areas exerted no influence on the hypertension induced by NA infusion. If morphine or naloxone was microinjected into the medial aspect of the parietal cortex, no effect was shown.

Therefore it is suggested that the NA infusion induced hypertension is not only caused by the direct vasoconstriction of NA, but is also due to the chemoreceptive pressor reflex. This is because NA could activate β receptors which increase the metabolism, O_2 consumption and CO_2 production, and stimulate the chemoreceptor. The depressor effect of EA is mainly due to the dilatation of splanchnic vessels caused by inhibition of the sympathetic vasomotor centre. This central inhibition was related to the activation of the opiate receptors in the PAG, HSM and dHPC etc., where plenty of opiate receptors existed.[15,14]

Depressor Effect of Acupuncture-Like Sciatic Nerve Stimulation in Spontaneously Hypertensive Rats (SHR)

Yao et al.[22] used awake adult SHRs and their normotensive control Wistar-Kyoto rats (WKY) to study the effect of acupuncture on them. The femoral arterial BP and HR were continuously recorded on a polygraph. In some rats, the splanchnic nerve discharge was also recorded. The sciatic nerve was stimulated with 3 Hz repetitive rectangular pulses of 0.2 ms duration for 30 minutes to mimic EA. The current intensity was started at a level of 4–8 times the twitch threshold (0.1 ± 0.05 mA) and then increased every 5–10 minutes, reaching 10–25 times that of the twitch threshold in the final 5–10 minutes of the stimulation period. A few minutes after the onset of stimulation, the rats showed relaxation and lay quiet in the cage. After the stimulation stopped, many rats fell asleep for hours but were easily woken up by light probing or pinching the tail.

LONG-LASTING DEPRESSOR EFFECT AFTER STIMULATION OF THE SCIATIC NERVE

In awake and free moving SHR, their BP and HR during the control period were about 160 mmHg and 400 beats/min. Stimulation of the sciatic nerve with a low frequency and low current for 30 minutes induced a light pressor response (about 10 mmHg) and increases of HR (about 35 beats/min). However, after the cessation of the sciatic nerve stimulation both the BP and HR decreased toward the pre-stimulation levels within a few minutes, followed by a further reduction in 1–3 hours. The lowest BP is about 20 mmHg below the pre-stimulation level. The BP did not fully recover to its high level until 12 hours after the termination of sciatic nerve stimulation. While in the WKYs, the same sciatic nerve stimulation also produced an increase in BP and HR. However, the post-stimulation depressor response was less pronounced and of shorter duration as compared with the response in SHR. The BP usually returned to the pre-stimulation control level within 2 hours.

This result demonstrated that prolonged low frequency acupuncture-like stimulation of the sciatic nerve induced a long-lasting depressor response that is more pronounced in hypertensive than in normotensive rats. This is again consistent with clinical observations that acupuncture lowers high blood pressure in hypertensive patients while it causes no significant BP alterations in normotensive subjects.

CHANGES OF SYMPATHETIC NERVE DISCHARGE DURING AND AFTER SCIATIC NERVE STIMULATION

The splanchnic nerve discharges of SHR increased by about 20% during the stimulation of sciatic nerve, but decreased along with the development of a depressor response after cessation of the sciatic nerve stimulation. The post-stimulation reduction of the splanchnic sympathetic outflow paralleled the fall in BP (correlation coefficient $r = 0.851$, $P < 0.01$). This implies that the post-stimulation depressor response is attributed to the sympathetic inhibition.

INFLUENCE OF ANAESTHESIA, STIMULUS PARAMETERS AND SINO-SORTIC DEAFFERENTATION ON THE DEPRESSOR RESPONSE

In SHR anaesthetised with chloralose and urethane (50 mg/kg and 500 mg/kg, respectively, iv), the elevation of BP and HR remained during the sciatic nerve stimulation. Nevertheless, after the stimulation stopped, BP and HR went back to the pre-stimulation control level, and no further decrease in BP was observed. However, in 1984 Shyu et al.[16] reported, that in SHR lightly anaesthetised with chloralose, the post-stimulation depressor response could appear.

The stimulus current intensity is another factor that influences the post-stimulation depressor response. In Yao's experiments, the post-stimulation depressor response was observed in the SHR only when the stimulus current intensity was strong enough to activate small myelinated (group III) fibres. Since the maximal current intensity used in their experiments was not higher than 25 times the twitch threshold, the group IV fibres (C fibres) were not activated.

The long-lasting post-stimulation depressor response remained in the SHRs in which the sino-aortic nerves had been sectioned on both sides. This means that the baroreceptor reflex mechanism is not involved in the above-mentioned depressor responses.

ENDOGENOUS OPIOIDS INVOLVED IN THE LONG-LASTING DEPRESSOR RESPONSE

It was shown that in the NA infusion induced hypertensive dogs, the depressor effect of EA was due to the release of endorphins, and activation of opiate receptors in the brain. So, is it similar in the SHR? Yao et al.[23] showed that when the post-stimulation depressor response had fully developed in SHR, naloxone (10–15 mg/kg, iv) almost completely reversed the depressor response for 15–30 minutes. If a bolus dose of naloxone was given 5–10 minutes before sciatic nerve stimulation, followed by a continuous intravenous infusion of naloxone in the following 2 hours, the post-stimulation depressor response was attenuated in a dose-dependent manner, whereas the pressor response and tachycardia were unaffected.

The dose of naloxone used here is much higher than that used to reverse the analgesic effect of EA, which is only 1 mg/kg in the tail flick experiments on rats. The mechanism of the difference needs further investigation.

PARTICIPATION OF CENTRAL SEROTONIN IN THE LONG-LASTING DEPRESSOR RESPONSE

In order to analyse whether the other neuro-transmitters were involved in this long-lasting depressor response, the following experiments were done. Parachlorophenylalanine methylester-HCl (PCPA), a tryptophan hydroxylase inhibitor that reduces the synthesis of serotonin, was used to pretreat the SHRs. The acupuncture-like sciatic nerve stimulation produces only a pressor response during the stimulation period, but no post-stimulation depressor response appeared. This indicates the possible participation of serotonin in the mechanism of the depressor response. If the rats were pretreated with benzerazid and peripheral decarboxylase inhibitors and 5-HTP, the precursor of serotonin, were given 30 minutes later, the acupuncture-like sciatic nerve stimulation was followed by a more marked post-stimulation depressor response. The magnitude of that was greater than that of the response induced by either 5-HTP alone or sciatic nerve stimulation alone, showing an additive effect. The effect of 5-HTP was attributable to an increase in the central serotonin, since the peripheral decarboxylase was inhibited by benezerazid. If the serotonin reuptake inhibitor zimelidine was admitted before the sciatic nerve stimulation, the post-stimulation depressor response was also enhanced. Therefore, there is much evidence to show that serotonin is also involved in the post-stimulation depressor response. The relationship between central endorphin and serotonin neurons in the cardiovascular centre will be discussed in Chapter 11.

The Depressor Effect of the Deep Peroneal Nerve (DPN) on Stress-Induced Hypertensive Rats

In modern society psychosocial stress is very serious, and it is noted that stress is closely related to the incidence of hypertension, heart attack etc. So we tried to make some stress-induced hypertensive models to study the effect of acupuncture and analyse its mechanism.

STRESS-INDUCED HYPERTENSIVE RATS

The method to make stress-induced hypertensive rats was previously introduced in Chapter 4. In this series of experiments, 22 SD rats were divided into stress and control groups at random.[8] The stress group was put into a cage, and foot shocks were given 2 hours/time, twice a day, and combined with an electric buzz as a conditional stimulus. The systolic blood pressure (SBP) was recorded from the tail artery by the tail cuff method during conscious. After 9–15 days stress, the SPB elevated from 110 ± 1 mmHg to 143 ± 5 mmHg ($P < 0.01$, n = 9). When these rats were anaesthetised, the SBP measured directly from the tail artery was $145 + 7$ mmHg, similar to the record of the tail cuff method ($P > 0.05$). It was proved that in this kind of hypertensive animal, the plasma catecholamine, angiotensin II, corticoid, glucose, cholesterol and triglycerine etc. all elevated.[26,30] This is related to the activation of the cholinergic system in the central nervous system, especially in the RVLM[8,28,29] and the corticoid had some positive feedback mechanism on the cardiovascular centre in the RVLM.[6,27]

THE DEPRESSOR EFFECT OF DPN STIMULATION

In 9 stressed rats[21] when the DPN underneath the acupoint Zusanli (St 36) was stimulated with a current of 250–300 mA (5 Hz, 0.5 ms duration) for 10 minutes, the SBP dropped markedly and decreased continuously after the cessation of stimulation. It reached its lowest level, 123 ± 10 mmHg ($P < 0.001$), one hour later. The diastolic BP (DBP) also decreased from $98 + 9$ mmHg to 72 ± 8 mmHg ($P < 0.01$). In the

6 control rats, stimulation of the DPN with the same parameters had no significant influence on the SBP and DBP.

THE DEPRESSOR EFFECT IS RELATED TO THE ACTIVATION OF OPIATE RECEPTORS IN THE ROSTRAL VENTRO-LATERAL MEDULLA (RVLM)

If naloxone (0.5 μg in 0.1 μl) was microinjected into bilateral RVLM from the dorsal aspect, stimulation of DPN with the same parameters had no depressor effect on this stress-induced hypertension. Their SBP and DBP stayed at 153 ± 4 and 99 ± 8 mmHg respectively. When normal saline was microinjected into RVLM instead of naloxone, stimulation of DPN still had a significant depressor effect. Dong et al.[2] reported that the depressor effect of stimulation of DPN on stress-induced hypertensive rats could be attenuated or blocked by injection of verapamil into the cerebroventricle. They suggested that this depressor effect might be related to the calcium influx of the neurons.

Therefore it is suggested that the depressor effect of DPN stimulation be related to the activation of opiate receptors in the cardiovascular centre of RVLM. Sun[20] reported that morphine could inhibit the cardiovascular response and renal sympathetic nerve activity induced by tail stimulation in conscious unrestrained rats. In 1996 Sun, et al.,[19] microinjected opioid agonists and naloxone into RVLM in normotensive and hypertensive rats, and found that μ and δ receptor agonists but not κ agonist had a depressor effect. So they suggested that the depressor effect of acupuncture or somatic nerve stimulation be related to the activation of μ and δ receptors in RVLM.

Physiological Significance and Clinic Application

It was shown that in all the experimental hypertension, including NA-induced hypertensive dogs, SHR, stress-induced hypertensive rats and even renal hypertension EA applied on Zusanli (St 36), Neiguan (Pe 6) or the somatic nerves underneath these acupoints had a significant depressor effect and is long-lasting. This effect could be demonstrated in conscious animals or in some urethane-chloralose anaesthetised animals, which suggested that anaesthetics could prevent this effect, and that it is centrally mediated. The afferent input might come from group III fibres, since in these experiments low current and low frequency stimulation were used effectively. It is known that the ergoreceptors in the skeletal muscles respond to muscle stretch and contractions with low frequency discharges conducted centripetally by the small myelinated (group III) fibres. Under physiological conditions these receptors are activated during muscle exercise. Maybe acupuncture can stimulate these receptors, while acupuncture-like somatic nerve stimulation directly activates the group III fibres. This hypothesis was supported by the reports of Shyu and Thoren.[17] In their experiment, the SHR was placed in a cage installed with a treadmill, the turning of which was measured automatically by a computer. Living in such a cage for several weeks, the SHR developed a spontaneous running in the treadmill, particularly at night. The rats used to run 5–7 kilometers every night and showed a decrease in blood pressure after running. The post running depressor response lasted for ½ to 2 hours and could be reversed by a large dose of naloxone, suggesting the involvement of endorphin in the mechanism. Hoffmann and Thoren[3] also showed that direct stimulation of the gastrocnemius muscle in an awake SHR causes a long-lasting post-stimulation reduction in blood pressure that is also naloxone-reversible. This kind of depressor response has much the similar characteristics as that produced by EA or prolonged somatic nerve stimulation.

In all these experiments, EA or somatic nerve stimulation inhibited the sympathetic outflow, caused vasodilatation, and exerted inhibition on the chemoreceptive pressor response in the NA induced hypertensive dogs. It is not a simple somatosympathetic reflex, but is some modification of the integrative function of the brain. It is mediated by the release of endogenous opioids in the central nervous system, and an activation of the opiate receptors in the RVLM, PAG, HSM and dHPC etc., a 5-HT mechanism might also be involved.

In clinic, when doctors or acupuncturists treat hypertensive patients, they will not only use Zusanli (St 36) or Neiguan (Pe 6), but also like to use more acupoints in one treatment, such as Quchi (LI 11), Sanyingjiao (Sp 6) etc. Underneath these acupoints are deep somatic nerves, which have more myelinated fibres. So to stimulate these points could release more endorphins, gaining a better depressor effect. However, if acupoints are stimulated too much, including acupoints innervated by superficial nerves and unmyelinated fibres, the patient will be overexcited, and no depressor effect can be obtained.

Since the depressor is long lasting (up to 12 hours) doctors treat hypertensive patients once a day or every other day. After treating them for a course (about 10 treatment) stable results are usual, especially in stages I and II.

It should be mentioned that the depressor effect of acupuncture is related to the release of endorphin, 5-HT etc. and activation of their receptors in the brain. Any medicine or chemicals that interfere with the neuro-transmitters or receptors in the brain will affect the effect of acupuncture. Of course any medicine or chemicals that help the release of endorphin and activation of opiate receptors etc. will increase the effectiveness of EA.

References

1. Acupuncture research group of An Hui Medical University (1961) Primary observation of 179 hypertensive cases treated with acupuncture. *Acta Acad Med An Hui* **4**: 6–13 (in Chinese).
2. Dong ,Y.F., Liao, S.Y. and Liang, Y.L. (1997) Effect of ventricular injection of verapamil on blood pressure decreasing action of acupuncture in stress rat. *Shanghai J. Acup Moxib* **16**: 30–31 (in Chinese).
3. Hoffman, P. and Thoren, P. (1988) Electric muscle stimulation int he hind leg of the spontansously hypertensive rat induces a long-lasting fall in blood pressure. *Acta Physiol Scand* **133**: 211–219.
4. Hu, X.C., Chen, W.L., Lu, S.Z., Gong, M.C. and Yong, Y.Q. (1960) The Normalization phenomenon of experimental abnormal blood pressure and some related observations. *A selection of Shanghai Science Technological Thesis (Biology)*. Shanghai Science and Technology Publisher **II**: 32–34.
5. Li, P., Lin, S.X., Xiao, Y.F., Wang, C.L. and Deng, Z.F. (1983) Action of buffer nerves on the depressor effect of electroacupuncture on acute experimental hypertension. *Acta Physiol Sin* **35**: 72–78 (in Chinese).
6. Li, P., Zhu, D.N., Gao, K.M., Lin, Q. and Sun, S.Y. (1995) Role of acetylcholine, corticoids and opioids in the rostral ventrolateral medulla in stress-induced hypertensive rats. *Biol Signals*, **4**: 124–132.
7. Lim, R.K.S., Lin, C.V. and Moffite, R.L. (1960) *A stereotaxic atlas of the dog's brain*. CC Thomas Publisher, Springfield.
8. Lin, Q. and Li, P. (1990) Rostral medullary cholinergic mechansisms and chronic stress-induced hypertension. *J. Auton Nerv Sys* **31**: 211–218.
9. Lin, S.X. and Li, P. (1981) Mechanism of inhibitory effect of electro-acupuncture on noradrenaline hypertension. *Acta Physiol Sin* **33**: 335–342 (in Chinese).
10. Lin, S.X., Zhang, W.Y. and Li, P. (1981) Influence of microinjecation of morphin and anloxone into brain on depressor effect of electroacupuncture. *Acta Physiol Sin* **33**: 351–357 (in Chinese).
11. Lin, S.X., Xui, G.Z. and Li, P. (1982) Effect of somatic afferent impulses on renal nerve activity and some interoceptive reflexes. *Acta Physiol SIn* **34**: 150–156 (in Chinese).

12. Malizia, E., Andrencci, G., Paolucci, D., Crescenzi, F. and Fabri, A. (1979) Electroacupuncture and peripheral B-endorphin and ACTH levels. *Lancet* **2** (8141): 535–536.
13. Qi, L.Z. (1994) Recent advance in the study of theraputic effect on hypertension by acupuncture and moxibustion. *Shanghai J. Acup Moxib* **13**: 87–89 (in Chinese).
14. Rossier, J. and Bloom, F. (1979) Central neuropharmacology of endorphins. In: Loh, H.H., Ross D.H. (eds.) *Neurochemical mechanisms of opiates and endorphins. (Adv Biochem Psychopharmacol)* Vol **20**: 165–185. Raven Prress, New York.
15. Simantov, R., Kuhar, M.J., Pastunak, C.W. and Snyder, S.H. (1976) The regional distsribution of a morphine-like factor enkephalin in monkey. *Brain Res* **108**: 189–197.
16. Shyu, B.C., Anderson, S.A. and Thoren, P. (1984) Circulatory depression following low frequency stimlulation of the sciatic nerve in anaesthetized rats. *Acta Physiol Scand* **121**: 97–102.
17. Shyu, B.C. and Thoren, P. (1986) Circulatory events following spontaneous muscle exercise in normotensive and hypertensive rats. *Acta Physiol Scand* **128**: 515–524.
18. Sjolund, B., Terenius, L., Eriksson, M. (1977) Increased cerebrospinall fluid levels of endorphins after electro-acupuncture. *Acta Physiol Scand* **100**: 383–384.
19. Sun, S.Y., Liu, Z., Li, P. and Ingenito, A.J. (1996) Central effecat of opioid agonists and naloxone on blood pressure and heart rate in normotensive and hypertensive rats. *Gen Pharmac* **27**: 1187–1194.
20. Sun, Z.J., Li, P. and Hayashida, Y. (1992) Inhibitory effect of morphine on cardiovascular response and renal sympathetic nerve activity induced by tail stimulation in conscious unrestrained rats. *Chin J. Physiol Sci* **8**: 326–332.
21. Xie, G.Z., Zhu, D.N. and Li, P. (1997) Effect of blood pressure decreasing on stress rat of hypertension treated by elecatroacupuncturing deep peroneal nerve under Zhsanli (St 36). *Shanghai J. Acup Moxib* **16**: 32–33 (in Chinese).
22. Yao, T., Andersson, S. and Thoren, P. (1982a) Long-lasting cardiovascular depression induced by acupuncture-like stimulation of the sciatic nerve in unanesthetized spontaneously hypertensive rats. *Brain Res* **240**: 77–85.
23. Yao, T., Andersson, S. and Thoren, P. (1982b). long-lasting cardiovascular depressor response following sciatric stimualtion in spontaneously hypertensive rats. Evidence for the involvement of central endorphin and serotonin systems. *Brain Res* **244**: 295–303.
24. Zhang, C.L. (1956) Clinical investigation of acupuncture therapy. *Clin J. Med* **42**: 514–517.
25. Zhang, A.Z., Huang, D.K., Zeng, D.Y., Zheng, L.M., Wang, D.L. and Zhu, C.G. (1981) The changes of endorphins in perfusate of certain brain nuclei in rabbits during acupuncture analgesia. *Acta Physiol Sin* **33**: 8–16.

26 Zhu, D.N., Cao, Q.Y., Qian, Z.W. and Li, P. (1994). The changes of plasma concentration of corticosterone, glusoce and lipids in the stress-induced hypertensive rat. *Chin J. Physiol Sci* **10**: 146–154.

27. Zhu, D.N., Xue, L.M. and Li, P. (1995) Cardiovascular, effects of microinjection of corticoids and antagonists into the rostral ventrolateral medulla in rats. *Blood Pressure* **4**: 186–194.

28. Zhu, D.N., Xue, L.M. and Li, P. (1996) Effect of central muscarine receptor blockade with DKJ-21 on the blood pressure and heart rate in stress-induced hypertensive rats. *Blood Pressure* **5**: 170–177.

29. Zhu, D.N., Xie, G.Z., Li, P. (1997) The cardiovoascular response to medullary cholinergic and corticoid stimulation is calcium channel dependent in rats. *Blood Pressure* **6**: 171–179.

30. Zhu, D.N. and Li, P. (1997) Changes of noradrenaline contents in plasma and brain homogenate of the rostral ventrolateral medulla in stress-induced hypertensive rats. *Chin J. Neurosci* **4**: 161–165 (in Chinese).

6 THE PRESSOR AND ANTI-SHOCK EFFECTS OF ACUPUNCTURE ON HYPOTENSION

Peng Li

Clinical Studies

In Chinese traditional medical practice, acupuncture is also used to treat symptoms caused by low blood pressure or circulatory shock, and has been proved to be effective. In 1973, the No. 2 Hospital of Hu Nan Medical College showed that acupuncture could raise blood pressure and had a therapeutic effect on shock.[7] Thus, acupuncture can be used to elevate low blood pressure in hypotensive patients as well as to lower high blood pressure in hypertensive patients. This chapter deals with the pressor effect of electroacupuncture (EA) and acupuncture-like somatic nerve stimulation in some experimental hypotension, in order to analyses its mechanism.

The Pressor Effect of EA on Nitroprusside (NP) Infusion Induced Hypotension in Dogs

In this series of experiments[15] both conscious and anaesthetised (pentobarbital 30 mg/kg iv) dogs were used. In conscious dogs the blood pressure (BP) was measured indirectly by the method described in Chapter 6, and in anaesthetised dogs femoral BP was recorded directly on a polygraph simultaneously with heart rate (HR) and blood flow.

EFFECT OF INTRAVENOUS INFUSION OF NP

In six conscious dogs, when NP was infused intravenously at a constant rate (10–30 μg/kg/min), the systolic blood pressure (SBP) decreased from 116 ± 6 mmHg to 78 ± 6 mmHg, and HR increased from 103 ± 8 beats/min to 189 ± 4 beats/min. No remarkable change of respiration was observed. During infusion the SBP could be maintained stably at a low level for more than one hour, and both SBP and HR returned to the control level 5–10 minutes after the cessation of NP infusion.

THE PRESSOR EFFECT OF EA ON NP INFUSION INDUCED HYPOTENSION

When acute experimental hypotension was produced in the six conscious dogs by intravenous infusion of NP, EA applied on Zusanli (St 36) or Neiguan (Pe 6) for 20 minutes could induce a significant pressor effect within 5–10 minutes. It was maintained at a higher level during EA, but dropped down quickly after the cessation of EA. There is no significant change in HR.

In contrast to the depressor effect of EA on NA induced hypertension, the pressor effect of EA could also be produced in the barbital anaesthetised dogs. The acupoints and parameters used to produce pressor effect were just the same as those to induce depressor effect in hypertensive dogs. Therefore the effect of EA is closely related to the level of BP, but not only to the site of acupoints and stimulation parameters. This problem will be discussed in Chapter 12.

CHANGES OF CARDIAC OUTPUT AND BLOOD FLOW IN DIFFERENT ORGANS DURING THE PRESSOR EFFECT OF EA

It is known that the depressor effect of NP infusion is due to its direct vasodilatation effect on vascular smooth muscle. We tried to analyse whether the pressor effect of EA came from the increase of cardiac output or vasoconstriction of some splanchnic or muscular vessels. In pentobarbital anaesthetised dogs, electromagnetic flow probes were implanted on the ascending aortic artery, renal, mesenteric and femoral arteries to measure the cardiac output, renal (RBF), mesenteric (MBF) and femoral blood flows (FBF) respectively.

The results showed that during intravenous infusion of NP, the cardiac output and RBF decreased markedly, but the MBF and FBF decreased only a little. When EA was applied to Zusanli (St 36) or Neiguan (Pe 6) and the pressor effect was produced, the cardiac output increased significantly. The RBF decreased further, while the MBF and FBF exhibited no remarkable change.

Therefore it is suggested that the pressor effect of EA in the NP induced hypotension is mainly due to the increase of cardiac output and further decrease of RBF. The decrease of RBF may decrease urine formation and increase water and sodium retention. This will increase the blood volume and so improve the cardiac output. Whether the renin-angiotensin system is involved in this response needs to be further investigated.

RESETTING OF BAROREFLEX DURING THE PRESSOR EFFECT OF EA

When the relationship between the dog's HR and BP was investigated, it was found that the HR-BP relation curve shifted to the right during EA, especially when BP was low. This means that there was a reset time of the baroreflex. Kumada et al.[6] reported that sciatic nerve stimulation in a cat could induce a reset of the baroreflex which attenuated the inhibitory action on cardiac sympathetic activity, leading to an increase in the HR and BP. In our experiment, maybe the reset of the baroreflex is there for the increase of cardiac output and BP by attenuating the inhibition of the cardiovascular sympathetic centre.

NALOXONE COULD NOT BLOCK THE PRESSOR EFFECT OF EA

Holiday et al.[6] showed the importance of endorphin in shock, because intravenous injection (iv) or intracerebroventricular injection (icv) of naloxone could reverse the hypotension. Nevertheless, in our study, naloxone (0.2 mg/kg iv) could not block the pressor effect of EA, and neither naloxone iv nor morphine (0.1 mg/kg iv) showed any significant influence on the NP induced hypotension. So it is suggested that the pressor effect of EA is not due to the release of endogenous opioids or activation of opiate receptors in the brain as it was in the depressor effect in hypertensive dogs.

CENTRAL CHOLINERGIC MECHANISMS INVOLVED IN THE PRESSOR EFFECT OF EA

When we tried the other way,[16] we applied atropine (0.15 mg/kg) or scopolamine (0.25 mg/kg) intravenously in other six conscious dogs. There was no influence on the hypotension induced by NP infusion, but both atropine and scopolamine could block the pressor effect of EA on NP infusion induced hypotension.

Brezenoff et al.[1] reported that the icv injection of acetylcholine (ACh) or microinjection of physostigmine into the posterior area of the hypothalamus could induce a pressor effect. Atropine could block this effect. To investigate the role of central cholinergic mechanisms in the pressor effect of EA, another series of experiments were carried out. Hypotension was also induced by intravenous infusion of NP. When EA was applied and showed a pressor effect, microinjection of scopolamine (20 μg dissolved in 2 μl isotonic saline) into the midbrain periaqueductal grey (PAG), midbrain reticular formation (MRF) or ventromedial hypothalamus (VMH) could block the pressor of EA. When ACh (200 μg dissolved in 2 μl isotonic saline) was microinjected into these areas, a pressor effect was elicited and lasted about 10 minutes.

If isotonic saline was microinjected into these areas, or the above drugs were micro-injected into the parietal lobe of the cortex, no influence on the hypotension and pressor effect of EA could be found. There are plenty of ACh receptors in the cerebral parietal lobe as well as in PAG, MRF and VMH.[4,13] However, in our experiments there was no significant influence on BP when ACh was microinjected into the cerebral parietal lobe. These findings suggested that the cholinergic receptors in the cerebral parietal lobe are not involved in cardiovascular regulation.

It is known that the action of ACh only lasts for a very short time. Nevertheless, the pressor effect of ACh microinjected into the PAG, MRF and VMH lasted about 10 minutes, and the pressor effect of EA persisted for several minutes after EA stopped. It is possible that in this situation, ACh is a modulator rather than a transmitter.[3] Other transmitters or long lasting neuropeptides might take part in the pressor effect of EA. This hypothesis needs to be further investigated.

The Pressor Effect of Deep Peroneal Nerve (DPN) Stimulation on Dogs with Hypotension and Shock

It was mentioned in Chapter 3 that the DPN is just beneath the acupoint Zusanli (St 36). In the above paragraph we talked about the pressor effect of EA on NP infusion induced hypotension. In this series of experiments, we tried to test whether stimulation of DPN with a current of 2–4 mA (20 Hz, 0.5 ms in duration) could also produce a pressor response in dogs anaesthetised with pentobarbital. In these experiments,[17] the mean arterial pressure (MBP) was recorded from the femoral artery. The left ventricular pressure (LVP), $\pm$ dp/dt max and the area of cardiac force loops (CFL) were recorded by inserting a catheter into the ventricle. The renal blood flow (RBF) and mesenteric blood flows (MBG) were measured by an electromagnetic flow meter.

THE PRESSOR EFFECT OF DPN STIMULATION ON NP INFUSION INDUCED HYPOTENSION

In the first group of dogs, when hypotension was induced by intravenous infusion of NP, the MBP, LVP, $\pm$ dp/dt max, and CFL decreased markedly. Stimulation of DPN produced a significant pressor response and an increase in LVP, ± dp/dt max and the area of CFL. After the cessation of DPN stimulation, all variables returned gradually to their prestimulation values.

THE PRESSOR EFFECT OF DPN STIMULATION ON DOGS WITH ENDOTOXIC SHOCK

In the second group of dogs, circulatory shock was produced by intravenous injection of E. Coli endotoxin (5 mg/kg). One hour after endotoxin injection, electrical stimulation was applied to the DPN, which resulted in significant increases in MBP, ± dp/dt max and the mesenteric vascular resistance derived from MAP/MBF, but there was no significant change in HR and renal vascular resistance (MAP/RBP). No such changes were observed in dogs with endotoxin shock without DPN stimulation.

These results indicate that stimulation of the DPN had the same pressor effect as EA in the hypotensive dogs induced by NP infusion or endotoxic shock. However, during the hypotension induced by NP infusion, the pressor effect of DPN stimulation was mainly caused by an increase of cardiac contractile force, that consistent with described in paragraph 2. In dogs with endotoxic shock, the pressor effect of DPN stimulation was not only mediated by the increase of the cardiac contractile force, but also by the increase of resistance of mesenteric vessels.

The Pressor Effect of Sciatic Nerve Stimulation in Haemorrhagic Hypotensive Rats

This series of experiments was performed by Sun et al. in 1983.[12] Hypotension was induced by hemorrhage in conscious male adult rats. The rats were divided into two groups: a stimulation group and a control group. The average body weights of the rats in these two groups were in the same range, being 301 ± 14g and 301 ± 7g (mean ± SE), respectively. According to the literature, the total blood volume of the rat is approximately 6 ml/100g of body weight. A volume of blood amounting to 50% of the total blood volume was thus withdrawn through a venous cannula over 5–10 minutes. In the control group, the HR increased and the BP decreased immediately after bleeding, being 55% of the control level. The BP gradually returned to a level about 66% of the control value within one hour after blood loss, but there was no further recovery. Of the 9 rats in the control group, all collapsed on the floor. After hemorrhage, only 1 rat drank water and 2 rats died after 30 minutes.

THE PRESSURE EFFECT OF SCIATIC NERVE STIMULATION

In the stimulation group, an acupuncture-like electrical stimulation was applied to the sciatic nerve 30 minutes after bleeding when the BP was 59.7% of the control value. The stimulation parameters were the same as were used in the SHR experiments (see Chapter 5). This stimulation caused an increase in the BP to a level of 81% of the control value. After cessation of the sciatic nerve stimulation, the BP was maintained at a level about 80% of the control value for at least 2 hours. There was a significant difference in the BP level between this group and the control group ($P < 0.05$).

Simultaneous recording of the splanchnic nerve activity showed an increase of discharge during and after the sciatic nerve stimulation. During the sciatic nerve stimulation there were also behavioural changes. The rats usually showed a normal posture and sometimes groomed. Five out of the nine rats drank water in the post-stimulation period. None of them died within the experimental observation period of 36 hours.

SCOPOLAMINE BUT NOT NALOXONE COULD BLOCK THIS PRESSOR EFFECT

In contrast to the depressor effect of EA or somatic nerve stimulation in hypertensive animals, the pressor effect of sciatic nerve stimulation in haemorrhagic hypotensive rats was not naloxone reversible, even when the dose of intravenous injection of naloxone was as high as 8 mg/kg. In naloxone-pretreated hypotensive rats, electrical stimulation of the sciatic nerve still produced a pressor effect similar to that in rats without naloxone treatment.

However, it has already been described that the pressor effect of EA or DPN stimulation on the NP infusion induced hypotension and endotoxic shock was related to the activation of the central cholinergic system. So, a scopolamine injection was also tried in the haemorrhagic hypotensive rats. Consequently, when an intravenous injection of scopolamine (8 mg/kg) was applied in these hypertensive rats, the same sciatic nerve stimulation-induced pressor response was much weaker than that in rats without scopolamine treatment. These observations imply that acetylcholine could be involved in the mechanism of the pressor response upon somatic nerve stimulation in hypotensive rats.

In conclusion, the hypotensive animals induced by NP infusion, endotoxic shock or haemorrhage, EA or stimulation of the DPN or sciatic nerve produced a marked pressor effect. An increase in cardiac contractile force, cardiac output, splanchnic nerve activity and mesenteric vascular resistance, and a further decrease of RBF, and resetting of baroreceptor reflex might accompany it. The activation of cholinergic M receptors in the PAG, MRF and VMH etc. is essential for the pressor effect. It is very interesting that the acupoints and parameters used to produce the pressor effect in hypotensive animals are the same as those used to produce depressor effect in hypertensive animals. This phenomenon will be discussed further in Chapter 12.

Role of the Brain's Cholinergic Mechanism in the Pressor Response of Acupuncture or Somatic Nerve Stimulation

The above paragraphs showed that the pressor effect of EA or somatic nerve stimulation in hypotensive animals is related to the activation of cholinergic receptors in hypothalamic and midbrain defence areas. In 1985 Brezenoff[2] reported that activation of the central cholinergic system could elevate BP accompanied by enhanced sympathetic activity. So, in this section we will discuss further the role of the brain's cholinergic mechanism in the pressor effect of somatic nerve stimulation. These experiments were performed on urethane-chloralose (700 mg/kg and 35 mg/kg, respectively) anaesthetised rabbits.

THE PRESSOR EFFECT OF BRAIN CHOLINERGIC ACTIVATION

This part of the work[18] was undertaken to observe the cardiovascular effect of icv injection of neostigmine (a cholinesterase inhibitor) and whether it evokes some effect on the BP and the survival time in animals with shock.

In normotensive rabbits when neostigmine (100 μg in 200 μl) was injected into the lateral cerebroventricle, the MBP, LVP and renal nerve discharge (RND) all increased, but HR decreased significantly within 5 minutes and was maintained for more than one hour. Therefore it is believed that this pressor effect is due to renal vasoconstriction and improvement of cardiac function, as with the pressor effect of EA. The animals also showed salivation, pupil dilation and behavior such as swallowing, raising their heads etc.

In another group of rabbits, the superior mesenteric artery (SMA) was occluded for one hour and then released to allow reperfusion. The MAP dropped slowly from 104 ±5 mmHg to 68 ± 5 mmHg within 5–20 minutes. This may have been due to the release of some toxic substances from the cyanotic and stinky intestine, causing peripheral arteriole paralysis and myocardial contractility. After icv neostigmine (100 μg in 200 μl), the MAP returned to 77 ± 5 mmHg 20 minutes later. The diastolic pressure did not increase markedly. HR decreased a little and RND increased slightly. There were no deaths 2 hours after icv injection of neostigmine, while in the control group (icv injection of saline) MAP went down continuously and two thirds of the rabbits died within 2 hours.

THE ROLE OF RVLM IN THE PRESSOR EFFECT OF BRAIN CHOLINERGIC ACTIVATION

In 1983 Hilton et al.[5] demonstrated that the RVLM is an important relay station in the pathway descending from the hypothalamic and midbrain defence areas to the cardiovascular effectors. It was also proved that neurons in RVLM projecting directly to the intermediolateral column (IML) of the spinal cord could be excited by hypothalamic and midbrain defence area stimulation.[8,10,11] Willette et al.[19] reported that a pressor response could be elicited by bilateral microinjection of cholinomimetic drugs into the RVLM. In the present study[14] we tried to investigate the role of the RVLM in the pressor effect of icv injection of some cholinomimetic drugs or acetylcholinesterase inhibitors.

After neostigmine (0.25 μg/0.5 μl on each side) or Carbachol (30 μg/ 0.5 μl on each side) was microinjected into the RVLM, the MAP and maximum blood pressure (MAPmax) induced by PAG stimulation increased significantly and was maintained for more than one hour. When atropine or scopolamine (0.25 μg/0.5 μl on each side) was microinjected into the RVLM, the MAP and MAPmax, HR, LVP and RND decreased significantly, but FBF and conductance increased slightly. No such effect could be obtained if the above drugs were microinjected into the caudal VLM. These results showed that the cholinergic receptors in the RVLM play an important role in maintaining cardiovascular sympathetic tone and BP.

Moreover, after atropine was microinjected into the RVLM, icv injection of neostigmine had no pressor effect at all. Therefore, it is suggested that the pressor effect of icv neostigmine is due to the activation of cholinergic M receptors in the RVLM.

THE PRESSOR EFFECT OF SUPERFICIAL PERONEAL NERVE (SPN) STIMULATION IS CHOLINERGIC RELATED

In the above paragraphs, we mentioned that atropine or scopolamine could block the pressor effect of DPN or sciatic nerve stimulation. It is suggested that in these nerves there are both myelinated type III fibres and type IV unmyelinated fibres. The pressor effect might be due to the activation of its unmyelinated fibres. Therefore, we tried to stimulate the superficial peroneal nerve, which contained more unmyelinated fibers, and tested its pressor effect and the cholinergic activation.

In this series of experiments,[20] the SPN was stimulated with a current of 100–300 μA, 0.5 ms duration at 5–10 Hz. After it was stimulated, the MAP and MAPmax increased significantly for about 30–35 minutes, indicating that stimulation of the SPN increased MAP and facilitated the pressor response of defence reaction. If atropine (0.25 μg each side) was microinjected into the RVLM bilaterally, both MAP and MAPmax decreased immediately and significantly, despite the SPN still being stimulated. Microinjection of atropine into the caudal VLM had no such effect.

Therefore, it is suggested that stimulation of SPN may excite the afferent fibres projecting to the hypothalamic and midbrain defence areas and their important central relay station RVLM, activating the brain cholinergic system, enhancing the sympathetic activity and eliciting the cardiovascular response of defence reaction. This is the mechanism whereby acupuncture or somatic nerve stimulation could have a pressor effect in hypotensive animals.

CHANGES OF BRAIN ACH CONCENTRATION DURING DEFENCE AREAS OR SPN STIMULATION

In this experiment, the ACh concentration in cerebroventricle push-pull perfusate was measured.[21] When the hypothalamic defence area was stimulated for 30 minutes and pressor responses were observed, the concentration of ACh in the perfusate increased markedly and nearly returned to the control level 30 minutes after the cessation of stimulation.

If SPN was stimulated and a pressor response was shown, the ACh concentration in the perfusate also increased significantly (n = 6 for each group, P < 0.01).

The ACh concentration in the push-pull perfusate of RVLM also increased significantly during stimulation of the hypothalamic defence area or SPN, and returned nearly to the control level 30 minutes after the stimulation was stopped (n = 6 for each group, P < 0.01).

Therefore, the parallel relationship between the cardiovascular activities and the release of endogenous ACh in the brain, especially in the RVLM, combined with the findings in the above paragraphs, directly confirmed our previous hypothesis. The release of endogenous ACh and activation of the cholinergic M receptors in the RVLM participated in the excitatory action on cardiovascular activities of the defence reaction and in the facilitatory effect of SPN input.

Clinical Application

The above experiments showed that acupuncture does have pressor and anti-shock effects on hypotensive animals, and that it is related to the activation of the cholinergic M receptors of the sympathetic cardiovascular centre of RVLM. This is the scientific base for the therapeutic efficacy of acupuncture in the treatment of some kinds of hypotension and shock in clinics. It will be more effective than using solely conventional treatment, e.g., intravenous infusion of fluid, etc. Acupuncture is surely better than using vasoconstriction agents, which have a lot of side effects.

The acupoints we used were Renzhong (Du 26), Chenjiang (Ren 24) and Shixuan, Zusanli(St 36) and Neiguan (Pe 6) can also be chosen. Although these acupoints are usually used for depressor effect when the patients have hypertension, in hypotensive patients stimulation of Neiguan or Zusanli also has pressor effect. Maybe underneath Zusanli (St 36) and Neiguan (Pe 6), there are DPN and MN that have some unmyelinated fibers, and by stronger current stimulation and under hypotensive status, they can activate the cholinergic receptors in RVLM and thus get pressor effect. The inputs from myelinated fibers may also have some beneficial effects on the cardioavascular sympathetic center, and modulate the cardiovascular function.

References

1. Brezenoff, H.F. and Giuliano, R. (1982) Cardiovascular control by cholinergic mechanism in the central nervous system. *Annu Rev Pharmocol Toxicol* **22**: 341–381.
2. Brezenoff, H.E. (1985) Brain acetylcholine and hypertension: a compelling association. *Trends Auto. Pharmocol* **3**: 203–212.
3. Brown, D.A. (1983) Slow cholinergic excitation—a mechanism for increasing neuronal excitability. *Trends Neuro-Sci* **8**: 302–307.
4. Fibizer, H.C. (1982) The organization and some projections of cholinergic neurones of the mammalian forebrain. *Brain Res Rev* **4**: 323–388.
5. Hilton, S.M., Marshall, J.M. and Timms, R.J. (1983) Ventral medullary relay neurons in the pathway from the defence areas of the cat and their effect on blood pressure. *J. Physiol (London)* **345**: 383–389.
6. Holady, J.W. and Faden, A.I. (1980) Naloxone acts at central opiate receptors to reverse hypotension, hypothermia and hypoventilation n spinal shock. *Brain Res* **189**: 295–300.
7. Hu Nan Med Col (1973) Analysis of 160 cases with shock treated by new acupuncture. *New Med J* **2**: 10 (in Chinese).
8. Huangfu, D.H. and Li, P. (1986) Defence reaction-related-neurons in ventral medulla of rabbits. *Acta Physiol Sin* **38**: 383–389.
9. Kumada, M., Nogami, K., Sagawa, K. (1975) Modulation of carotid sinus baroreceptor reflex by sciatic nerve stimulation. *Am J. Physiol* **228**: 1535–1540.
10. Li, P. and Lovick, T.A. (1985) Excitatory projections from hypothalamic and midbrain defence regions to nucleus paragantocellularis lateralis in the rat. *Exp Neurol* **89**: 543–553.
11. Lovick, T.A., Smith, P.R. and Hilton, S.M. (1984) Spinally projecting neurons near the ventral surface of the medulla in the cat. *J. Auton Nerv Syst* **11**: 27–33.
12. Sun, X.Y., Yu, J. and Yao, T. (1983) Pressor effect produced by stimulation of somatic nerve on haemorrhagic hypotension in conscious rats. *Acta Physiol Sin* **35**: 264–270 (in Chinese).
13. Totter, A., Bindsall, N.J.M., Field, P.M. and Raisman (1979) Muscarinic receptors in the central nervous system of rat. II. Distribution of binding of (^{3}H)-propylberzilylholine mustard in the midbrain and hindbrain. *Brain Res Rev* **1**: 167–183.
14. Xia, Q.G., Lu, L. and Li, P. (1989) Role of rostral ventrolateral medulla in the pressor response to intracerebroventricular injection of neostigmine. *Acta Physiol Sin* **41**: 19–29 (in Chinese).
15. Xiao, Y.F., Lin, S.X., Deng, Z.F. and Li, P. (1983) Mechanism of pressor effect of electroacupuncture on nitroprusside hypotension in dogs. *Acta Physiol Sin* **35**: 257–263 (in Chinese).
16. Xiao, Y.F. and Li, P. (1985) Influence of microinjection of scopolamine into various brain areas on pressor effect of electroacupuncture in nitroprusside induced hypotensive dogs. *Acta Physiol Sin* **37**: 31–36 (in Chinese).

17. Xiao, Y.F., Sun, X.Y., Yao, T. and Li, P. (1985) Cardiovascular effects of deep peroneal nerve stimulation in hypotensive or shock dogs. *Chin J. Appl Physiol* **1**: 269–273 (in Chinese).
18. Xiao, Y.F., Xia, Q.G., Zhong, G.Q. and Li, P. (1989) Pressor response to intracerebroventricular injection of neostigmine in normotensive and hypotensive rabbits. *Chin J. Physiol Sci* **5**: 26–32.
19. Willete, R.N., Pennen, S., Kreigh, A.J. and Sapru, H.N. (1984) Cardiovascular control by cholinergic mechanism in the rostral ventrolateral medulla. *J. Pharmacol Exp Ther* **231**: 457–463.
20. Zhu, D.N., Guo, X.Q. and Li, P. (1990) Relationship between the rostral medullary cholinergic mechanism and the cardiovascular component of the defence reaction. *Chin J. Physiol Sci* **6**: 86–99.
21. Zhu, D.N., Guo, X.Q. and Li, P. (1991) Influence of hypothalamic or superficial peroneal nerve stimulation on the release of intracerebral acetylcholine. *Chin J. Physiol Sci* **7**: 18–26.

7 THE INHIBITORY EFFECT OF ACUPUNCTURE ON ARRHYTHMIA

Peng Li

Clinical Studies

In traditional Chinese medicine, it was said that acupuncture could cure arrhythmia. In 1979 Lin[40] first reported at the Chinese Physiological Congress that in his recent years of clinical observation acupuncture could be used to treat arrhythmia. 1981 Gao et al.[14] reported a clinical observation on the treatment of 220 cases of arrhythmia with acupuncture. Usually they used one or two of the following acupoints: Neiguan (Pe 6), Shenmen (He 7), Jianshi (Pe 5), Jueyinshu (UB 14), or Xinshu (UB 15). They claimed that the patients' symptoms disappeared and the pulse and electrocardiogram (ECG) turned out to be normal, the effective rate being as high as 86.4%. In our own experience, we saw that acupuncture could inhibit some kinds of arrhythmia quickly and effectively. So we tried to set up some experimental models to investigate the mechanism of the modulatory effect of acupuncture on different kinds of arrhythmia.

The Inhibitory Effect of Acupuncture on Ventricular Extrasystoles Induced by Hypothalamic Stimulation

EXPERIMENTAL ARRHYTHMIA INDUCED BY HYPOTHALAMIC STIMULATION IN RABBIT

Many authors reported that stimulation of various central nervous structures electrically or chemically elicited a diversity of ventricular arrhythmia.[54,69] Hall et al.[29] showed that electrical stimulation of an area near the midline of the posterior hypothalamus caused a variety of cardiac arrhythmia with the T wave of ECG reversed. Evans[11] reported that the region of the rabbit hypothalamus is partly homologous with that hypothalamic area associated with the defence reaction in the cat. In 1980, Fu et al.[12] induced arrhythmia in rabbits by stimulation of the midline area of the hypothalamus. Guo et al.[74] started to use this model for studying the mechanism of acupuncture.

Experiments were carried out on rabbits of both sexes with a body weight of 2.5–3.0 kg. Animals were anaesthetised with urethane and chloralose (700 mg/kg and 35 mg/kg, respectively, iv). The CO_2 concentration in the expired air was maintained at 3.55–4.0%. The rectal temperature was kept at 37–38°C. Femoral BP, HR and ECG (lead II) were monitored and recorded on an SJ-42 polygraph (Shanghai Medical Instrumental Factory). Stimulation of the vicinity area of the dorsal medial hypothalamic nucleus, ventral medial hypothalamic nucleus and fornix of the medial and posterior hypothalamus could induce pupil dilation and an increase in BP and LVP. When the pressor response was pronounced, bradycardia, missing of beats, ventricular extrasystoles and ventricular tachycardia etc. were commonly observed. After vagotomy, the bradycardia and missing of beats disappeared, but the extrasystoles still existed. However, the latter could be abolished with the attenuation of pressor response by stellalectomy or administration of phentolamine or propranolol. Thus, it is believed that the extrasystoles were due to cardiac sympathetic excitation, adrenergic β-receptor activation and the rise of arterial pressure caused by hypothalamic stimulation. Xia et al.[76] also showed that stimulation of the medial portion of the hypothalamus evoked pupillary dilation, pressor effect, splanchnic vasoconstriction, increases in the femoral blood flow and other effects similar to the defence reaction in the cat. The only difference to cats is that the increase of femoral blood flow could not be blocked by atropine. It also increases the cardiac sympathetic activity. Bilateral stellectomy abolished the ventricular extrasystoles and pressor response, induced by stimulation of the hypothalamus, while vagotomy produced the opposite effects. So the hypothalamus stimulation induced ventricular extrasystoles (HVE) are mainly due to an increased activity of the cardiac sympathetic nerves and vagus exerting an inhibitory effect on HVE. Our results are very similar to those described by Azevodo et al. in cats.[1] So we called the vicinity area of the fornix as the hypothalamic defence area.

Stimulation of the hypothalamus also increased the blood and plasma viscosity. Bilateral section of the cervical vagi could not block it. However, after an intravenous injection of propranolol or bilateral adrenalectomy, the BP dropped, and the pressor response, the number of HVE and the blood viscosity induced by hypothalamic stimulation diminished. Therefore the increase of blood or plasma viscosity is similar to HVE, and is probably due to the over excitation of the sympathetic-adrenaline system.[24]

THE INHIBITORY EFFECT OF ACUPUNCTURE ON THE HVE

In this series of experiments, HVE were induced by stimulation of the hypothalamus (in the vicinity of the dorsomedial nucleus, ventromedial nucleus or fornix) for 5 seconds every 5 minutes. The number of HVE after each stimulation did not vary significantly for more than one hour. In such cases, electroacupuncture (EA) was applied to the leg areas analogous to Zusanli (St 36) or Neiguan (Pe 6), and the HVE were obviously inhibited (P < 0.01). If we stimulated the deep peroneal nerve (DPN) or median nerve (MN) which is just underneath the Zusanli and Neiguan acupoints, respectively, it had the same inhibitory effect on HVE. The current used should be less than 500 μA, while the frequency is 5 Hz and pulse duration 0.5 ms. Stimulation of the superficial peroneal nerve (SPN) or superficial radial nerve (SRN) had no such inhibitory effect. During DPN or MN stimulation, the pressor effect of hypothalamus stimulation did not change significantly while the HVE was inhibited. Section of both vagus nerves could not block such inhibition. So it is assumed that EA or deep nerve stimulation might exert some kind of inhibitory effect on the cardiac sympathetic centre.[16] In our further analysis we usually used deep nerve stimulation instead of EA.

INFLUENCE OF CHEMORECEPTOR AND BARORECEPTOR REFLEXES

Spyer[57] reported that defence reaction could be facilitated by chemoreceptor reflex and inhibited by baroreceptor reflex. Li et al.[39] showed that the chemoreceptor reflex could be inhibited by somatic nerve stimulation. Here we tried to study the influence of chemoreceptor and baroreceptor reflexes on HVE, and whether the inhibitory effects of EA or somatic nerve stimulation depend on these reflexes.

Xia et al.[73] reported that intravenous injection of KCN (0.3 mg/kg) could induce ventricular extrasystoles and facilitate the HVE. This phenomenon was abolished after bilateral section of the carotid sinus nerves. HVE was diminished by stimulation of the depressor nerve, and increased markedly accompanied by the elevation of BP after buffer nerves were cut. So it is certain that HVE could be facilitated by chemoreceptor excitation and inhibited by baroreceptor activation. However, the inhibitory effect of DPN stimulation on HVE did not depend on the chemoreceptor or baroreceptor reflex; it still existed even when the buffer nerves were cut.

ROLES OF THE MIDBRAIN PERIAQUEDUCTAL GRAY (PAG) IN THE INHIBITORY EFFECT OF EA ON HVE

Stimulation of dorsal PAG could also induce a pressor effect, defence reaction and ventricular extrasystoles as well as stimulation of the hypothalamic defence area. It is also known that there were projections from the hypothalamic defence area to dorsal PAG.[43] In this section we will talk about the influence of application of opiates, 5-HT and noradrenaline and their antagonists into PAG on the HVE and the inhibitory effect of DPN stimulation.

When morphine (2 μg/μl) was microinjected into the PAG, HVE could be inhibited instantaneously. While naloxone (2 μg/1μl) was injected into PAG, the HVE increased markedly and could no longer be inhibited by DPN stimulation. So it is suggested that endogenous opiate receptor activation was related to the inhibitory effect on sympathetic outflows by EA or DPN stimulation.[16]

Microinjection of 5-HT (2 μg/1 μl) into PAG could inhibit the HVE instantaneously, whereas microinjection of normal saline (1 μl) or LSD (0.2 μg/1 μl) had no significant effect. The inhibitory effect of DPN stimulation on HVE could be reduced or abolished by microinjection of PCA (4 μg/2 μl), LSD (0.2 mg/1 ml) or cinanserine (4 mg/2 ml) into PAG. Hence, it was indicated that normal activity of 5-HT neurons was necessary for the inhibitory effect on HVE by DPN stimulation.

The inhibitory effect on the HVE by microinjection of morphine into PAG could be reduced by microinjection of LSD into PAG beforehand, but the inhibitory effect of 5-HT microinjected into PAG could not be blocked by previous microinjection of naloxone. So it is suggested that the inhibitory effect of endogenous opiate is mediated in part by a serotonergic pathway.[17]

Microinjection of NE (4 μg/2 μl) into the ventral PAG resulted in a facilitory effect, and increases in the number of HVE. In contrast, microinjection of β-adrenoceptor antagonist practolol (2 μg/2 μl) into the same area produced a marked decrease in the number of HVE, and blocked the facilitatory effect of NE on the HVE. However, α-adrenoceptor antagonist phentolamine (2 μg/2 μl) had no such effect. After microinjection of NA into PAG, the inhibitory effect of morphine (4 μg/2 μl) microinjected into the PAG still existed, but the inhibitory effect of DPN stimulation was attenuated or abolished.

In these primary observations, the volume of microinjection is up to 1–2 μl and seems too large. Nevertheless, the results suggested that the activation of β-adrenoceptors in the PAG might facilitate the HVE, and the inhibitory effect of DPN stimulation on HVE at least in part via endogenous opiates, which inhibit NA release in PAG.[38]

ROLES OF ARCUATUS AREA (ARC) IN THE INHIBITORY EFFECT OF SOMATIC NERVE STIMULATION ON HVE

It is known[2,70] that met-enkephalin neurons exist in the lower brain stem, whereas β-endorphin neurons are clustered in the vicinity of the arcuate nucleus and the basal tuberal area. Projections were sent through the anterior hypothalamic area into the dorsal midline thalamus and innervated the median eminence and other circumventricular organs. In our experiments, it was shown that the ARC area might play an important part in the inhibitory effect of DPN stimulation on HVE. So we tried to analyse the role of ARC in this inhibition.

The ventricular extrasystoles could be induced not only by stimulation of the hypothalamic defence area, but also by stimulation of a dorsal portion of the midbrain periaqueductal gray (dPAG) and the rostral ventrolateral medulla (RVLM). The inhibitory effect of DPN stimulation on ventricular extrasystoles induced by dPAG or RVLM was still evident after an oblique transaction of the brain stem from the anterior border of the superior colliculi to the preoptic chiasma. However, it could be abolished by a transaction from the anterior border of superior colliculi to the rostral end of the pons. The inhibitory effect of DPN stimulation on HVE and all the ventricular extrasystoles induced by stimulation of dPAG or RVLM was still evident after an electrolytic lesion of the pituitary, but was abolished after an electrolytic lesion of the ARC. So the ARC but not the pituitary is important in the inhibitory effect of DPN stimulation on HVE.

Our experiments further showed that the HVE could be inhibited by a microinjection of morphine (2 μg/1 μl) into the ARC, and increased by a microinjection of naloxone (2 μg/1 μl) into the same area. In the latter case, the inhibitory effect of DPN stimulation on HVE was no longer in evidence. Therefore, the activation of opiate receptors in the ARC is essential for the inhibitory effect of DPN stimulation. Further analysis showed that with a lesion of the RVLM a microinjection of naloxone (2 μg/1 μl) into the ventral PAG, the inhibitory effect on HVE by microinjection of morphine (2 μg/1 μg) into ARC was abolished. So it is suggested that the ventral PAG and RVLM (18) might mediate the inhibitory effect on HVE by microinjection of morphine into the ARC area.

INFLUENCE OF THE ACTIVITY OF LOCUS COERULEUS COMPLEX (LC–SC) ON THE HVE

The Lc-Sc also has some influence on the HVE. Microinjection of morphine (4 μg/2 μl) into the Lc-Sc could decrease the number of HVE, while microinjection of ACh into the same area facilitated HVE. This facilitatory effect of ACh could be blocked by microinjection of propranolol (2 mg/1 ml) into the ventral PAG or medial portions of the medulla, but microinjection of phentolamine (10 μg/1 μl) into the same area had no blocking effect.

The inhibitory effect of DPN stimulation on HVE was diminished by a microinjection of naloxone (4 μg/2 μl) or ACh (50 μg/2 μl) into the Lc–Sc. Stimulation of the LC–Sc with a weak current had the same effect. A bilateral lesion of LC–SC could enhance the inhibitory effect of DPN stimulation. These results suggested that activation of the Lc–Sc might have an antagonistic effect on the inhibition of HVE induced by DPN stimulation. Activation of opiate receptors in Lc–Sc had an inhibitory effect, and activation of cholinergic receptors had a facilitory effect on HVE, probably mediated via PAG and the medial portion of the medulla.[19]

Further experiments showed that activation of the α_2-adrenorceptor by microinjection of norepinephrine (NE, 4 μg/2 μl) or clonidine (10.6 μg/ 2 μl) into the Lc–Sc also reduced the number of HVE. Whereas microinjection of the α_1-adrenoceptor agonists methoxamine (20 μg/1μl), phenylephrine (20 μg/2 μl), and α_2-adrenoceptor antagonist yohimbine (4 μg/2 μl), opiates receptor antagonist naloxone (4 μg/2 μl) or β-adrenoceptor antagonist propranolol (2 μg/2 μl) into the same area had no such effect. However, the inhibitory effect of microinjection of NE into the Lc–Sc on HVE could be prevented or reversed by microinjection of yohimbine (4 μg/2 μl) or intravenous injection (2 mg in 1 ml saline) into the same area. Microinjection of naloxone (4 mg/2 ml) into the Lc–Sc could also reverse the inhibitory effect of clonidine on HVE, but propranolol had no effect.

These results suggest that the inhibitory effect of HVE by microinjection of NE or clonidine into the Lc–Sc is mediated by activation of its α_2-adrenoceptor. Endogenous opioids might be also involved.[20]

ROLES OF THE MEDIAL MEDULLA IN THE INHIBITORY EFFECT OF DPN STIMULATION ON HVE

The medial medullary area includes the nucleus raphe obscure (NRO) and nucleus raphe parvus. In 1985, Xia et al.[75] reported that the number of HVE was decreased by stimulation of the midline area of the medulla oblongata 0–2 mm rostral to the obex. After destroying this area, the inhibitory effect of DPN stimulation on HVE ended. Microinjection of cinanserine (4 μg/2 μl) into this area attenuated the inhibitory effect of DPN stimulation on the HVE, while microinjection of naloxone (4 μg/2 μl) into this area completely blocked the inhibitory effect. The number of HVE was be reduced if 5-HT or morphine was microinjected into the ventral PAG. This effect could be abolished by destroying the medial portion of the medulla. These results suggest that the inhibitory effect of DPN stimulation on HVE is mediated by activation of opiate and serotonin receptors in the medial medulla.

ROLES OF THE ROSTRAL VENTROLATERAL MEDULLA (RVLM) IN THE EFFECT OF SOMATIC NERVE STIMULATION ON HVE

Guo and Li[21,22] showed that the pressor response and HVE induced by stimulation of the hypothalamic and midbrain defence areas could be abolished by electrolytic lesion of the bilateral RVLM. This result suggests that the RVLM might receive convergent inputs from the hypothalamic and midbrain defence areas and is an essential link in the efferent pathway for HVE.

Destroying the contralateral RVLM could abolish the inhibitory effect of DPN stimulation on extrasystoles induced by stimulation of the unilateral RVLM. This suggests that the RVLM also plays a part in the inhibitory effect of DPN stimulation.[40]

NEUROTRANSMITTERS OF RVLM IN THE INHIBITORY EFFECT OF DPN STIMULATION ON HVE

Endogenous opioids
Our experiments showed that the inhibition of HVE by DPN stimulation was less obvious or abolished by microinjection of naloxone (2 μg in 0.5–1 μl) into RVLM; while microinjection of morphine (5 μg in 0.5–1 μl) into the RVLM bilaterally decreased the number of HVE. In another experiment, electrical stimulation of the caudal raphe nuclei or microinjection of L-sodium Glutamate (50 mmol/L, 0.5–1 μl) into the same area caused a decrease in the number of HVE. However, these effects were diminished following bilateral microinjection of naloxone into the RVLM. So it is suggested that the activation of opiate receptors in the RVLM may inhibit HVE. The inhibitory effect of DPN stimulation

on HVE is possibly mediated by the excitation of the caudal raphe nuclei, which in turn activates the opiate receptors in the RVLM.[22,23]

Gamma-aminobutyric acid (GABA)

Bousquets et al.[5] and Keeler et al.[37] reported that application of GABA and muscimol (a GABA receptor agonist) could inhibit the neuronal activity in RVLM and result in a decrease of BP and HR. Our results showed that microinjection of GABA into the RVLM bilaterally caused a fall of BP, and decreased the number of HVE, while microinjection of the GABA receptor antagonist bicuculline into the same area facilitated HVE.[26]

Our study also showed that the inhibition of HVE by DPN stimulation was less obvious or even abolished by bilateral microinjection of bicuculline or picrotoxin into the RVLM, but microinjection of strychnine into the same area had no effect. If picrotoxin was microinjected into the caudal ventrolateral medulla (CVLM), the inhibitory effect of DPN stimulation was not blocked. This may be due to the different cardiovascular function of neurons in the CVLM as Blessing and Peis suggested.[3]

The inhibitory effect of a microinjection of morphine into the RVLM on HVE was reduced, when bicuculline was microinjected into the RVLM first. On the other hand, the inhibitory effect of GABA microinjected into the RVLM was still evident, even when naloxone was microinjected into the RVLM first. Therefore, it is believed that the inhibitory effect of morphine-like substance on HVE is mediated in part through the GABAergic pathway in the RVLM.[27]

Acetylcholine

Acetylcholinesterase was found in RVLM.[31] Our results showed that bilateral microinjection of carbachol (30 ng in 0.5 μl) or neostigmine (0.25 μg in 0.5 μl) into the RVLM could elevate the mean arterial pressure (MBP) and facilitate the pressor response and HVE evoked by stimulation of the hypothalamic defence area. On the other hand, microinjection of the cholinergic M-receptor blocker scopolamine (0.15 μg in 0.5 μl) or atropine (0.25 μg in 0.5 μl) could cause a decrease of MBP, inhibition of pressor response and HVE. Electrical stimulation of the unilateral superficial peroneal nerve (SPN) with low frequency and low intensity (0.1–0.3 mA, 5–10 Hz, 0.5 ms duration) for 15 minutes could elevate MBP and facilitate pressor response and HVE. Bilateral microinjection of atropine (the same dose as mentioned above) into the RVLM could reduce the MBP, pressor response and HVE and block the facilitatory effect of SPN stimulation. All these results suggested that the activation of cholinergic sensitive neurons in RVLM could elevate the MBP and facilitate the pressor response and HVE. The facilitatory effect of SPN stimulation is also related to the activation of cholinergic M-receptors in the RVLM.

Further evidence was obtained with the techniques of push-pull perfusion and redioimminoassay of acetylcholine (ACh). Zhu et al.[78,79] found that the ACh content in the perfusate from the cerebroventricule (CV) or RVLM increased significantly during the stimulation of the hypothalamic defence area or the SPN. After cessation of the stimulation, it returned nearly to the control level (see Chapter 6). These results showed that the release of endogenous ACh in the RVLM is involved in the cardiovascular component of the defence reaction evoked by stimulation of the hypothalamic defence area, and so is the facilitatory effect of SPN stimulation.

Serotonin

Central serotonin neurons are believed to play a role in the neural control of circulation. Baum et al.[4] reported that a decrease of cardiac sympathetic efferent discharge correlated to an increase of 5-HT in the brain. Coote et al.[9] showed that the depressor response to icv administration of 5-HT was due to its action on the hindbrain. Lovick and Li[44] reported that microinjection of 5-HT (10–100 nmol) bilaterally into the RVLM in rats produced a long lasting depressor response. Guo et al.[17] found that HVE could be inhibited instantaneously by microinjection of 5-HT (2 μg/1 μl) into the central grey. The pressor response and HVE induced by electrical stimulation of the hypothalamic defence area were attenuated by bilateral microinjection of 5-HT into the RVLM, but were not affected by vagotomy. These results suggest that the activation of 5-HT receptors in the RVLM could inhibit HVE. This inhibitory effect might be mediated by an inhibition of the cardiac sympathetic centre. It is also suggested that 5-HTergic mechanisms in the RVLM are tonically active, because bilateral microinjection of the 5-HT receptor blocker cinanserine into the RVLM facilitated HVE.

Guo et al.[28] further showed that icv injection of 5-HT or microinjection of L-sodium Glutamate into NRO resulted in a significant decrease in the number of HVE. These effects could be prevented by bilateral microinjection of the 5-HT receptor antagonist cinanserine into the RVLM; so, it is thought that 5-HT pathways may be involved in the inhibition of RVLM by NRO.

In summary, electric needling of Zusanli or Neiguan or stimulation of the DPN or MN (with repetitive pulses of low frequency and low current)

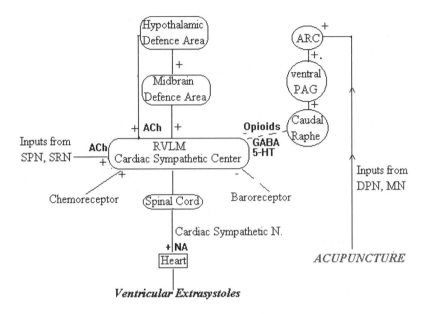

Fig. 7.1   Mechanism of the inhibitory effect of acupuncture or somatic inputs on HVE ... excitation, ... inhibition.

could significantly reduce the HVE in rabbits. This effect might be mediated by an inhibition of the cardiac sympathetic centre. The RVLM is an essential link in the efferent pathway for the inhibitory effect of DPN stimulation on HVE. The activation of opiate, GABA and 5-HT receptors in the RVLM were involved (Fig. 7.1).

Blocking Effect of the Somatic Inputs on the Evoked Vagal Bradycardia

The above section discussed the inhibitory effect of somatic stimulation on the experimental extrasystoles induced by hypothalamic stimulation that increased cardiac sympathetic outflow. However, few experiments have been performed concerning the modulatory effect of somatic inputs on the arrhythmia originated from the over-excitation of the central parasympathetic component. In this series of experiments, an attempt was made to find out whether there is any modulatory effect of various somatic inputs on the evoked vagal bradycardia induced by electrical stimulation of the aortic nerve (AN) in rabbits. If so, further study would be carried out to explore the putative mechanisms underlying the effect of somatic inputs on the evoked bradycardia. All these studies were performed on rabbits anesthetized intravenously with urethane (700 mg/kg) and chloralose (35 mg/kg).

THE EVOKED VAGAL BRADYCARDIA (EVB)

It has been identified that the AN of rabbits is solely barosensory,[53] and that electrical stimulation of the AN invariably produced a decrease in heart rate and a depressor response. The bradycardiac response induced in this approach was attributed primarily, if not solely, to an excitation of parasympathetic outflows.[51,58] This notion was strongly supported by the observations in our experiments that showed that the evoked bradycardia was completely abolished by systemic administration of the cholinergic receptor antagonist atropine or bilateral vagotomy. Likewise, application of the β-adrenergic receptor antagonist propranolol or removal of bilateral stellate ganglia failed to affect the AN stimulation evoked bradycardia.[59] In the present study, the vagal bradycardia evoked by stimulation of the AN or, in a few cases, nucleus tractus solitarii (NTS) was used as a regular model to assess the further influence of somatic inputs on it.

THE EFFECTS OF VARIOUS SOMATIC AFFERENT NERVE STIMULATION ON THE EVB

Prolonged electrical stimulation of the cutaneous nerve, i.e., the superficial peroneal (SPN) or superficial radial nerve (SRN), with low intensity (100–300 μA) and low frequency (5 Hz) produced a partial blockade of the EVB induced by the AN stimulation.[59] The blocking effect usually existed throughout the 10–15 minutes stimulation period and was maintained for 10–35 minutes after the termination of somatic nerve stimulation. However, the somatic nerve stimulation does not appear to affect the decrease of BP induced by AN stimulation.

The partial inhibition of EVB can be also produced by electrical stimulation of the deep muscular nerve, i.e., DPN or MN. However, in order to achieve the same inhibition, the intensity for stimulating deep nerves should be increased up to 600–800 μA. Low intensity stimulation (100–300 μA) of deep nerves only produced a very slight influence on the EVB without statistical significance.

The activation of C fibres in various somatic afferent nerves seems necessary for producing the effect of somatic input. Measurement of the conduction velocity of the peroneal nerve fibres revealed that the A_α (96–100 m/s), A_β (40–44 m/s) and A\delta(18–22 m/s) afferents were activated by stimulation of deep nerves with low intensity while the C fibres (<1 m/s) were, only activated by stimulation of the cutaneous nerves with low intensity or deep nerves with high intensity. Stimulation of deep nerves with low intensity, which did not activate the C fibres, did not affect the EVB. On the other hand, stimulation of the deep nerves with high intensity or cutaneous nerves with low intensity, which activate C fibres, blocked the EVB. So, it is reasonable to say that the blocking effect of somatic inputs on the EVB might be related to the activation of the C fibres.

THE BRAIN AREAS MEDIATING THE BLOCKING EFFECT OF SOMATIC INPUTS

In terms of the traditional transacting technique at different levels of the brain, one can explore the neural substrate that may process the effect of somatic inputs. In the experiments in which the cerebral cortex, septum and hippocampus were disconnected from the lower brain structures the blocking effect of the SPN on the EVB still remained. Transaction made just in front of the midbrain also had almost no effect on the bradycardiac response by somatic inputs. These results suggest that brain structure organising the somatic input effect is most likely to be located in the lower brainstem.[59]

In the study of neural regulation of cardiovascular activity, much attention has been focused on the RVLM. The neurons within this region have been confirmed not only to play an important role in maintaining resting HR and BP, but also to be important in cardiovascular reflexes. In the present study, we were interested in the observation of the neurons within the RVLM, which served as a key link in the circuitry. These neurons mediate the blocking effect of the somatic inputs on the bradycardia produced by stimulation of AN. Direct electrolytic lesions of the RVLM region resulted in an almost total attenuation of the effect of somatic input. Similar results were also obtained following microinjection of lidocaine into the same area within RVLM.[25] Also, direct electrical stimulation of the RVLM or microinjection of the excitant aminoacid DL-homocysteic acid (DLH, 0.2M in 100 nl), which has been shown to affect cell bodies but leave was passing fibres unaffected, into the RVLM produced the same blocking effect on EVB as revealed during somatic afferent nerve stimulation.[65] Together, the neurons within the RVLM play an important role in processing somatic input, effects. However, it could be argued that the results obtained after the RVLM lesion were an abnormal response, since a profound fall in both BP and HR took place after the RVLM lesion. To rule out this possibility, a series of experiments were set up. In the animals receiving the RVLM lesion, a phenylephrine hydrochloride was infused intravenously to maintain mean BP with a normal physiological limit. Under such conditions, an attempt to examine the blocking effect of somatic inputs on the EVB was repeated. The results showed that no significant inhibition of the bradycardiac response to the AN stimulation occurred although BP was recovered to the normal level. On the contrary, in the animals in which the RVLM regions remained intact but BP was artificially decreased to the same lower level as that in RVLM lesioned animals by means of bleeding, the blocking effect of somatic inputs was still evident. From the results shown above, we can come to the conclusion that the neurons within the RVLM indeed act as a crucial relay in the inhibitory pathway of somatic inputs on the EVB.

The neuropharmacological studies also strongly support the notion that the RVLM is an important substrate integrating somatic inputs. Microinjection of atropine into the bilateral RVLM completely abolished all the effects of SPN stimulation on the EVB. In the spines of the animals (C_1 or C_2 transacted), application of both the cholinomimetic agent physostigmine salicylate and DLH into the same areas within the bilateral RVLM exerted a blocking effect on the EVB.[66] These results show that endogenous cholinergic mechanisms in the RVLM appear to contribute to the inhibitory effect of somatic afferent stimulation on the EVB.

NEURAL MECHANISMS UNDERLYING THE INHIBITORY EFFECT OF SOMATIC INPUTS

Central organisation of the baroreceptor reflex

The baroreceptor of the carotid sinus and aortic arch send information to the central nervous system via the IXth and Xth cranial nerves respectively. The distribution of their projection has been a matter of intense study over many years.[56] In all species investigated so far, it appears that the control projection is restricted to the nucleus tractus solitaries (NTS) which is located in the dorsomedial medulla.[57] The baroreceptor sensitive neurons within the NTS in turn send their efferent projections to the nucleus ambiguous (NA) and dorsal vagal nucleuses (DVN) and have connections with the preganglionic vagal cardiomotor neurons within both of these medullary nuclei. The vagal cardiomotor neurons finally send their axons descending in the vagus nerve to achieve the baroreceptor control of the heart. However, it should be admitted here that the complexity of this segment of the parasympathetic reflex pathway is not resolved. There is data showing that the connections between the NTS and NA or DVN are polysynaptic rather than monosynaptic.[57] The study of this question is still underway.

With the central vagal reflex pathway stated above, there are at least four neural mechanisms that merit being considered in exploring the possible explanation for the influence of somatic inputs on the cardiac vagal reflex. Firstly, somatic inputs activate the neurons within the RVLM which have direct connections with the spinal preganglionic sympathetic neurons, which then increase sympathetic outflows and antagonise cardiac vagal activity. Secondly, primary afferent depolarisation of the baroreceptor afferent, i.e., presynaptic inhibition of the primary baroreceptor afferent, occurred during the somatic afferent stimulation, which accounts for the suppression of the baroreceptor reflex. Thirdly, postsynaptic inhibition of the baroreceptor-sensitive neurons within the NTS leads to a blockade of the EVB. Lastly, postsynaptic inhibition may also bring about in the NA and DVN an inhibition of the baroreceptor reflex.

Changes in cardiac sympathetic effect during RVLM or somatic afferent stimulation

The AN stimulation-produced baroreceptor reflex was still suppressed by the SPN stimulation in animals whose cardiac sympathetic effect was blocked by an intravenous injection of propranolol.[59] Also, in the animals whose spinal cords were transacted at C_1 or C_2 level the inhibition of vagal bradycardia was still observed following electrical stimulation of the RVLM or microinjection of DLH into this area.[66] In addition, RVLM and somatic inputs failed to modify the bradycardiac responses induced by electrical stimulation of the central cut end of the vagus. Therefore, under the conditions of our experiments, the suppression of the evoked baroreceptor reflex was caused by the inhibition of the central parasympathetic components and was mediated by the cardiac vagal nerve, rather than by increasing the sympathetic outflow. This means there is no evidence to show the first suggestion in the above section is true.

The inhibition of NTS neurons induced by RVLM and somatic afferent stimulation

In this series of experiments, the orthodromic excitatory responses of the NTS neurons were recorded extracellularly following the ipsilateral stimulation of the AN.[61] From the histogram of these recordings we can see that the onset latency of these responses is variable, ranging from 3–5 ms, indicating a postsynaptic response to the primary afferent of the baroreceptor. Their ability to follow low frequency stimulation and multiple response characteristics are also in agreement with the suggestion that these units are postsynaptic to baroreceptor nerve stimulation. They were identified as baroreceptor sensitive neurons. The anatomical locations of various recording units were plotted onto the representative sections of the medulla, and were distributed mainly in the medial part of the NTS, within 1 mm caudal to 1.5 mm rostral to the obex.

In most of the baroreceptor sensitive neurons examined within the NTS, the excitatory responses elicited by a test stimulus delivered to the ipsilateral AN were significantly inhibited by a conditioning stimulus previously applied to the ipsi or contra-lateral RVLM. In some particularly stable unit recordings, the evoked activities were suppressed not only by application of a conditional stimulus to the RVLM, but also by prolonged electrical stimulation of the central cut end of the SPN with low intensity.

Similar inhibition of the excitatory responses of the NTS neurons to the aortic nerve input was also seen after microinjection of DLH into the ipsi- or contra-lateral RVLM region.

The preceding results showed that the activation of neurons within the RVLM could inhibit the evoked activities of NTS cells. Therefore, the neurons in the RVLM are capable of modulating the baroreceptor reflex by affecting the baroreceptor input to the NTS cells. The most important finding is that the excitatory responses of some NTS neurons were suppressed by stimulation of both the RVLM and somatic afferent nerve. This led us to speculate that inhibition of the transmission of the baroreceptor input to the NTS cells following RVLM or somatic nerve stimulation is most likely responsible for the blockade of AN stimulation-produced cardiac slowing. This fits with the observations in electro-physiology[8] and morphology, demonstrated in our (see below) and other laboratory results[42,50] which showed bilateral projections from the RVLM to the NTS.

It is well known that the presynaptic inhibition of the primary afferent input is a major mechanism contributing to the control of peripheral input means of central structures. There is evidence showing that the presynaptic inhibition contributes at least in part to the powerful suppressive effect of the hypothalamic stimulation on the baroreceptor reflex.[71] Since the activity of the baroreceptor-sensitive neurons within the NTS are subject to considerable modification by electrical activation of the RVLM as well as the somatic afferent nerve, it seems important to clarify whether the presynaptic control mechanism is involved in the suppression of the baroreceptor reflex during the RVLM and somatic stimulation. By observing the influence of the RVLM or somatic afferent nerve stimulation on the magnitude of antidromically evoked responses recorded in the buffer afferent, detecting the involvement of the presynaptic control mechanism in the suppression of the baroreceptor reflex is possible. In brief, a change in the antidromic excitability of buffer afferent endings within the NTS produced by the conditioning stimulus given to the RVLM was reflected as a change in the amplitude of the antidromic potential of the buffer nerve evoked by the NTS test stimulus. An increase in the excitability, i.e., an increase in the amplitude of the evoked field potentials, was an indirect measure of primary afferent depolarisation that is considered related to the presynaptic inhibition. A decrease in the amplitude of the evoked field potentials reflected primary afferent hyperpolarization.

Under the conditions of our experiment, although the RVLM conditioning stimulation could reduce the excitatory responses of the NTS baroreceptor sensitive neurons to AN test stimulation, stimulation with the same parameters delivered to the same RVLM region had no significant influence on the magnitude of the antidromically evoked field potentials recorded either in the carotid sinus nerve or in AN.[62] Nor did somatic afferent inputs. This suggests the lack of primary afferent depolarisation of the baroreceptor afferent fibres during RVLM or somatic afferent nerve stimulation. Therefore, the presynaptic inhibition appears not to be responsible for the suppression of the baroceptor reflex.

Afferent projection to the intermediate NTS
The intermediate region of the NTS is an important area for the control of circulation and serves to integrate many important cardiovascular reflexes.[33,52] Functionally, this region has been designed as the cardiovascular NTS. While most investigators have described the innervation of the NTS from peripheral and central structures, there is as yet no systemic analysis of the sites of the origin of the projections directed toward the intermediate portions of the nucleus in this species of rabbit. With the horseradish peroxidase retrograde tracing method, we found that the most extensive retrograde labelling was present in the bilateral RVLM region as well as the other brain area.[67] This provides an anatomical support for the modulatory effect of the RVLM on the baroreceptor reflex.

GABAergic and opiate systems present in the NTS processing the inhibition of the evoked baroreflex

The ipsilateral microinjection of γ-aminobutyric acid (GABA) into the NTS markedly blocked the evoked bradycardia produced by the AN stimulation. This blocking effect was greatly antagonized by the pretreatment of the GABA receptor antagonist bicuculline into the same medullary area.[62] In the electrophysiological study, iontophoretic application of GABA inhibited the evoked responses of the baroreceptor sensitive neurons in the NTS to the AN stimulation, which was reversed when bicuculline was given simultaneously. From these data, it appears that GABA may be an important transmitter or modulator which inhibits the activity of the NTS neurons relaying the baroreceptor inputs from the baroreceptor afferent. This fits with Maley and Elde's observations[45] which showed the dense presence of a significant amount of GABA in the NTS area and the existence of high affinity binding sites for GABA at this medullary site.

The administration of bicuculline alone into the NTS resulted in a decrease of basal HR and a slight potentiation of the baroreceptor response.[62] Iontophoretic application of bicuculline alone enhanced the spontaneous discharges of baroreceptor sensitive neurons within the NTS and their excitatory responses to the AN stimulation. These results are according to those reported by Mifflin and his co-workers in cats,[48] indicating that the baroreceptor sensitive neurons within the NTS are normally inhibited by some tonic inputs. These tonic inputs which inhibit the NTS cells have been verified mainly from the hypothalamic defence area[47,48] and the peripheral somatic afferent to the brainstem. Since bicuculline can take central and peripheral tonic inhibition away, we tentatively propose that these inhibitory inputs may tonically stimulate a release of GABA at the NTS region, and thus inhibit the baroreceptor sensitive neurones in this nucleus. Further speculation we can make is that excitation of the baroreceptor afferent by the AN stimulation may then result in either inhibition of GABA released at the NTS and/or cause a release of a substance that excites the neurons comprising this nucleus. The effect of the excitatory substance on the cell bodies of the baroreceptor-sensitive neurons would override the inhibitory effect of GABA on the baroreceptor reflex.

The GABAergic mechanism present at the NTS region might mediate the inhibition of the baroreceptor reflex during somatic afferent and RVLM stimulation. This is proved by the fact that administration of bicuculline into the NTS abolished the RVLM and that somatic inputs induced suppression of the excitatory responses of the baroreceptor sensitive neurons within the NTS to baroreceptor afferent stimulation.[60] These observations suggest that GABA is an important transmitter responsible for the inhibition of the evoked bradycardia. Consistent with this idea are the findings that the inhibition of evoked bradycardia produced by RVLM or somatic input are not modified by administration of larger doses of strychnine,[63] a glycine blocker.[10]

Another putative neurotransmitter probably working in the NTS for suppressing the baroreceptor reflex was an endogenous opiate substance. It is generally agreed that opiate peptides often act as an inhibitory transmitter on most of the central neurons.[30] From the observation of this laboratory, direct microinjection of the opiate receptor agonist morphine into the intermediate NTS region attenuated the bradycardia produced by AN stimulation on which naloxone had a disinhibitory effect.[67] Further evidence demonstrating the role played by an opiate substance in the control of the operation of the baroreceptor reflex comes from the observation of Miura et al.[49] who found that iontophoretic administration of naloxone enhanced the field potential evoked in the NTS by electrical stimulation of the carotid sinus nerve. The anatomical finding that opiate neurons concentrate in the medial area of the intermediate NTS region[35] provides further evidence that opiate peptides may be involved in the modulation of the baroreflex. However, it is noticeable that the morphine induced inhibitory effect on the evoked bradycardia was dramatically antagonised by a preceding injection of bicuculline. This suggests that the action of opiate peptides in the modulation of the baroreceptor reflex is mediated by GABA receptor.

Since application of naloxone into the NTS attenuated the inhibitory effect of the RVLM and somatic nerve stimulation-evoked bradycardia, the release of an endogenous opiate substance in the NTS is an important link in processing the inhibition of the baroreflex. According to the finding that bicuculline blocked the effect of morphine, it appears that an application of naloxone blocked the RVLM and somatic nerve stimulation induced inhibition of the baroreceptor reflex, possibly through the mechanism of reducing the release of GABA.

The inhibition of preganglionic vagal cardiomotor neurons in the DVN and NA

The previous statements have pointed out that the RVLM-NTS inhibiting pathway is an important neural mechanism in managing the inhibitory effect of somatic inputs. Since the electrophysiological and morphological findings of the neurons in DVN and NA receiving afferent projections from the RVLM, examining the influence of somatic inputs and RVLM on DVN and NA neurons is important.

The antidromically firing neurons in DVN and NA could be recorded following electrical stimulation of the ipsilateral cervical vagus.[60] Antidromically evoked responses were identified by the all or nothing nature of the response; the constant latency at a specific frequency of stimulation; its ability to follow high frequency (up to 150 Hz) stimulation: and cancellation of the evoked responses by collision with a spontaneous spike. On the basis of axonal conduction velocity calculated from the latency of the recorded antidromic impulse and the straight horizontal distance between the recording and the stimulating electrodes, these neurons showed that a cardiac modulation had axons in the range of B fibres referring to the conduction velocity 3.7–12.5 m/s in the DVN and 44.1–11.6 m/s in the NA. In addition to the antidromic response of these neurons to the cervical vagus stimulation, they were also orthodromically excited by the stimulation of the contralateral NTS area, or the ipsi-or contralateral AN. These neurons recorded in two medullary areas (DVN and NA) were then classified as preganglionic vagal cardiomotor neurons (PVCN). The electrophysiological properties of PVCN tested in the current study are very similar to those revealed by Ciriello and Calaresu in the cat,[6,7] Katana et al., in the dog,[36] as well as Jorden, et al. in the rabbit.[34] In addition, it is conceivable that these units, antidromically activated from the cervical vagus, are cell bodies rather than passing axons of cells situated elsewhere, since most of the units had a clear inflexion on the rising phase of the spike, i.e., the IS-SD inflexion.[41] Furthermore, the antidromic spikes could be recorded over a depth of 100 μm or more.[13]

Our results showed that the excitatory responses of the identified PVCN in the DVN areas were significantly inhibited during prolonged electrical stimulation of the SPN with low intensity. Similar results were obtained by DPN stimulation with high intensity, but not with low intensity.[60] A conditioning stimulus applied to the ipsi- or contralateral RVLM produced a powerful suppression of evoked discharges of PVCN induced by a test stimulus to the AN.[63] In some units tested, the evoked activities were not only suppressed by application of a conditional stimulus to the RVLM, but could also be inhibited by stimulation of the SPN. Using the excitant amino acid DLH to affect cell bodies rather than passing fibres in RVLM, evoked activity of most neurons tested were instantaneously suppressed after an injection just as those observed during electrical stimulation of RVLM.[63] These electrophysiological data imply that the suppression of the baroreceptor reflex during the RVLM or somatic afferent stimulation is related to the activation of neurons of the RVLM area, which in turn inhibit the PVCN.

The stimulating sites within the RVLM, which could inhibit the neurons in PVCN, were mainly localised in an area corresponding well with the region where stimulation resulted in an inhibition of the baroreceptor sensitive neurons in the NTS. The fact that the neurons within the same RVLM area appear to mediate two different components of the central cardiac vagal reflex raises the following question: whether the neurons in the RVLM responsible for the modulation of different vagal components are functionally specific or non-specific. The resolution of this question remains to be investigated. Nevertheless, it is consistently thought that structures in the ventro-lateral medulla contain a subpopulation of neurons that can readily exert a more discrete, differential control over cardiac, vascular and even non-cardiovascular activities.

In exploring the pharmacological mechanism underlying the inhibition of vagal cardiomotor neurons in DVN and NA induced by RVLM or somatic afferent stimulation, Williford et al.[72] have shown that a GABAergic mechanism within the NA of cats which contains the preganglionic vagal cardiomotor neurons[7,8] exerts a profound influence on the parasympathetic outflow to the heart. This was shown by the observation that microinjection of the GABA receptor agonist muscimol into the NA completely prevented the bradycardia reflexively evoked by the pressor effect of phenylephrine. In this laboratory, the effect of GABA directly microinjected into the DVN that contains preganglionic vagal cardiomotor neurons in rabbits[34] on the brady-cardia induced by AN stimulation was studied.[63] The results showed that microinjection of GABA blocked the bradycardia, while bicucul-line administered into the same medullary area after GABA restored most of the evoked bradycardiac response. Besides the antagonising effect of bicuculline on GABA, administration of bicuculline into the bilateral DVN regions also substantially prevented the inhibitory effect of somatic inputs. However, larger doses of strychnine (up to double the dose of bicuculline) failed to affect the somatic input-induced inhibition.

In high spinal (C_1 or C_2 transacted) animals whose mean BP was maintained at a normal level with intravenous infusion of phenylephrine, the bradycardiac response was also observed by aortic nerve stimulation, and could be blocked by electrical stimulation of the RVLM area. The RVLM induced inhibition of evoked bradycardia was partially blocked after microinjection of bicuculline into the unilateral DVN area.

However, larger doses of strychnine did not affect RVLM induced inhibition of evoked bradycardia.[63]

From the observation listed above, one can infer that the GABAergic system present at the DVN is perhaps involved in the inhibition of evoked bradycardia during somatic afferent and RVLM stimulation. Since larger doses of strychnine exhibited no influence on the inhibition of bradycardia produced by RVLM or somatic inputs, it is reasonable to propose that GABA may be a special transmitter responsible for the inhibition of the baroreceptor reflex at the DVN area.

In summary, in the anesthetized rabbits, using the bradycardiac response to the aortic nerve stimulation as an observation model, we found that inputs from the peripheral somatic afferent to mimic acupuncture are capable of suppressing the EVB. This inhibitory effect was achieved by the activation of neurones within the RVLM, which in turn suppressed postsynaptically both baroreceptor sensitive neurons within the DVN and NA. The GABAergic and opiate mechanism present at the NTS, and DVN and NA play an important role in the mediation of the baroreflex inhibition (Fig. 7.2).

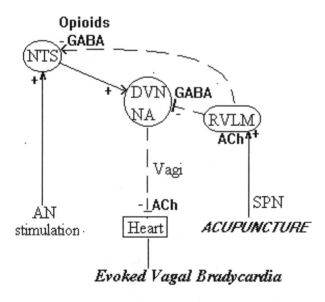

Fig. 7.2   Mechanism of the inhibitory effect of acupuncture or somatic inputs on EVB ... excitation, ... inhibition.

Clinical Application

In clinic, once a patient got arrhythmia, either due to coronary heart disease, myocarditis or other pathogenesis, doctors logically concentrate their attention to the patient's heart itself, and offer a lot of drugs to these patients, e.g., β-blocker, Na^+ channel blocker, Ca^{++} channel blocker etc. All are effective, but have a series of side effects. In China, in some Traditional Chinese Medical Hospitals, they have tried to use acupuncture to treat the patients with different kinds of arrhythmia, and gained some good results. In this chapter, the above experimental data showed that treating arrhythmia with acupuncture has a scientific base. Different kinds of arrhythmia require the use of different acupoints and different stimulation parameters. Needling on Neiguan (Pe 6) or Zusanli (St 36) could inhibit the ventricular extrasystoles due to sympathetic over-excitation. This is because needling these acupoints could excite type II and III fibres in MN and DPN, and release opioids, GABA and 5-HT etc. which inhibit the cardiac sympathetic centre. The evoked vagal bradycardia could be inhibited by the inputs from SPN and SRN or stronger stimulation of deep nerves, which release ACh to excite RVLM and in turn, inhibit the cardiac vagal centre via GABA and opioids. All the effects are due to the modulation of the cardiac sympathetic or parasympathetic centre. It is effective and has no side effects. These facts again showed that cardiac diseases are not only the problems of the heart. The nervous system also had big influence. Doctors should look at the patient as a whole, and not concentrate on a small part of the body.

References

1. Azevedo, A.D., Hilton, S.M. and Timms, R.J. (1980) The defence reaction elicited by midbrain and hypothalamic stimulation in the rabbit. *J Physiol*, **301**: 56.
2. Bloom, F.E. (1978) Neurons containing β-endorphin in rat brain exist separately from those containing enkephalin: Immunocytochemical studies. *Proc Natl Acad Sci USA,*, **75**: 1591–1595.
3. Blessing, W.W. and Peis, D. (1982) Inhibitory cardiovascular function of neurons in the caudal ventrolateral medulla of the rabbit: Relationship to the area containing A1 noradrenergic cell. *Brain Res*, **253**: 161–171.
4. Baum, T. and Shropshire, A.T. (1975) Inhibition of efferent sympathetic nerve activity by hydroxytrytophan and centrally administered 5-hydroxytryptamin, *Neuropharmacol*, **14**: 227–233.

5. Bousquet, P., Feldman, T., Bloch, R. and Schwartz, J. (1981) The ventromedullary hypotensive effect of muscimol in the anesthetized cat. *Clin Exp Hypertension*, **3**: 195– 205.

6. Ciriello, J. and Calaresu, F.R. (1982) Medullary origin of vagal preganglionic axons to the heart of the cat. *J Auton Nerv Syst*, **5**: 9–22.

7. Ciriello, J. and Caverson, M.M. (1986) Bidirectional cardiovscular connections between ventrolateral medulla and nucleus of the solitary tract. *Brain Res*, **367**: 273–281.

8. Ciriello, J. and Calaresu, F.R. (1980) Distribution of vagal cardioinhibitory neurons in the medulla of the cat. *Am J. Physiol*, **238**: Rs57–64.

9. Coote, J.H., Dalton, D.M., Feniuk, W. and Humohrey, P.P.A (1987) The central site of action of 5-hydroxytryptamine in the cat. *Neuropharmacol*, **26**: 147–154.

10. Curtis, O.R., Duggan, A.M. and Johnston, G.A.R (1971) The specificity of sstrychnine as a glycine antagonist in the mammalian spinal coard. *Exp Brain Res*, **12**: 547–565.

11. Evans, D.E. and Gillis, R.A. (1978) Reflex mechanism involved in cardiac arrhythmias induced by hypothalamic stimulation. *Am J. Physiol*, **234**: H 199–209.

12. Fu, X.W., Yu, J., Su, Q.F. and Li, P. (1980) Effect of hypothalamic stimulation on the cardiac funcation in the rabbit. *Acta Physiol Sin*, **32**: 37–43 (in Chinese).

13. Fussey, I.F., Ridd, C. and Whitwan, J.S. (1970) The differentiation of zxonal and soma dentritic spike activity. *Pflugers Arch*, **321**: 283–292.

14. Gao, Z.W., Yu, X.Z., Shen, A.X., Bao, L.E. and Ling, X.C. (1987) Clinical observations on treatment of 220 cases of arrhythmia with acupuncture. In: *Compilation of the abstract of acupuncture and moxibustion papers. The first World Conference on Acupuncture-Moxibustion*. 13–14.

15. Gong, Q.L. and Li, P. (1989) The inhibitory effect of nucleus raphe obscurus on defence pressor response. *Chin J. Physiol Sci*, **5**: 311–318.

16. Guo, X.Q., Jia, R.J., Cao, Q.Y., Guo, Z.D. and Li, P. (1981) Inhibitory effect of somatic nerve afferent impulses on the extrasystole induced by hypothalamic stimulation *Acta Physiol Sin*, **33**: 343–350 (in Chinese).

17. Guo, X.Q,. Wang, Q.M., Li, L.H. and Li, P. (1982) Effect of 5-HT on extrasystole induced by hypothalamic stimulation. *Acta Physiol Sin*, **34**: 253–259 (in Chinese).

18. Guo, X.Q., Xia, Y. and Li, P. (1984) Role of arcuatus area in inhibitory action of somatic nerve stimulation on ventricular extrasystoles induced by hypothalamic stimulation in rabbits. *Acta Physiol Sin*, **36**: 9–15 (in Chinese).

19. Guo, X.Q. (1984) Influence of the activity of locus coeruleus complex on the ventricular extrasystoles induced by hypothalamic stimualtion in the rabbit. *Acta Physiol Sin*, **36**: 431–439 (in Chinese).

20. Guo, X.Q. (1985) Effect of microinjection of norepinephrine into the locus coeruleus area on the ventricular extrasystoles induced by hypothalamic stimulation. *Acta Physiol Sin*, **37**: 346–352 (in Chinese).

21. Guo, X.Q. and Li, P. (1986) Inhibitory effect of deep peroneal nerve input on the ventricular extrasystoles induced by hypothalamic stimulation of the defence area in the rabbit. *Acupunct Res*, **3**: 174.
22. Guo, X.Q., Liu, N.A. and Li, P. (1986) Role of the ventral medullary area on the ventricular extrasystoles induced by hypothalamic stimulation in the rabbit. *Acupunct Res*, **3**: 174.
23. Guo, X.Q., Liu, N.A. and Li, P. (1987) Inhibitory effect of microinjection of morphine into the ventral medulla on extrasystoles induced by hypothalamic stimulation in the rabbit. *Acta Physiol Sin*, **39**: 132–138 (in Chinese).
24. Guo, X.Q. (1988) Changes of blood viscosity during arrhythmia induced by hypothalamic defence area stimulation in the rabbit. *Chin J. Appl Physiol*, **4**: 57–61 (in Chinese).
25. Guo, X.Q., Wang, Q., Zang, X.H. and Li, P. (1988) Involvement of ventrolateral medulla in the blocking effect of somatic inputs on NTS stimulation induced bradycardia in rabbits. *Chin J. Physiol Sci*, **4**: 327–336.
26. Guo, X.Q. and Xu, N.S. (1989) Mechanism of depressing effect of Diazepam on the blood presure and on ventricular extrasystoles induced by hypothalamic stimulation in the rabbit. *Acta Physiol Sin*, **41**: 10–18 (in Chinese).
27. Guo, X.Q., Chen, C.F., Liu, Y. and Li, P. (1989) A GABAergic mechanism in the RVLM mediates the inhibitory effect of DPN stimulation on HVE. *Chin J. Physiol Sci*, **5**: 203–209.
28. Guo, X.Q., Gao, K.M. and Zhu, D.N. (1990) Effect of microinjection of 5-HT into the rostral ventrolateral medulla on ventricular extraqsystoles induced by hypothalamic stimulation in the rabbit. *Chin J. Physiol Sci*, **6**: 129–137.
29. Hall, R.E. (1974) Myocardial alterations following hypothalmic stimualtion in the intact conscious dog. *Am Heart J*, **88**: 770–776.
30. Hassen, A.H., Feuerstein, G. and Faden, A.I. (1983) Differential cardiovascular effects mediated by mu and kappa opiate receptors in hindbrain nuclei. *Peptides*, **4**: 621–625.
31. Helke, C.J., Sohl, B.D. and Jacobowitz, D.M. (1980) Choline acetyltansferase activity in discrete brain nuclei of DOCA-salt hypertensive rats. *Brain Res*, **193**: 293–298.
32. Hokfelt, T., Terenius, L., Kuypers, abd Dann, O. (1979) Evidence for enkephalinimmunoreactive neurons in the medulla oblangata projecting to the spinal cord. *Neurosci Lett*, **14**: 55–60.
33. Huangfu, D.H., Huang, Q. and Li, P. (1987) Afferent connection of the vemtrolateral medulla in the rabbit studied with HRP technique. *Chin J. Physiol Sci*, **3**: 86–95.
34. Jordon, D., Khalid, M.E.M., Schneiderman, N. and Spyer, K.M. (1982) The location and properties of preganglionic vagal cardiomotor neurons in the rabbit. *Pflugers Arch*, **395**: 244–250.
35. Kalia, M. (1984) Distribution of neuropeptide immunreactive nerve terminals within the subnuclei of the nucleus solitarius of rabbit. *J. Comp Neurol*, **222**: 409–444.

36. Katona, P.G., Poitras, J., Barnett, O. and Terry, B. (1970) Cardiac vagao efferent activity and heart period in the carotid sinus reflex. *Am J. Physiol*, **218**: 1030–1037.
37. Keeler, J.R., Shults, C.W., Chas, T.N. and Helke, C.J. (1984) The ventral surface of the medulla in the rat: Pharmacologic and autoradiographic localization of GABA induced cardiovascular effect. *Brain Res*, **297**: 271–224.
38. Li, L.H., Guo, X.Q., Jia, R.L., Fan, S.D. and Li, P. (1984) Effect of noradrenaline injected into central gray on ventricular extrasystoles induced by hypothalamic stimulation in rabbit. *Acta Physiol Sin*, **36**: 247–254 (in Chinese).
39. Li, P. (1983) Mechanism of the modulatory effect of acupuncture on acute experimental hypertensin, hypotension and extrasystole. *Acupun Res*, **8**: 241–248.
40. Li, P., Huangfu, D.H., Guo, X.Q. and Liu, N.A. (1986) Role of ventrolateral medullary area in the inhibitory effect of electro-acupuncture on experimental pressor response and arrhythmia. *Acupun Res*, **3**: 166–173.
40. Lin, J.M. (1979) A study of the acupuncture therapy on arrhythmia. *Abstract of the national symposium of acupuncture-moxibustion and acupuncture analgesia*. 39.
41. Lipsiki, J. (1981) Antidromic activation of neurons as an analytic tool in the study of the central nervous system. *J Neurosci Methods*, **4**: 1–32.
42. Loewy, A.D., Wallaach, J.H. and McKeller, S. (1981) Efferent connection of the ventral medulla oblongata in the rat. *Brain Res Rev*, **3**: 63–80.
43. Lovick, T.A. (1988) Convergent afferent inputs to neurons in nucleus paragigantocellularis lateralis in the cat. *Brain Res*, **456**: 483–487.
44. Lovick, T.A. and Li, P. (1989) Integrative function of neurons in the rostral ventrolateral medulla. *Prog. Brain Res*, **81**: 223–231.
45. Maley, B. and Elde, R. (1982) Immunohistochemical localization of putative neurotransmitters within the feline nucleus tractus solitarii. *Neuroscience*, **7**: 2369–2490.
46. Maley, B. and Newton, B.W. (1985) Immunohistochemistry of aminobutyric acid in the cat nucleus tractus solitarri. *Brain Res*, **330**: 364–368.
47. McAllen, R.M. (1971) Inhibiton of the baroreceptor input to the medulla by stimulation of the hypothalamic defence area. *J. Physiol (London)*, **257**: 45–46.
48. Mifflin, S.W., Jordon, D. and Spyer, K.M. (1987) Hypothalamic defence area (HDA) inhibition of carotid sinus nerve (CSN) inputs is GABA mediated. *Fed Proc*, **46**: 494.
49. Miura, M., Takayama, R. and Okada, J. (1982) Study of possible transmitters in the carotid sinus baro- and chemoreceptor reflex. *J. Auton Nerv Syst*, **19**: 179–188.
50. Onai, T., Kiuoshige, T. and Miura, M. (1987) Projections to areas of the nucleus tractus solitarii related to circulatory and respiratory response in cats. *J. Auton Nerv Syst*, **18**: 363–375.

51. Quest, J.A. and Gebber, Q.L. (1972) Modulation of baroreceptor reflexes by somatic afferent nerves stimulation. *Am J. Physiol*, **222**: 1251–1259.
52. Ross, C.A., Ruggier, D.A. and Reis, D.J. (1981) Afferent projections to cardiovascular portions of the nucleus of the tractus sollitarius in the rat. *Brain Res*, **223**: 402–408.
53. Schwaber, J. and Schneiderman, N. (1975) Aortic nerve activated cardioinhibitory neurons and interneurons. *Am J. Physiol*, **229**: 783–789.
54. Stainsky, J., Kosowsky, B., Lown, B. and Kerzner, J. (1971) Ventricular fibrillation induced by hypothalamic stimulation during coronary occlusion. *Circulation*, **44**: 11–60.
55. Steinbush, H.W.M. (1981) Distribution of serotonin immunoreactivity in the central nervous system of the rat cell bodies and terminals. *Neurosci*, **6**: 557–618.
56. Spyer, K.M. (1981) The neural organisation and control of the baroreceptor reflex. *Rev Physiol Biochem Pharmacol*, **88**: 23–124.
57. Spyer, K.M. (1984) Central control of the cardiovascular system. In Baker PF ed. *Recent Adv Physiol* Churchill Livingstone, Edingburgh 163–199.
58. Stornetta, R.L., Guyenet, P.G. and McAllen, R.C. (1987) Autonomic nervous system control of heart rate during baroreceptor activation in conscious and anesthetized rat. *J Auton Nerv Syst*, **20**: 121–127.
59. Wang, Q., Guo, X.Q. and Li, P. (1987) The blocking effect of somatic inputs on bradycardia induced by stimulation of the nucleus tractus solitarius in rabbits. *Chin J. Physiol Sci*, **3**: 336–371.
60. Wang, Q., Guo, X.Q. and Li, P. (1988) The inhibitory effect of somatic inputs on the excitatory responses of vagal cardiomotor neurons to stimulation fo the nucleus tractus solitarii in rabbits. *Brain Res*, **439**: 350–356.
61. Wang, Q. and Li, P. (1988a) Stimulation of the ventrolateral medulla inhibits the baroreceptor input to the nucleus tractus solitarius *Brain Res*, **473**: 227–235.
62. Wang, Q. and Li, P. (1988b) Is presynaptic inhibiton responsible for the suppression of baroreceptor reflex during rostral ventrolateral medulla stimulation. *Chin J. Physiol Sci*, **4**: 361–368.
63. Wang, Q. and Li, P. (1988c) Inhibition of baroreflex following microinjection of GABA or morphine into the nucleus tractus solitarii in rabbits. *J. Auton nerv Syst*, **25**: 165–172.
64. Wang, Q. and Li, P. (1988d) The inhibitory effect of ventrolateral medulla on excitatory responses of the vagal cardiomotor neurons in rabbits. *Chin J. Physiol Sci*, **4**: 126–136.
65. Wang, Q. and Li, P. (1988e) A GABAergic mechanism in the inhibition of cardiac vagal reflexes. *Brain Res*, **457**: 367–370.
66. Wang, Q. and Li, P. (1989a) A cholinergic mechanism in the rostral ventrolateral medulla mediates the somatic afferent stimulation produced inhibition of baroreflex in rabbits. *Chin J. Physiol Sci*, **5**: 108–115.

67. Wang, Q. and Li, P. (1989b) Afferent projections to area of the nucleus tractus solitarii related to circulatory responses in the rabbit. *Chin J. Physiol Sci*, **5**: 195–202.
68. Wang, Q. and Li, P. (1989c) Bicuculline- and naloxone-sensitive inhibiton of baroreflexes during the somatic afferent stimulation in the rabbit. *Chin J. Physiol Sci*, **5**: 155–163.
69. Verrier, R.L., Calvert, A. and Lown, B. (1975) Effect of posterior hypothalamic stimulation on the ventricular fibrillation threshold. *Am J. Physiol*, **228**: 923–927.
70. Wastoon, S.J., Akil, H., Richard, C.W. and Barchas, J.D. (1978) Evidence for two separate opiate peptide neuronal systems. *Nature*, **275**: 226–228.
71. Weiss, G.K. and Crill, W.E. (1969) Carotid sinus nerve: primary afferent depolarization evoked by hypothalamic stimulation. *Brain Res*, **16**: 269–272.
72. Williford, D.J., Hamilton, B.L. and Gillis, R.A. (1980) Evidence that a GABAergic mechanism at nucleus ambiguus influence reflex-induced vagal activity. *Brain Res*, **193**: 584–588.
73. Xia, Y., Guo, X.Q. and Li, P. (1983) Action of buffer nerves on the ventricular extrasystoles induced by hypothalamic stimulation in rabbits. *Acta Physiol Sin*, **35**: 250–256 (in Chinese).
74. Xia, Y., Guo, X.Q. and Li, P. (1984) Defence reaction and ventricular extrasystoles induced by hypothalamic stimulation in rabbits. *Acta Physiol Sin*, **36**: 133–141 (in Chinese).
75. Xia, Y., Guo, X.Q. and Li, P. (1985) Role of medial medulla in the inhibitory effect of somatic afferent nerves stimulation on ventricular extrasystoles induced by hypothalamic stimulation in the rabbit. *Acta Physiol Sin*, **37**: 37–43.
76. Xia, Y., Guo, X.Q., Zhang, A.D. and Li, P. (1985) Inhibitory effect of analogous electro-acupuncture on experimental arrhythamia. *Acupunct Electrother Res*, **10**: 13–34.
77. Xu, N.S., Guo, X.Q. and Zhang, J.R. (1989) Inhibitory effect of diazepam or flurazepam on pressor response of defence reaction by stimulation of midbrain. *Chin J. Physiol Sci*, **5**: 276.
78. Zhu, D.N., Guo, X.Q. and Li, P. (1990) Relationship between the rostral medullary cholinergic mechanism and the cardiovascular comoponent of the defence reaction. *Chin J. Physiol Sci*, **6**: 86–94.
79. Zhu, D.N., Guo, X.Q. and Li, P. (1991) J. Auton Nerv Influence of hypothalamic or superficial peroneal nerve stimulation on the release of intracerebral acetylcholine. *Chin J. Physiol Sci*, **7**: 18–26.

8 THE INHIBITORY EFFECT OF ACUPUNCTURE ON MYOCARDIAL ISCHEMIA

Peng Li

Clinical Studies

In 1977 Diao, et al.[6] reported that electroacupuncture was effective for coronary heart disease. In 1981, Wang, et al.[24] conducted further studies on acupuncture therapy for coronary heart disease and pointed out that both short and long term therapeutic effects of acupuncture were proven. Besides clinical symptoms and ECG, the patient's BP, serum lipid and blood viscosity etc. were improved. It was also reported that acupuncture had a good effect on congestive heart failure, arrhythmia and sick sinus syndrome. In 1987 Xu, et al.[25] analysed the effect of acupuncture on patients with coronary heart disease. They showed that in 106 normal subjects, left ventricular function measured with systolic time intervals (STI) did not show any marked changes after acupuncture; while in 135 cases of patients suffering from coronary heart disease, their pre-ejection period (PEP), and its ratio to left ventricle ejection time (LVET), i.e., PEP/LVET and HR decreased after acupuncture was applied to Neiguan (Pe 6), which indicated improvement of the left ventricular contractile function. The scientists therefore believed that acupuncture therapy was easily mastered, inexpensive and without side effects. It was worth being popularised. Bao, et al.[4] and the Nan Ning Institute of Acupuncture[2] also reported the therapeutic effect of acupuncture on acute myocardial infarction and coronary heart disease. In recent years, acupuncture therapy has spread to western countries. In 1986 Ballegaard, et al.[3] observed that electroacupuncture, administered 20 minutes per day for 3 weeks, increased the maximal rate-pressure product for patients with severe, stable angina during exercise. In 1991, Richter, et al.[20] demonstrated that acupuncture administered three times per week for 30 minutes reduces the number of anginal attacks compared with a placebo and increases the threshold for angina during exercise. These data suggested clinical efficacy of acupuncture in patients with coronary heart disease. As such, it is important to study this technique and explain the underlying mechanisms.

Experimental Studies on the Inhibitory Effect of Acupuncture on Reflex-Induced Myocardial Ischemia

There are some reports related to the effect of acupuncture on myocardial ischemia or infarction. However, these studies used hypothalamic stimulation or ligation of the whole left anterior descending branch of the coronary artery, or decreased ventilation to induce myocardial ischemia and infarction as measured by ECG ST-segment deviation or myocardial necrosis. Each of these models has limited applicability to clinical ischemia, which generally is the result of an imbalance between myocardial oxygen supply and demand. Also, measurement of myocardial ischemia was inexact, relying primarily on ECG changes.

REFLEX-INDUCED MYOCARDIAL ISCHEMIA

In view of the limited information on the mechanisms that underlie the potentially beneficial effects of acupuncture and electroacupuncture, a feline model of provocable myocardial ischemia was developed in Longhurst's lab, in which myocardial oxygen supply and demand could be evaluated independently.[14] Adult cats of either sex (3–7 kg) were anaesthetised with ketamine (40 mg/kg) and α-chloralose (50–75 mg/kg). Arterial Po_2 and Pco_2 were kept within normal limits (Po_2 100 mmHg, Pco_2 30-35 mmHg), and the arterial pH was kept between 7.35–7.45. Body temperature was maintained at a range of 36°–38°C.

System arterial BP, left ventricular pressure (LVP) and LV dP/dt were monitored. To produce a controlled reduction in regional coronary blood, the proximal left anterior descending branch (LAD) coronary artery was isolated and partially occluded by an occluder. Conversely a small high diagonal branch of the LAD on the anterior left ventricular wall was tied with a 4–0 silk suture to induce regional ischemia.

Measurement of left ventricular wall thickness was performed with a modified 20 MHz single-transducer sonomicrometer system. The reliability and accuracy of this ultrasonic single-transducer sonomicrometer system has been published previously.[19] The transducer was secured on the epicardium with 4–0 silk sutures or was glued using medical grade cyanoacrylate glue. It was positioned within the ischemic zone by using a few brief test occlusions of the LAD.

Reflex-induced sympathetic stimulation was used as a physiological trigger of myocardial ischemia. We applied BK to the gallbladder because this maneuver simulates the clinical conditions of inflammation and ischemia or cholecystitis and reflexively activates the sympathetic nervous system to increase arterial BP, myocardial contractility and to a lesser extent, HR, all of which serve to augment myocardial oxygen demand.[17,18] Less commonly, chemical activation of the abdominal visceral organs causes sympathetically mediated coronary arterial vasoconstriction. When a 1 cm^2 pledget soaked with BK solution (mostly 1–10 μg/ml) was applied on the serosal surface of the gallbladder, a pressor response was reflexively induced. After the maximum pressor reflex (> 20 mmHg) was observed, the filter paper was removed and the gallbladder was washed twice with normal saline from cotton-tipped applicators to remove BK. To prevent tachyphylaxis, recovery periods of at least 15 minutes were provided between applications.

The application of BK to the gallbladder resulted in pronounced activation of the cardiovascular system, as evidenced by increased BP, double product and wall thickening (WTh). After partial occlusion, the coronary blood velocity was reduced by 47% (5.8 ± 0.4 to 3.1 ± 0.3 cm/d; n = 6, P < 0.05). This degree of flow reduction was not associated with significant changes in resting values of double product, regional LV wall function, or diastolic BP. However, when BK was reapplied to the gallbladder, the normalized WTh was significantly reduced and became negative (10.7 ± 4.2 versus -23.6 ± 2.9%; control versus ischemia; n = 7; P < 0.05), despite increments of coronary blood velocity, diastolic BP, and double product that did not differ from the increments induced by BK before occlusion. The calculated index of coronary resistance was increased from 17.2 ± 2.3 to 32.5 ± 5.7 mmHg/cm per second by partial coronary occlusion. The change in the coronary resistance index during reflex stimulation by BK before occlusion (0.3 ± 0.6 mmHg/cm per second) was not significantly different from that observed during occlusion (–2.1 ± 2.9 mmHg/cm per second). The risk and infarct areas were also measured by the method described before.[1] In the partial occlusion group, the risk area was 14.3 ± 1.9% (range 7.1% to 21.4%) of the left ventricle, whereas in the small branch complete occlusion group, the risk area was 2.8 ± 1.5% (range 0.5% to 8,5%) of the left ventricle (P < 0.05). There was no evidence of infarction in any animals subjected to partial occlusion. In the small branch complete occlusion group, there were small infarctions in two of the five animals; the infarct sizes were 12.2% and 0.9% of the risk areas, or 0.4% and 0.005% of the left ventricle, respectively.

It is well known that normal cardiac mechanical function is associated with a high rate of aerobic metabolism, a condition that makes myocardial contractile function particularly vulnerable to reductions in oxygen supply. The balance between coronary blood supply and myocardial oxygen demand is crucial for maintenance of normal cardiac contractile function. In the present study, reduction of coronary blood supply by partial occlusion of the LAD tended to decrease resting regional contractile function, but the decline in function did not attain statistical significance. This finding suggests that the coronary supply/demand ratio at rest was not seriously compromised, and was perhaps related to the delivery of additional coronary blood flow to the region at risk by collateral blood vessels, increased extraction of arterial oxygen, and/or reduction of myocardial oxygen requirements. We believe the latter explanation is unlikely because there was no change in double product, a parameter related closely to myocardial oxygen demand.[10] However, because contractility tended to decrease and because the double product does not account for changes in contractile function, a determinant of myocardial oxygen demand,[8] we cannot absolutely discount a decrease in the myocardial oxygen requirement. It is likely that an increase in oxygen extraction played a minor role because oxygen extraction in the heart is near maximal at rest.

When bradykinin was applied to the gallbladder to augment sympathetic stimulation of the heart and vasculature reflexively, and, in this way, to increase arterial BP, LVP, LV dP/dt, and HR, it generally led to increased myocardial oxygen demand and increased coronary blood flow and oxygen extraction.[17] The elevated sympathetic drive exacerbated the imbalance in coronary supply and demand, as evidenced by a marked reduction in regional LV function when coronary blood flow was restricted. The use of BK to reflexively induce a transient increase in sympathetic stimulation provides a model of physiological stress similar to that occurring during surgical manipulation of the biliary tract, inflammatory conditions involving abdominal organs,[15] exercise[23] and mental stress[21] some of which have been shown to provoke angina when coronary blood flow is limited by a stenosis.

EFFECT OF ACUPUNCTURE-LIKE MEDIAN NERVE (MN) STIMULATION ON MYOCARDIAL ISCHEMIA

Since, in clinical reports, Neiguan (Pe 6) has been used to treat coronary heart disease, and because this acupoint was positioned over the median nerve that could be located in animals, we tried to use MN stimulation to mimic electroacupuncture, and observed its effect on a reflex induced model of myocardial ischemia. The median nerves in both forelimbs were exposed carefully, and flexible stainless steel bipolar electrodes were placed around each nerve. Resin-enforced vinyl polysiloxane was applied around the nerves and electrodes to prevent damage and desiccation of the nerves. The electrodes were then connected to a constant current stimulator with a stimulus isolation unit.

Before the first application of BK to the gallbladder, the animals were allowed to stabilise for one hour after all the surgical procedures. When the cardiovascular response to BK was constant, the LAD was occluded partially to reduce flow by ~50% or a small proximal diagonal branch of the LAD was ligated and completely occluded. Partial or complete occlusion was maintained throughout the remainder of the experiment. BK was applied twice during the next 30–40 minutes. MN stimulation was initiated for 30 minutes. The stimulation frequency was 5 Hz, similar to that used in clinical electroacupuncture, and the current was 0.43 ± 0.07 mA (0.5 ms duration), a level of intensity sufficient to produce moderate paw twitches. This level of current is much less than that used in electroacupuncture, because the nerve was stimulated directly. During MN stimulation, BK was applied twice, while after cessation of MN stimulation, BK was applied every 15 minutes for the next hour. Thus, BK was applied during the control (2 repeatable responses), coronary arterial occlusion (2 responses), MN stimulation (2 responses), and recovery after MN stimulation (4 responses) yielding a total of 10 data points.

Because the responses in the partially occluded and the small branch complete occlusion groups were not significantly different, they were combined into a single group and compared with a time-control group that did not receive MN stimulation. The results showed that coronary occlusion was associated with a significant decrease in the BK-induced change in regional LV wall function in both the time-control (n = 4) and the MN stimulation groups (n = 15), whereas the decrement in regional LV wall function evoked by BK was virtually constant for all subsequent repeat applications of BK during the control period, and stimulation of the MN significantly improved wall thickening to a level above the controls for an hour after cessation of MN stimulation. The improvement in regional LV wall function with stimulation of the MN was accompanied by a diminished pressor response, including significant smaller increments of diastolic BP and double product (n = 18). The increase in systolic BP during administration of BK was not significantly different during occlusion (38.2 ± 4.5 mmHg) compared with the baseline (42.8 ± 4.6 mmHg). However, stimulation of the MN significantly diminished the increment of systolic BP (23.6 ± 2.8 mmHg), and after one hour it did not differ significantly (31.5 ± 4.1 mmHg) from the increase observed during MN stimulation. The increase in LV dP/dt during BK stimulation at a baseline (1111 ± 330 mmHg/s) was reduced during ischemia (951 ± 311 mmHg/s) and MN stimulation (591 ± 149 mmHg/s), but these changes did not differ significantly (n = 8). The small increases in heart rate produced by BK before occlusion (5 ± 2 bpm) and during occlusion (4 ± 2 bpm), MN stimulation (2 ± 1 bpm), and at 1 hour (2 ± 3 bpm) were not significantly different. Stimulation of the MN did not change the resting value of HR, arterial BP, LV dP/dt, double produce, or wall thickening.

Our finding that both the resting and the reflex-induced increments in coronary blood velocity were unchanged during MN stimulation suggests that an increase of coronary blood flow is not produced by MN stimulation. Because our index of coronary resistance showed no change during stimulation with BK in the MN stimulation group, our results suggest that MN stimulation did not increase myocardial blood flow and hence oxygen supply, but rather reduced myocardial oxygen demand.

In the present study, both myelinated (Aδ) and unmyelinated (C) fibres in the median nerve were activated by the low frequency, low-intensity parameters we used. However, a larger proportion (63%) of finely myelinated fibres were stimulated, suggesting that the depressor effect observed was related to the predominance of the activation of Aδ-fibres.

The important new findings in the present study were that MN stimulation, used to mimic electroacupuncture, significantly improved regional cardiac dysfunction produced reflexively by increased sympathetic stimulation in the context of restricted coronary flow. The mechanism of this salutary effect was related to diminished cardiac oxygen demand rather than improved blood supply. These results provide a physiological basis for the reputed therapeutic efficacy of acupuncture in the management of myocardial ischemia and angina.

ACTIVATION OF OPIATE RECEPTORS IN THE RVLM BY MN STIMULATION

As noted above MN stimulation could diminished sympathetically mediated myocardial ischemia by reducing cardiac oxygen demand, secondary to a diminished pressor response during reflex activation of the cardiovascular system. In these experiments we analysed the mechanism of the central neural inhibitory effect of EA on myocardial ischemia. The RVLM is known to be an important brainstem region for maintaining BP and integrating cardiovascular reflexes.[16] It is also is a key area for the modulatory effect of acupuncture on abnormal cardiovascular function.[11] Our previous work showed that the depressor effect of acupuncture at certain acupoints or stimulation of the deep nerves beneath them is caused by activation of opiate receptors in RVLM.[12] Therefore, we studied the role of RVLM in the inhibition of EA on myocardial ischemia and pressor response. Our results showed that when EA applied to bilateral Neiguan (Pe6) acupoint or MN was stimulated with low current and low frequency, the pressor response to BK was inhibited, and regional myocardial function was significantly improved. We observed that this inhibitory effect of EA could be reversed by naloxone, either injected intravenously (0.4 mg/kg, n = 9) or microinjected (10 nM, 0.1ml/site, n = 14) into RVLM bilaterally from the ventral approach.[5] Therefore, the inhibition of EA on the myocardial ischemia and pressor reflex appears to be related to the activation of opiate receptors in the RVLM.

There are three major subtypes of opioid receptors in the central nervous system: m, d, k receptors. The physiological effects resulting from their structure is different.[8,9] In 1996, Sun, et al.[22] found that in normotensive, spontaneous hypertensive and stress induced hypertensive rats microinjection of μ and δ receptor agonists, DAGO and DADLE, led to significant depressor and bradycardia response; while a k receptor agonist, U50488H was not so effective. With this information in mind, we tried to clarify the subtypes of opiate receptors in RVLM that were related to the inhibitory effect of acupuncture on the pressor reflex induced by application of BK on the gallbladder.[14] The experimental preparations and protocols were similar to before. Usually a five-barrelled micropipet was inserted into the RVLM from the dorsal aspect of the medulla to reach the RVLM. In some experiments two five barrelled micropipets were inserted into the RVLM bilaterally to check the effect of bilateral microinjections. Instead of direct stimulation of MN, in this study we used acupuncture needles inserted into the Neiguan (Pe 6) and Jianshi (Pe 5) points (overlying the median nerves) on both forelimbs of the cat. The stimulation parameters were 0.5 ms, 5 Hz, 10–20 V, representing levels sufficient to produce moderate paw twitches for 45 minutes.

The results of this study showed that unilateral microinjection of a μ or δ receptor antagonist, CTOP or ICI174864, into the RVLM by a micropritzer blocked the inhibitory effect of EA on the pressor reflex induced by application of BK on the gallbladder. In other cats, microinjection of a κ receptor antagonist, nor-BNI, also blocked the inhibitory effect of EA, but the inhibition was weaker and lasted for a shorter time.

Unilateral microinjection of μ receptor agonist, DAGO, or δ receptor agonist, DALDO, into the RVLM inhibited the pressor reflex induced by application of BK on the gallbladder, but did not significantly influence resting MBP or HR. However, microinjection of a k receptor agonist, U50488H, into the same area had little affect on the resting MBP and HR or the pressor reflex induced by BK.

The results of this study indicated that inhibition of EA or stimulation of MN could activate the opiate receptors in the RVLM, inhibit sympathetic outflow, thereby blunting the BK reflex effects. This represented the mechanism underlying EA and demonstrated a therapeutical effect on several kinds of hypertension as well as improvement of myocardial ischemia. The receptors activated appeared to be mainly μ and δ receptors. The κ receptor plays a smaller role in this inhibition. Whether there are fewer κ receptors in RVLM or whether is this receptor simply less effective will require future study.

Further Studies

The above result represents simply the beginning of our research work. Many studies will be needed in future both in basic research and clinical areas. With regard to the mechanism of the inhibitory effect of acupuncture on the myocardial ischemia, there are many questions remaining:

(1) Is the effect of stimulation of other somatic nerves similar to the MN? Stated differently, is the effect of acupuncture of other acupoints similar to Neiguan (Pe 6)?

(2) Does transcutaneous electrical nerve stimulation (TENS) have a similar effect to EA or acupuncture?

(3) In clinic and hospital, doctors usually use a set of acupoints to treat patients with angina pectoris rather than only the Neiguan (Pe 6) point. Is this approach necessary? If such an approach is more effective, what is the underlying mechanism?

(4) Can all patients with myocardial ischemia and angina pectoris be treated by acupuncture or EA? If not, how should physicians select patients for acupuncture therapy? Is acupuncture helpful in treating myocardial infarction?

(5) What is the central pathway that input from the acupoint into the RVLM, which inhibit the cardiovascular neurones? Is this the same pathway as that which inhibits this hypertension and arrhythmias?

(6) Are there neurotransmitters other than opioids related to the inhibitory effect of EA on myocardial ischemia? What are the interactions between neurotransmitters?

(7) Why is the inhibitory effect of EA so long-lasting? Is it a result relating to the release of opioids, or there are other mechanisms involved?

(8) Does EA also influence the humoral factors in patients with myocardial ischemia, e.g., plasma catecholamines, angiotensin, corticosteroids, vasopressin, endothelin, etc.?

These questions and more deserve study in the near future. We believe that if acupuncture is used more commonly in clinics and hospitals, it may assist in the effective treatment of patients.

References

1. Amsterdam, E.A., Sthl, G.L., Pan, H.-L., Rendig, S.V., Fletcher, M.P., Longhurst, J.C. (1995) Limitation of reperfusion injury by a monoclonal antibody to C5a during myocardial infarction in pigs. *Am J. Physiol*, **268**: H448–457.

2. Anonymous, (Nanning Institute of Acupuncture and Moxibustion, Guangxi) (1981) Clinical Observations on acupuncture treatment of coronary artery diseases. *Chin Acupun Moxib*, **1**: 5–8 (in Chinese).

3. Ballegaard, S., Jensen, G., Peterson, F., Nissen, V.H. (1986) Acupuncture in severe stable angina pectoris: a randomized trial *Acta Med Scand*, **220**: 307–313.

4. Bao, Y.X., Yu, G.R., Lu, H.H., Zhen, D.S., Cheng, B.H. and Pan, C.Q. (1982) Acupuncture in acute myocardial infarction. *Chin Med J*, **95**: 824–828.

5. Chao, D.M., Shen, L.L., Cao, Y.X., Pitsillides, K.F., Longhurst, J.C. and Li, P. (1998) Naloxone reverses the inhibitory effect of electroacupuncture on sympathetic cardiovascular reflex responses. (In submission)

6. Diao, C.L., Zu, Q., Wang, S.P. and Yang, S.J. (1977) Clinical therapeutic effect of electro-acupuncture on 110 cases of coronary heart disease. *Chin J. Intern Med*, **2**: 70. (in Chinee).

7. Graham, T.P., Ross, J. Jr, Covell, J.W., Sonnenbick, E.H., Clancy, R.L. (1967) Myocardial oxygen consumption in acute experimental cardiac depression. *Cir Res*, **21**: 123–138.

8. Holzgrabe, U., Natchtsheim, C., Siener, T., Drosihn, S. and Brandt, W. (1997) Opioid agonists and antagonists, opioid receptors. *Pharmazie*, **52**: 4–22.

9. Jimenez, I., Iglesias, T. and Fuentes, J.A. (1990) Steroselectivity and subtype of the opiate receptor involved in stress-induced hypertension. *European J. Pharmacal*, **182**: 155–160.

10. Kiamura, K., Jorgensen, C.R., Gobel, F.L., Taylor, H.L. and Wang, Y. (1972) Hemodynamic correlates of myocardial oxygen consumption during upright exercise. *J Appl Physiol*, **32**: 516–522.
11. Li, P. (1991) Modulatory effect of somatic inputs on medullary cardiovascular neuronal function. *News Physiol Sci*, **6**: 69–72.
12. Li, P. and Yao, T. eds. (1992) *Mechanisms of the modulatory effect of acupuncture on Abnormal cardiovascular functions.* Shanghai Med Univ Press, Shanghai, China.
13. Li, P., Pitsillides, K.P., Stephen, V.R., Pan, H.L. and Longhurst, J.C. (1998) Reversal of refelx-induced myocardial ischemia by median nerve stimulation—a feline model of electroscupuncture. *Circulation*, **97**: 1186–1194.
14. Li, P., Tien-A-Looi, S., Holt, R.R., Rendig, S.V., Pitsillides, K.F. and Longhurst, J.C. (1998) Opioid receptor subtypes of rostral ventrolateral medulla in inhibition of gallbladder pressor response by electroacupuncture. (In submission).
15. Longhurst, J.C. (1991) Reflex effects from abdominal visceral afferents. In: Zucker, I.H., Gillmore, J.P. eds: *Reflex control of the circulation.* Caldwell, NJ: Telford Press. 551–577.
16. Lovick, T.A. (1987) Differential control of cardiac and vasomotor activity by neurons in nucleus paragigantocellularis lateralis in the cat. *J Physiol*, **389**: 23–35.
17. Martin, S.E., Pilkington, D.M. and Longhurst, J.C. (1989) Coronary vascular responses to chemical stimulation of abdominal visceral organs. *Am J. Physiol*, **256**: H735–744.
18. Orday, G.A. and Longhurst, J.C. (1983) Cardiovascular reflexes arising from the gallbladder of the cat: effects of capsaicin, bradykinin, and distension. *Circ Res*, **52**: 26–35.
19. Pitsillides, K.F. and Longhurst, J.C. (1995) An ultrasonic system for measurement of absolute myocardial thickness using a single transducer. *Am J. Physiol*, **37**: H358–367.
20. Richter, A., Herlitx, J. and Hjalmarson, A. (1991) Effect of acupuncture in patients with angina pectoris. *Eur Heart J*, **12**: 175–178.
21. Rozanski, A., Bairey, C.N., Krantz, D.S., Friedman, J., Resser, K.J., Morell, M., Hilton-Chalfen, S., Hestrin, L., Bietendorf, J. and Berman, D.S. (1988) Mental stress and the induction of silent myocardial ischemia in patients with coronary artery disease. *N Engl J. Med*, **318**: 1005–1012.
22. Sun, S.Y., Liu, Z., Li, P. and Ingenito, A.J. (1996) Central effects of opioid agonists and naloxone on blood pressure and heart rate in normotensive and hypertensive rats. *Gen Pharmac*, **27**: 1187–1194.
23. Victor, R.G., Seals, D.R. and Mark, A.L. (1987) Differential control of heart rate and sympathetic nerve activity during dynamic exercise: insight from intraneural recordings in humans. *J Clin Invest*, **79**: 508–516.

24. Wang, H.R., et al. (1981) A further study on the treatment of coronary artery arteriosclerotic heart disease with acupuncture. *Chin Acupun Moxib*, 1: 1–5 (in Chinese).
25. Xu, H.K. and Jiang, W.P. (1987) A morphological observation on the influence of acupuncture on the ischemic myocardial injury. *Compilation of the abstract of acupuncture and moxibustion papers. The First World Conference of Acupuncture-Moxibustion*. Abstract 377.

9 THE MECHANISMS OF ACUPUNCTURE THERAPY ON OTHER DISEASES

Peng Li

Clinical Studies

Besides pain and cardiovascular diseases acupuncture was reported to treat gastrointestinal diseases, including the peptic ulcer, diarrhoea, constipation, chronic gastritis, indigestion of children, the hiccup, nausea, etc.[11-p 155]. It was also used to treat urinary diseases, endor-criopathy, neurological and immunological diseases, such as urination difficulties, enuresis, asthma, insomnia, prostatitis, overweight and obesity, stroke, nerve paralysis, epilepsy, diabetes, hyperthyroidism, dysmenorrhoea and hypermenorrhea, etc. It is even used to stop smoking and drug addiction.[20-p 29]

GASTROINTESTINAL DISEASES

In 1995, Zhang, et al.,[35] performed 150 cases of gastroscopic observation and saw that needling on Neiguan (Pe 6) and Zusanli (St 36) could markedly improve patients' symptoms such as nausea and vomiting, and modulate their gastric peristalsis and regurgitation of the bile and duodenum fluid etc. Zhen, et al.[40] reported that in patients with irritable bowel syndrome, their plasma gastrin levels are much higher than in healthy people. After needling Zusanli (St 36) the gastrin level decreased significantly and their symptoms were much improved. Guan[8] reported that ear acupuncture and combined acupuncture applied on Zusanli (St 36), Zhongwan (Ren 12), Tianshu (St 25), Yinglinquan (Sp 9) or Yanlingquang (GB 34) could cure 64% of patients with postoperative enteroparalysis, and another 24% were improved. All together 88% were effective.

URINARY DISEASE

Wang, et al.[22] showed that acupuncture and moxibustion could decrease the female urethral syndrome by decreasing the urethral pressure. Its effectiveness is 88%, while in the control group treated by drugs it is only 33%. Chen et al.[39] observed that acupuncture could release spasm of the ureter. Liu et al.[39] reported that acupuncture applied on Qugu (Ren 2), Guanyuan (Ren 4), Zhongji (Ren 3), Pangguangshu (UB 28), Jimen (Sp 11) etc. could induce contraction of the bladder in patients with urine retention. Shi et al.[39] showed that acupuncture applied on Zusanli (St 36) could increase intra-abodominal pressure and inhibit the contraction of the bladder. Acupuncture on Sanyingjiao (Sp 6) had a similar effect, and could increase both intra-abodominal pressure and contraction of the bladder. Kubista, et al.,[11−p151] also reported twenty cases of female urethral incontinence treated with electroacupuncture. Seventeen patients (85%) showed a positive closing pressure of the urethra. They suggested that acupuncture could increase the tonus of the entire sphincter area of the urethra and strengthen the muscles by increasing blood flow in the submucosal region of the urethra. Ellis, et al.,[6] showed that in treating incontinence in the elderly, 90% of the acupuncture group had reduced nocturnal voiding, while only 11% of the placebo (mock transcutaneous nerve stimulation, TENS) showed an effect.

ASTHMA

Yang, et al.[30] treated asthma with acupuncture and moxibustion, and the effectiveness reached as high as 85%. In these patients, their eosinophilic granulocytes and the counts of peripheral activated T-lymphocytes were elevated markedly. After treatment, both decreased significantly ($P < 0.001$). So the allergic responses of these patients were much suppressed.

ENDOCRINOPATHY

Zhen[38] reviewed the research progress in acupuncture treatment of diabetes neuropathy, and showed that acupuncture could much improve the syndrome and neuropathy.

Chen, et al.,[4] did a series of studies for more than ten years on the effect of acupuncture and moxibustion on Hashimoto's thyroiditis and hyperthyroidism. Their results showed that acupuncture and moxibustion had a favorable regulating effect on the immune and thyroid functions of these patients.

In patients with Hashimoto's thyroiditis,[25] they made moxibustion on the following acupoints: Tanzhong (Ren 17), Zhongwan (Ren 12), Gaunyuan (Ren 4), or Dazhu (Du 14), Shenshu (UB 23) and Mingmen (Du 4), once a day (or the other day) for 50 times. After about two months, they saw that the combination rate of plasma thyroglobulin antibodies (TGA and MCA) in these patients decreased markedly; their serum T4 and T3 increased significantly (P < 0.05, 0.001 respectively); while the TSH decreased significantly (p < 0.001). In 10 cases, they followed the patients for three months and found that their serum TGA and MCA combination rate remained at a low level. In six cases they followed patients for six months and they still showed a low level of TGA and MCA. In the control group, who were treated with ordinary drugs (thyroid 40–120 mg/day) patients had no significant change of their high TGA and MCA level. Further work[26] showed that moxibustion could modulate the function and ratio of the subgroup of T-lymphocytes, and thus inhibit the secretion of TGA and MCA from B-lymphocytes. So moxibustion had a therapeutic effect on the thyroiditis.

Their work[9,10] also showed that in patients with hyperthyroidism, 86.3% could improve their syndrome and symptoms after acupuncture was applied on Neiguan (Pe 6), Jianshi (Pe 5), Shenmen (He 7), Zusanli (St 36), Taichong (Liv 3), Taixi (Ki 3) and Guanyuan (Ren 4) etc. Patients' serum T4, T3 and the TSH receptor antibody activity decreased, but the serum TSH increased.

Being overweight and obesity are mainly a dietary problem. It was reported[11−p 196] that acupuncture was applied on Liangqui (St 34) and Gongsun (Sp 4) twice a week for ten times a course. After three courses of treatment an average weight reduction of seven and one-half kilograms was obtained. The mechanism is not completely understood.

GYNECOLOGICAL AND OBSTETRIC DISEASES

Dunn, et al.[5] used TENS at acupoints to improve the uterine contractions in pregnancies past the due date, and saw that it produced a much greater increase in strength and frequency of uterine contractions than the sham TENS group.

It was reported that acupuncture applied on Hegu (LI 4) and Tanzhong (Ren 17) could cure 94,7% of patients with oligogalactia after labour.[11−p 152]

Yu, et al.,[31,32, and 42] did a series of studies on the effect of electroacupuncture (EA) induced ovulation. In 1987 they reported that in 59 chronically anovulatory patients, acupuncture applied on Quanyuan (Ren 4), Zhongji (Ren 3), Zigong (Ren 19), and Sanyinjiao (Sp 6) could induce ovulation in 33.9% patients. When additional Chinese herbs were added according to the differential diagnosis of Traditional Chinese Medicine, the rate of ovulation increased to 52.5%. Further observation showed that in most successful patients, after EA their hand skin temperature increased, the plasma level of β-endorphin-like immunoreactive substances decreased, and their plasma FSH and LH value increased. So Yu, et al., suggested that in many anovulatory cases EA could inhibit the excessive sympathetic activity, decrease plasma β-endorphin and increase FSH, and LH, thus inducing ovulation.

NEUROLOGICAL DISEASES

Yu, et al.[33] reported that in 50 cases of facial nerve paralysis, EA plus moxibustion could cure 80% of the patients, and improve 20%. It was noted by Pomorenz that in China more than 100,000 cases of Bell's palsy were treated with acupuncture and had a success rate of 92%.

Acupuncture was used to treat paralysis resulting from stroke. Naser et al.,[16] showed that acupuncture was only effective in those patients in whom less than half the motor pathway was damaged, suggesting that plasticity of the surviving half was responsible for the recovery. Zhen[37] reviewed the mechanism of acupuncture therapy on the stroke, and showed that acupuncture could decrease blood pressure, blood viscosity and plasma cholesterol and lipids; improve microcirculation, increase the amplitude of somatic evoked potential and shorten its latency, and thus improve their clinical syndromes.

In many clinics it was reported that acupuncture was also used to treat anxiety, insomnia and epilepsy, etc.[11–p181]

SMOKING, ALCOHOLISM AND DRUG ABUSE

Acupuncture was also used to stop smoking. Zhou[41] speculated that smoking could inhibit the release of endogenous opioids, and acupuncture could increase the opioids in the brain and help the smokers not to become addicted. They also believed that auricular acupuncture is much better than acupuncture on other acupoints of the body.

Bullock et al.[1,2] treated chronic alcoholics with ear acupuncture and saw that of 50 patients 25 received three needles in true ear points, and 25 received three needles in the wrong ear points. 42% of alcoholics remained alcohol free for three months, and an additional 28% drank much less when given true acupuncture, while sham acupuncture had no effect.

Wen et al.[23,24] reported that prolonged daily ear acupuncture treatments for eight days helped patients withdraw from opium. It would be more rapid and effective with if combined with the antagonist naloxone with EA given for 30 minutes a day for three days.

One of the authors, Dr. Lily Cheung, has successful experience of treating various diseases, including Menière's disease, smoking addiction, alcoholism, rhinitis, hay fever and herpes zoster, etc. (see next section).

Experimental Studies

GASTROINTESTINAL

Jin, et al.[12] showed that EA in conscious dogs could inhibit gastric acid secretion after a meal, and this effect was mediated by β-endorphins, somatostatin and VIP. However, Noguchi and Hayashi[16] reported that EA in anesthetized rats increased gastric acidity via the vagal nerve.

Lei et al.[15] needling Zusanli (St 36) of rats bilaterally for 50 minutes found that the immune-reactive substance of enkephalin (Enk-IR) decreased markedly, while those of substance P increased significantly. They suggested that acupuncture on Zusanli (Sp 36) could increase the release of enkephalin in the gastrointestinal tract, cause the decrease of Enk-IR, and inhibit the release of ACh and SP. They thought that this was why acupuncture on Zusanli (St 36) could inhibit the motion of the gastrointestinal tract.

URINARY

Zhen[39] reviewed the effect of acupuncture on the urinary system. She reported that Tang et al. made EA on bilateral Sanyingjiao (Sp 6) and Zhaohai (Ki 6) of rabbits and discover a marked increase of renal blood flow, urine excretion and peristalsis of the ureter. Chai et al.[36] also found a marked increase of urine excretion and renal nerve discharge after EA on Shenshu (UB 23) of rabbits. Wu et al.[39] watched the effect of acupuncture on bladder and urethral function. They saw that acupuncture on Pangguangshu (UB 28) could induce contraction of the bladder and increase intrabladder pressure. Wu's work showed that acupuncture on Pangguangshu (UB28) could evoke unit discharge in the posterior hypothalamus and medullary reticular formation, while acupuncture on non-acupoints had no such effect. All their experiments proved that the posterior hypothalamus and medulla are important in the facilitatory effect of acupuncture on bladder function.

ENDOCRINOLOGICAL

Kang, et al.[13] observed the influence of acupuncture on blood sugar tolerance in normal Wistar rats at different times. They found that if acupuncture was applied on bilateral Feishu (UB 13), Yishe (UB 49), Weishu (UB 21), Neiguan (Pe 6), Zusanli (St 36), etc., the rise of blood sugar after intravenous injection of 50% glucose (1.75g) was smaller and recovered to a normal level faster. In addition, acupuncture did not affect sugar tolerance if applied before glucose loading.

Li, et al.[14] reported that the non-insulin-dependent diabetic rats had a series of problems, including obvious obesity, impaired glucose tolerance, marked increases of serum triglyceride (TG), total cholesterol (Tch), very low density lipid-cholestrol (VLDL-ch) and hepatic cholesterol, and a marked decrease of high density lipid cholesterol (HDL-CH) and high density lipid$_2$ cholesterol (HDL$_2$-ch). Their serum insulin level was significantly elevated. Acupuncture and moxibustion applied on Ganshu (UB 18), Pishu (UB 20) and ShenShu (UB 23) could significantly decrease their body weight, serum insulin level, TG, Tch, VLDL-ch, and hepatic cholesterol, and increase the serum HDL-ch, and HDL$_2$-ch. Therefore acupuncture and moxibustion could decrease all the risk factors that would induce arteriosclerosis.

Zhao, et al.[36] found many changes in old rats: their noradrenaline (NE) in the cortex, the thyroid releasing hormone (TRH) in the hypothalamus, serum T_3, T_4, FT_3, FT_4 and spleen IL-2 were all markedly lower than the young rats, while their serum TRH, TSH and rT3 were higher than the young rats'. Moxibustion applied on Guanyuan (Ren 4) three times a week for ten times could increase the NE in the cortex, TRH in hypothalamus, Serum T_4, and spleen IL-2, and increase the serum TRH. They suggested that moxibustion on Guanyuan (Ren 4) could modulate the hypothalamic-pituitary-thyroid axis and immunity, and thus delay the ageing.

GENITAL

After a series of clinical observations Yu, et al., suggested that EA could inhibit the release of β-endorphin, increase FSH and LH, and thus induce ovulation. Their further experiments[28,29] proved that the decrease in activity of hypothalamic β-ebdorphin and decrease of the hypothalamic μ opioid receptor are important for inducing the preovulatory LH surge. The changes in gene expression of hypothalamic prepropiomelanocortin during preovulatory LH surges may be regulated by estrogen and its receptors.

Ou, et al.[18] reported that auricular acupuncture could promote the contraction of the uterus. Wu, et al.[27] applied moxibustion on Shenque (Ren 8) of gerontal mice five minutes per day for one month, and showed that the diameters of convoluted seminiferous tubules were much bigger than the control group (P < 0.05), thus suggesting that moxibustion could delay ageing.

IMMUNOLOGICAL

Gong, et al.[7] reported the effect of needling Zusanli on immunologic function. They showed that EA could increase the synthesis of DNA and RNA of lymphocytes in the spleen, and also the content of IL-2 in these lymphocytes.

Zhai, et al.[34] studied the mechanism of moxibustion on immune function in mice, and showed that when HAC cancer was loaded, the cellular immune function decreased. Their adrenal glands markedly shrank. However, in those with moxibustion their cellular immune function could be maintained at a higher level, and their pituitary and adrenal glands enlarged. The content of β-Endorphin in these glands increased. The receptors of β-endorphin in the lymphocytes of the spleen also increased markedly. They suggested that moxibustion could increase the synthesis and secretion of β-endorphin and the β-endorphin receptor on immune cells and thus improve the immune function.

Chen, et al.[3] observed the effect of EA on cellular immune function in normal free-moving rats, and showed that EA could enhance the turnover of lymphocytes in the spleen, and markedly elevate the inducement of IL-2. So, they believe that EA could enhance the cellular immune function of normal rats.

Sato, et al.[19] showed in anesthetized rats the enhanced lytic activity of splenic natural killer cells after acupuncture.

NEUROLOGICAL

Pomeranz, et al.[20] found that EA markedly enhanced motor-nerve regeneration and sensory nerve sprouting in adult rats after sciatic nerve injury.

Wang and Cheng[21] saw that during convulsion dynorphin released from the hippocampus decreased. When EA was applied on Fengfu (Du 16) and Jinsuo (Du 8), it had an anticonvulsive effect, and increased the dynorphin released from the hippocampus.

Comments

The above data showed that acupuncture and moxibustion could be used to treat many diseases, including gastrointestinal, urogenital, neurological, endocrinological and immune diseases, etc. Usually it has a modulatory effect on this dysfunction. So, if patients come to see doctors early and the disease is in its early stages and not very severe, it is better to use acupuncture and other alternative medication instead of drugs, which often have many side effects. The acupoints chosen depends on the differential diagnosis of Traditional Chinese Medicine; either needling by hand or EA, they all have an effect. Doctors who like to use acupuncture should learn more about the basic ideas of Traditional Chinese Medicine, and the knowledge of integrative physiology and neuroscience. Sometimes auricular acupuncture is quite effective, especially for some gastrointestinal and endocrinological dysfunction, smoking and alcoholism, etc. It is also interesting that acupuncture can improve the paralysis of peripheral nerves and stroke, which indicates that it might promote neural regeneration. The mechanism of these effects is not very clear. It is a big area that needs further investigation.

References

1. Bullock, M., et al. (1987) Acupuncture treatment of alcoholics. *Alcoholism Clinical and Exp Res*, 11: 292–295.
2. Bullock, M., et al. (1989) Controlled trial of acupuncture for severe recidivist alcoholic *Lancent*, 1: 1435–1439.
3. Chen, X.D., Du, L.N., Jiang, J.W. and Cao, X.D. (1995) The effect of electrical zcupuncture on cellular immune function in rats. *Shanghai J. Acup Moxib*, 14: 128–129 (in Chinese).
4. Cheng, H.P., Wu, G.S., He, J.S., et al. (1991) Characteristics of the effect of acupuncture on auto-immuno hyperthyroidism. *Chin Acup*, 6: 33–36.
5. Dun, P.A., Rogers, D. and Halford, K. (1989) Transcutaneous electrical nerve stimulation at acupuncture pints in the nduction of uterine contractions. *Obstet Gynecol*, 73: 286–290.
6. Ellis, N., Briggs, R., et al. (1990) The effect of acupuncture on nocturnal urinary frequency and incontinence in the elderly. *Compl Med Res*, 4: 16–17.
7. Gong, B., Muo, Q.H. and Xiong, X.L. (1994) The effect of needling Zusanli on immunoloogic function in rat. *Shanghai J. Acup Moxib*, 13: 34–35 (in Chinese).
8. Guan, J.M. (1996) Ear-acupuncture combined with body acupuncture for postoperative enteroparalysis. *Shanghai J. Acup Moxib*, 15: 17 (in Chinese).

9. He, J.S., Jin, S.B., Hen, J.S., Chen, H.P., et al. (1990) Influence of acupuncture on the serum TSH receptor antibody activity of patients with hyperthyroidism and its clinic significance *Chin Acup*, **6**: 19–21 (in Chinese).
10. He, J.S., Jin, S.B., Hen, J.S., Chen, H.P., et al. (1994) A clinical observation on the effect of acuuncture on 136 cases of patients with hyperthyroidism and had side effect by using anti-thyroid drugs. *Shanghai J. Acup Moxib*, **13**: 54–55 (in Chinese).
11. Huang, K.C. (1996) *Acupuncture, the past and the present*. Vantage Press, New York.
12. Jin, H.O., Zhou, L., et al. (1992) Inhibition of acid secretion by electrical acupuncture is mediated via beta endorphin and somatostatin. *Amer J. Physiol*, **271**: G524–530.
13. Kang, S.Y., Xiong, X.H., Lin, J. and Sun, G.J. (1996) Effect of acupuncture on normal rats' sugar tolerance at different time. *Shanghai J. Acup Moxib*, **15**: 33–34 (in Chinese).
14. Li, S.L., Chen, H.P., Zhen, H.T., et al. (1995) The effect of acupuncture and moxibustion on lipostrophy in experimental rats with diabetes. *Shanghai J. Acup and Moxib*, **14**: 80–81 (in Chinese).
15. Lei, Y.N., Hu, D.S. and Ru, L.Q. (1995) Effect of electroacupuncture Zusanli (St 36) on ENK-energic nerves and SPenergic nerves in rats' small intestine. *Shanghai J. Acup Moxib*, **14**: 268–271 (in Chinese).
16. Naser, M.A., Alexander, M.P., et al. (1994) Acupuncture in the treatment of hand paresis in chronic and acute stroke patients. Improvement obersved in all cases. *Clin Rehabil*, **8**: 127–141.
17. Noguchi, E. and Hayashi, H. (1996) Increase in gastric acidity in response to electroacupuncture stimulation of the hindlimb of anesthetized rats. *Jap J. Physiol*, **46**: 53–58.
18. Ou, G.Z., Zhang, Z.T. and Wang, S.Y., et al (1996) Experimental observation of implication of electroacupuncture upon auricle of rabbits' uterine funcation. *Shangha J. Acup Moxib*, **15**: 35. (in Chinese).
19. Sato, T., Usami, S. and Takeshige, C. (1986) Roel of the arcuate nucleus of the hypothalamus as the descending pain-inhibitory system in acupuncture point and non-point produced analgesia. In: Takeshige, C. (ed) *Studies on the emchanism of acupuncture analgesia based on animal experiments*. Showa University Press, Tokyo P. 627 (in Japanese with English abstract).
20. Stux, G. and Pomeranz, B. (1998) Basics of acupuncture. 4th edition. Springer, Berlin.
21. Wang, B. and Cheng, J.S. (1995) The change of dynorphin released from rat's hippocampus during electrofit and anticonvulsion by electrical acupuncture. *Shanghai J. Acup Moxib*, **14**: 33–34.
22. Wang, S.Y., Zhen, H.T., Huang, C., et al. (1997) Research of high urethral pressure decreasing of female urehtral syndrome treated by acupuncture and moxibustin. *Shanghai J. Acup Moxib*, **16**: 4–6 (in Chinese).

23. Wen, H.L. (1977) Fast detoxification of heroin addicts and electrical stimulation in combination with naloxone. *Comp Med East West*, 5: 257–263.
24. Wen, H.L. and Cheung, S.Y.C. (1973) Treatment of drug addiction by acupuncture and electrical stimulation. *Asian J. Med*, 9: 138–141.
25. Wu, G.S., Chen, H.P., Hen, J.S., et al. (1987) A clinical study of moxibustion therapy on Hashimoto's throiditis. *Acta College Trad Med Sin Shanghai*, 1: 16–21 (in Chinese).
26. Wu, G.S., Chen, H.P., He, Y.J., et al. (1990) An immunological observation on the moxibustion therapy of Hashimoto's thyroiditis. *Shanghai J. Acup Moxib*, 4: 4–6.
27. Wu, Z.C., Wang, L.L., Xu, L.F., et al. (1996) The effect of moxibustion of Shench'uch (Ren 8) on the diameter of convoluted seminiferous tubule in gerontal mice. *Shanghai J. Acup and Moxib*, 15: 31 (in Chinese).
28. Yang, S.P., He, L.F. and Yu, J. (1997) Changes in densities of hypothalamic u opioid receptor during cupric acete-induced prevulatory LH surge in rabbit. *Acta Physio Sin*, 49: 354–358 (in Chinese with english abstract).
29. Yang, S.P., He, L.F. and Yu, J. (1998) Levels of hypothalamic proopiome-lanocortin mRNA and estrogen binding sites during prevulatory GnRH surge in rat. *Acta Zoolog Sin*, 44: 67–73 (in Chinese with English abstract).
30. Yang, Y.Q., Chen, H.P., Wang, A.Q., et al. (1994) Analysis of the curative effect of acupuncture on 174 cases of asthma. *Shanghai J. acup muxib*, 13: 153–154 (in Chinese).
31. Yu, J., Zheng, H.M. and Chen, B.Y. (1986) Relationship of hand temperature and blood b-endorphin = like immunoreactive substance with electroacupuncture induction of ovulation. *Acup Res*, 2: 86–90 (in Chinese with English abstract).
32. Yu, J., Zheng, H.M. and Bing, S.M. (1989) An observation on the plasma FSH and LH level, follicle growth and ovulation induced by electroacupuncture. *J. comb of Chin and Western Med*, 9: 199–202. (in Chinese).
33. Yu, J.F. (1994) Analysis of the curative effect of acupuncture on facial paralysis. *Shanghai J. Acup Moxib*, 13: 165 (in Chinese).
34. Zhai, D.D., Chen, H.P., Wang, R.Z., et al. Endorphin mechanism of the regulating effect of direct moxibustion on immunity. *Shanghai J. Acup Moxib*, 13: 223–224 (in Chinese).
35. Zhang, Z.I., Chen, J.L., Zhu, S.L., et al. Gastroscopic observation of the reaction to needling points Neiguan (Pe 6) and Zusanli (St 36) in 150 cases. *Shanghai J. Acup Moxib*, 14: 11 (in Chinese).
36. Zhao, W.K., Zhang, H.D., Jin Guoqing, et al. (1996) The effect of moxibustion of Guanyuan (Reb 4) on hypothalamus-pituitary throid axis and IL-2 in gerontal rats. *Shanghai J. Acup Moxib*, 15: 28–29 (in Chinese).
37. Zhen, C.L. (1995) The progress of the study of acupuncture therapy on stroke and its mechanism. *Shanghai J. Acup Moxib*, 14: 225–227 (in Chinese).
38. Zhen, W.T. (1994) The research progress in acupuncture treatment of diabetic neuropathy. *Shanghai J. Acup Moxib*, 13: 180–181.

39. Zhen, W.T. (1995) Regulatory effects of acupuncture on function of urinary system. *Shanghai J. Acup Moxib*, **14**: 185–186 (in Chinee).
40. Zhen, G.Y. and Chen W.M. (1996) Clinicall observation of needling Zusanli (St 36) in the treatment of IBS. *Shanghai J. Acup Moxib*, **15**: 20–21 (in Chinese).
41. Zhou, J.W. (1997) The progress of investigation on stop smoking by acupuncture *Shanghai J. Acup Moxib*, **16**: 36–37 (in Chinese).
42. Zuo, X.D., Wang, W.Y. and Yu, J. (1987) An observation on 59 cases with ovulation induced by a combined treatment of acupuncture and Chinese medicine. *Shanghai J. Chinese Med*, **3**: 12–13 (in Chinese).

10 THE EFFECTS OF ACUPUNCTURE ON DEFENCE REACTION, BARO- AND CHEMO-RECEPTOR REFLEXES

Peng Li

In the previous chapters, the modulatory effects of electroacupuncture (EA) have been described. For instance, acupuncture decreases blood pressure (BP) in hypertensives while increasing BP in hypotensives; it also reduces the extrasystoles induced by hypothalamic or midbrain defence areas stimulation while increasing the heart rate (HR) during bradycardia produced by vagal excitation. It could inhibit myocardial ischemia, stop pain etc. It is therefore important to perform further studies to clarify the mechanism behind the above phenomena. This chapter will deal with the work done in our laboratory that helps us to understand more profoundly the essence of the acupuncture effects, especially on the cardiovascular system.

Inhibitory Effect of EA on Defence Reaction

In chapter 7, we talked about the pressor response and ventricular extrasystoles induced by stimulation of the hypothalamic and midbrain defence areas which could be inhibited by acupuncture. In chapter 5, we demonstrated that acupuncture had a depressor effect and inhibited the splanchnic sympathetic nerve activities in SHR, which had a stronger sympathetic activity and defence reaction than their normotensive control Wistar-Kyoto rats. So, experiments were carried out in our laboratory to examine the effect of acupuncture on defence reaction induced by hypothalamic or midbrain stimulation, and we analysed its mechanism.

In 11 rabbits, when low frequency EA was applied to Zusanli (St 36) for 20 minutes, the defence reaction induced by hypothalamic stimulation attenuated. The pressor response decreased to 52%, and the renal nerve discharge, pupillary, respiratory and other behavioural responses were all significantly attenuated.[12]

THE ROLE OF ENDORPHIN IN THE INHIBITORY EFFECT OF EA

Interestingly, this inhibitory effect of EA on the defence reaction was naloxone-reversible. Following iv of naloxone (0.4 mg/kg), the amplitude of the pressor response and other components of the defence reaction returned immediately to the pre-acupuncture control level. However, bilateral lesion or local application of naloxone (1 μg in 1 μl of saline on each side) into the ventral portion of the periaqueductal grey matter (PAG) could block the inhibitory effect of EA on the pressor response. This observation shows that the activation of the opiate receptors in the ventral PAG is essential for the acupuncture-induced inhibition of the defence reaction.[13]

A bilateral lesion of the basomedial portion of the hypothalamus (including the arcuate nucleus, ARC) also abolished the inhibitory effect of acupuncture on the pressor response and the other components of the defence reaction induced by dorsomedial hypothalamic stimulation. After microinjection of L-sodium glutamate (50 mM in 1 μl) into the ARC of the hypothalamus, the pressor response and other components of the defence reaction produced by stimulation of the hypothalamus attenuated markedly. However, microinjection of saline (1 μl) into the ARC had no such effect. If L-sodium glutamate was injected into the third ventricle or the dorsolateral portion of the anterior hypothalamus, there was no effect. The inhibition of the hypothalamic stimulation-induced defence reaction by the microinjection of L-sodium glutamate into the ARC was reversed as well as prevented by iv naloxone (0.5 mg/kg). It has long been known that the β-endorphin-containing neurons are mainly located in the ARC of the basomedial hypothalamus, and send axons ending in the thalamic nuclei, the PAG in the midbrain and the locus coeruleus. These results suggest that the inhibitory effect of acupuncture on the defence reaction may be mediated by activating the β-endorphin-containing neurons in the ARC. Moreover, after bilateral lesions of the ventral PAG, or microinjection of naloxone (1 μg in 1 μl of saline on each side) into the ventral PAG, the subsequent microinjection of L-sodium glutamate into the ARC only had a small effect on the pressor response. Therefore, it is suggested that the activation of the β-endorphin containing neurons in ARC might exert an inhibition on defence reaction via the mediation of opiate receptors in the ventral PAG.[14]

THE ROLE OF SEROTONIN IN THE INHIBITORY EFFECT OF EA

In 10 rabbits pretreated with parachlorophenylaline methylester-HCl (PCPA), and an inhibitor of tryptophan hydroxylase, by icv for 3 days

(7 mg/day), stimulation of the hypothalamic defence area still caused a pressor response and the other components of defence reaction. However, following microinjection of L-sodium glutamate into the ARC (50 mg in 0.5 μl of saline), the pressor response was not reduced as much as that in control animals which received an icv injection of saline. In another experiment, after a serotonin receptor antagonist ketanserin (20 mg in 50 ml of saline) was administered icv, microinjection of L-sodium glutamate into the ARC could not affect the defence reaction induced by stimulation of the hypothalamic defence areas. These results imply that the brain serotonin is likely to participate in the mechanism of ARC stimulation-produced inhibition of the defence reaction.[14]

INHIBITION OF CARDIOVASCULAR COMPONENT OF DEFENCE REACTION BY DPN STIMULATION

For further analysing the mechanism of the inhibition on defence reaction by acupuncture, experiments were performed by stimulation of the deep peroneal nerve (DPN) to mimic acupuncture on Zusanli (St 36).[3] In urethane (700 mg/kg)-chloralose (35 mg/kg) anesthetized rabbits, stimulation of the hypothalamic perifornical area (HYP) or the dorsal portion of PAG with a current of 150–300 μA (3 sec trains of 0.5 ms pulses at 70 Hz) evoked a characteristic cardiovascular pattern of defence reaction, including a pressor response, tachycardia, an increase in left ventricular pressure (LVP), LV dP/dt, femoral blood flow (FBF) and pupillary dilatation etc. Stimulation of the HYP and PAG were repeated every 10 minutes. When the cardiovascular responses were kept stable for 3 times, the DPN was stimulated for 10–20 minutes with a current of 400 μA (0.5 ms at 10 Hz) to excite groups II and III fibres. The pressor response of HYP or PAG stimulation attenuated to about half the control value. In some animals the pressor response was completely abolished. The response of HR, LVP, LV dP/dt and FBF were also inhibited and recovered gradually after 1–6 hours. This inhibitory effect of DPN stimulation could be blocked by iv of naloxone (0.4 mg/kg).

When two pieces of morphine-moistened filter paper were applied onto the rostral ventromedial medulla (RVLM) surface bilaterally, the pressor response evoked by HYP or PAG stimulation could also be inhibited to about 70% of their control level. Stimulation of the RVLM (30–100 μA) also evoked characteristic cardiovascular responses of defence reaction, but these responses could not be inhibited by DPN stimulation.

While this work was done on rabbits in Shanghai in 1986 and 1987, later in 1995, Lovick, et al.[10] in Birmingham, UK got similar results in rats. It is suggested that the RVLM may be the final integrating area where the DPN inputs suppress the defence reaction, and opioids in this area may take part in this inhibitory process.

THE INHIBITORY EFFECT OF DPN STIMULATION ON RVLM NEURONS

The above suggestion was supported by electrophysiological examinations.[4] 40% of the neurons in the RVLM excited by single or double shocks applied to the PAG could be inhibited when the DPN was stimulated for 5–20 minutes. This inhibitory effect recovered within 20–120 minutes after the cessation of DPN stimulation, and could be reversed when naloxone was applied iontophoretically. These units firing could also be inhibited by iontophoresis of morphine.

In some experiments, the antidromic responses of RVLM neurons were recorded by stimulation of the lateral horn of the tenth thoracic spinal cord. It was shown that the antidromic latencies of RVLM neurons could be prolonged by stimulation of DPN for 10–30 minutes, and then returned to their original level gradually within 30–120 minutes. Therefore it seems that the inhibitory effect of DPN ideas on the RVLM neurons may be due to the hyperpolarization of the cell membrane. So it is shown that the spread of antidromic invasions in initial segment-soma delay was slowed down, and the latency was prolonged.

THE NEURONAL PATHWAY BY WHICH THE DPN INPUT INHIBITS THE DEFENCE REACTION-RELATED NEURONS IN THE RVLM

This series of experiments was designed to analyse the pathway of the DPN input which inhibits the defence reaction-related neurons in RVLM.[5,6,7,8] Results showed that the inhibitory effect of DPN inputs occurred even after decerebration at the level rostral to the ARC. However, it was abolished by decerebration at the level caudal to the ARC or electrolytic lesion of this nucleus. The cardiovascular responses of the defence reaction were also inhibited by microinjection of DL-homocysteic acid (DLH) into the ARC. The inhibitory effect was blocked by microinjection of naloxone or anti-β-endorphin serum into the ventral part of PAG. On the other hand, microinjection of morphine or DLH into the ventral part of PAG attenuated the pressor response induced by stimulation of the midbrain defence area. Therefore, it is suggested that the higher autonomic centre above the

ARC is not essential for the inhibitory effect of the DPN inputs on the cardiovascular responses of defence reaction. Nevertheless, the excitatory endorphinergic projection from ARC to the ventral part of the PAG is involved in this effect.

The pressor response elicited by stimulation of the midbrain defence area was attenuated following microinjection of morphine into the ventral portion of the PAG. The inhibitory effect of either DPN stimulation or morphine microinjection into the PAG could be blocked after lidocaine or naloxone was microinjected into the nucleus raphe obscurus (NRO). So it is suggested that the NRO is involved in the inhibition produced by the DPN inputs on the cardiovascular response of defence reaction.

Electrophysiological study showed that stimulation of the ARC by single or paired pulses resulted in synaptic responses of many neurons in the ventral PAG. 83% of the neurons were excited and responded with a single spike or a burst of 2–4 spikes, usually superimposed on a field potential, with latencies ranging from 1.5 to 25 ms. Most of the responsive units fired spontaneously with a mean frequency of 1–70 (21.9 ± 2.9) spikes/sec. Increasing the intensity of the stimulus usually decreased the latency of the response and increased the number of spikes during a burst response. Their frequency of spontaneous firing also increased after stimulation of the DPN for 5 minutes (0.5 ms in pulse width, 400 μA in 10 Hz), and returned to the control level after variant periods ranging from seconds to minutes.

Stimulation of the ventral PAG mainly resulted in synaptic activation of cells in the NRO. 64% of the NRO units activated orthodromically by stimulation of the ventral PAG were also activated orthodromically by stimulation of the dorsal PAG (defence area of the midbrain). Their spontaneous firing also increased after stimulation of the DPN. In 1994, Zhang, et al.[27] further showed that the inhibitory effect of ventral PAG on RVLM neurons will be blocked, if lidocaine is microinjected into NRO. Therefore it is further proved that this inhibition passes through NRO.

Recordings in the RVLM showed that 73% of the neurons excited orthodromically by dorsal PAG stimulation could also be inhibited orthodromically by DPN stimulation. These results support the view that the inhibitory effect of DPN stimulation may activate the ARC neurons, which has excitatory projections to neurons in the ventral PAG; from the ventral PAG there are excitatory projections to NRO, which in turn inhibits the defence reaction-related neurons in the RVLM.

In summary, application of EA or DPN stimulation could inhibit the defence reaction induced by stimulation of HYP or PAG. This inhibitory effect is due to the excitation of group II and III afferent fibres, which activates the endorphin containing neurons in ARC of the hypothalamus. The latter send excitatory projections to the ventral PAG, and then in turn to the NRO in medulla. From NRO there are inhibitory projections to the defence reaction related neurons in the RVLM. Evidence showed that except opioids, the serotonergic neurons might also be involved.

Baroreceptor Reflex Resetting by EA

In conscious rabbits, EA applied on Zusanli (St 36) and Shangjuxu (St 37) elicited no changes in basal mean blood pressure (MAP) level and heart (HR), but caused a significant increase in the slope of the MAP-HR regression line, showing an enhancement of the baroreflex sensitivity.[21]

In urethane-chloralose anesthetized rabbits, stimulation of DPN for 20 minutes resulted in an increase in the slope of the intrasinusal pressure (ISP)-MAP curve, and a marked decrease in the threshold of the baroreflex.[16] The MAP was higher than control at a given ISP when the ISP was below 110 mmHg, while the MAP was lower than control at a given ISP when the ISP was above 110 mm Hg. Thirty minutes after the cessation of the DPN stimulation, the ISP-MAP response curves were returned to their original values. This experiment shows that EA or acupuncture-like DPN stimulation could modulate or reset the function of the baroreflex. It increases the gain of the baroreflex. That means when the MAP is higher the baroreflex will be more sensitive, and when the MAP is lower the baroreflex will be less sensitive, therefore it is in favour of the maintenance of BP homeostasis. It is interesting that weak stimulation of DPN (0.1–0.16 mA) is inadequate to reset the baroreflex. Maybe excitation of group III fibres is important in resetting the baroreflex. If the anaesthesia is too deep, DPN stimulation also had no effect. Stimulation of the superficial peroneal nerve (SPN) with the same parameters as used in DPN stimulation got different results. The basal MAP level elevated markedly, and the whole ISP-MAP curve was displaced upwards without significant change in the slope of the curve. According to Iriki and Korner,[9] this is due to a direct excitation of the sympathetic neurons by incoming impulses.

THE ROLE OF CENTRAL ENDORPHIN IN THE BAROREFLEX RESETTING INDUCED BY DPN STIMULATION

Naloxone iv (0.4 mg/kg), icv (20 μg/kg) or microinjected into ventral PAG (20 μg in 1 μl saline on each side) caused no significant change in the shape of the ISP-MAP response curve. However, after administration of naloxone, stimulation of DPN displaced the whole ISP-MAP curve upwards, instead of downward displacement at high ISP as happened in the control animals. Microinjection of β-endorphin antiserum (1:3000) into ventral PAG produced the same effect. These results imply that the downward displacement of the ISP-MAP curve at high ISP is possibly mediated by the endogenous opioid peptides, which is of benefit in decreasing MAP during hypertension.[19,20]

THE ROLE OF CENTRAL SEROTONIN IN THE BAROREFLEX RESETTING INDUCED BY DPN STIMULATION

If a tryptophan hydroxylase inhibitor PCPA (10 mg/day) was icv for 3 days, or a serotonin receptor antagonist, ketanserin (20 μg) was icv, stimulation of DPN resulted in a significant increase in the basal MAP level. Meanwhile, there was a marked upward shift of the ISP-MAP curve at low ISP range but only a slight downward displacement of the curve or no change in the position of the curve at the high ISP range. These results imply that the central serotonergic neurones also play an important role in the baroreflex resetting induced by DPN stimulation, leading to a significant downward displacement of the ISP-MAP curve mainly at the high ISP range.[22] The relations between the central endophinergic and serotonergic neurons remains to be investigated.

THE ROLE OF CENTRAL ACH IN THE BAROREFLEX RESETTING INDUCED BY DPN STIMULATION

It is well known that central cholingeric activity has a pressor effect. In this series of experiments, when scopolamine (12.5 μg/kg in 100 μl of saline) was given icv, there was no significant change in the basal MAP and the baroreflex function curve. However, in such a situation, stimulation of DPN meant the upward shift of the ISP-MAP curve (at low ISP range) remained at its original position; while the downward-shift portion (at high ISP range) of the curve remained at the depressed position. On the other hand, icv injection of neostigmine, or microinjection of carbachol into the posterior hypothalamus or the dorsal PAG, produced a pressor effect and a significant upward shift of the ISP-MAP curve, particularly at a low ISP. These results show that the central cholinergic mechanism is also involved in the baroreflex resetting induced by DPN stimulation, leading to an upward displacement of the ISP-PAP curve mainly at a low ISP. This shift contributes to the increase of MBP during hypotension.[23]

THE ROLE OF VASOPRESSIN IN THE BAROREFLEX RESETTING INDUCED BY DPN STIMULATION

Intracisternal vasopressin displaced the ISP-MAP curve upward at low ISP and significantly increased the steepness of the curve. This effect of vasopressin was prevented by vasopressin antagonist pretreatment. If the animal were pretreated intracisternally with a vasopressin antagonist, d$(CH_2)_5$Tyr(Me)AVP (2 μg in 50 μl of saline), there was no change of the ISP-MAP curve. However, stimulation of DPN produced only a downward shift of the ISP-MAP curve at high ISP, and no displacement of the curve at low ISP range. These results imply that endogenous vasopressin exerts no tonic modulatory action on the baroreflex. Nevertheless, it plays a role in the baroreflex resetting produced by DPN stimulation, mainly related to the upward displacement of the ISP-MAP curve at low ISP, that aids the elevation of MAP during hypotension.[24]

THE ROLE OF CERVICAL SYMPATHETIC NERVE ACTIVITY IN THE BAROREFLEX RESETTING INDUCED BY DPN STIMULATION

Physiological studies have shown that the activity of the carotid sinus baroreceptor can be modulated by cervical sympathetic nerve stimulation.[26] It is interesting to know whether the cervical sympathetic nerve activity also mediates the baroreceptor resetting induced by DPN stimulation. In the first series of experiments,[17] after cervical sympathetic trunks were sectioned, stimulation of DPN caused an upward shift of the low ISP range of the ISP-MAP curve, while the high ISP range of the curve remained unaltered. This is different from the controls when the sympathetic nerves were intact.

The second series of experiments were to record the single baroreceptor afferent fibre discharges.[25] During DPN stimulation, the basal MAP was almost unchanged; however, the frequency of the single baroreceptor afferent fibre discharge was significantly increased at an ISP level higher than 80 mmHg. The firing threshold of the fibres was lower and the slope of the intrasinusal pressure-baroreceptor response curve at ISP 80 mmHg was steeper than their respective pre-stimulation values. In the cervical sympathectomized preparations, the above-mentioned changes in baroreceptor activity during the DPN stimulation did not appear.

These experimental results imply that the DPN stimulation-produced baroreflex resetting also takes place at the carotid sinus baroreceptor level. Stimulation of the DPN results in an increase in the cervical sympathetic nerve activity, which in turn sensitises the carotid sinus baroreceptor. This mechanism may be of significant importance when the intrasinusal pressure is higher than normal. Probably, the increase of the baroreceptor activity during DPN stimulation may induce the downward shift of the ISP-MAP curve at high ISP level, and thus help to decrease the high MAP.

In summary, this study shows that acupuncture as well as certain somatic afferent impulses may reset the baroreflex, enhancing the reflex sensitivity. This type of resetting can improve the performance of the baroreflex and is in favour of the maintenance of BP homeostasis. The central endorphin and serotonin with an increase in the sensitivity of the carotid sinus baroreceptor might be responsible for the downward displacement of the ISP-MAP response curve at high ISP and help the decrease of high MAP, while central ACh and vasopressin might play an important role in the upward shift of the curve at low ISP, which benefits the pressor response during hypotension.

Modulatory Effect of EA or Somatic Nerve Stimulation on Chemoreceptor Pressor Reflex

In chapter 5 we mentioned that the depressor effect of acupuncture on noradrenaline infusion-induced hypertension was due to the inhibition of the chemoreceptor pressor response. In this series of experiments the effect of acupuncture-like DPN stimulation on the chemoreceptor pressor response was examined and its mechanism was analysed.

EFFECT OF DPN STIMULATION ON CAROTID CHEMORECEPTOR PRESSOR RESPONSE

In urethane-chloralose anesthetized rabbits, stimulation of DPN (300 μA, 7 Hz) for 15 minutes had no marked influence on the resting MAP, while having a marked effect on the carotid chemoreceptor pressor response induced by a bolus injection of NaCN (40 μg) into the common carotid bifurcation region. There were two types of effect: The pressor response induced by NaCN injection was enhanced by DPN stimulation if its initial amplitude was small, but was reduced while it was large. The maximum facilitatory effect usually appeared at 10–30 minutes during and after DPN stimulation, then returned to its prestimulation level within 30 minutes after the cessation of stimulation. However, the inhibitory effect was maintained for more than 60 minutes. These results show that DPN stimulation can modulate the amplitude of the carotid chemoreceptor pressor reflex. It seems likely that the effect of DPN stimulation is related to the sensitivity of the central cardiovascular neurons.[1]

THE ROLE OF VAGI AND BUFFER NERVES IN THE EFFECT OF DPN STIMULATION ON CAROTID CHEMO-RECEPTOR PRESSOR RESPONSE

When the vagi were intact usually the magnitude of the pressor response induced by NaCN injection was small and could be enhanced by DPN stimulation. If the vagi were cut, the magnitude of the pressor response became larger, which might be due to the loss of inhibitory inputs from the cardiopulmonary area and the excitability of the sympathetic centre increasing. In such cases the chemoreceptor pressor response could be reduced by DPN stimulation.

If the bilateral aortic nerves and the contralateral sinus nerve were cut to abolish most of the baroreceptor inputs, there was no significant change in the effect of DPN stimulation on the carotid chemoreceptor response.

These results show that DPN stimulation can modulate the carotid chemoreceptor pressor response, and this effect depends on the functional state of the cardiovascular neuronal activity.

EFFECT OF DPN STIMULATION ON THE SYMPATHETIC RESPONSE UNDER DIFFERENT LEVELS OF SYMPATHETIC ACTIVITY

To examine how the functional state of the sympathetic centre influences the effect of DPN stimulation, the renal sympathetic discharges, cervical sympathetic trunk activity and ganglio-glomerular nerve activity were recorded and the following experiments were carried out.[2]

When the sympathetic activity was increased by hypoventilation, bilateral vagotomy, sino-aortic deafferentation or high PCO_2 in the artery, stimulation of DPN (3V, 10 Hz) for 15 minutes produced a decrease in the spontaneous renal nerve discharge; the response of renal nerve discharge to carotid chemoreceptor stimulation also decreased. However, the same DPN stimulation caused an increase in renal nerve discharge when the sympathetic activity was inhibited by hyperventilation, unilateral aortic depressor nerve stimulation or deep anaesthesia.

Further experiments showed that the inhibitory effect of DPN stimulation on the carotid chemoreflex was attributed to the release of endorphin, because it could be blocked by naloxone iv. Meanwhile the facilitatory effect of DPN stimulation was due to the activation of the central cholinergic system, since it could be blocked by scopolamine iv.

EFFECT OF DPN STIMULATION ON THE CHEMORECEPTOR AFFERENT DISCHARGES

Su, et al.[11] reported that a section of the cervical sympathetic nerve could significantly attenuate the facilitatory effect of DPN stimulation on the carotid chemoreceptor pressor response elicited by NaCN; while stimulation of the cervical sympathetic nerve produced an excitatory influence on the carotid chemoreceptor activity. When the sinus nerve and ganglioglomerular nerve activities were recorded, it showed that the DPN stimulation had an excitatory effect on both the spontaneous and evoked activities of the carotid chemoreceptor. Therefore, the excitation of sympathetic efferent to the chemoreceptor might be one mechanism of the facilitory effect of DPN stimulation on the carotid chemoreceptor activity.

In summary, stimulation of DPN could modulate the chemoreceptor pressor reflex mainly by activation of type II and III fibres. It had an inhibitory effect when the chemoreceptor pressor reflex is high and a facilitatory effect when the chemoreceptor pressor reflex is low. The former is related to the release of endorphin and the latter is due to the activation of the central cholinergic system and the sympathetic outflow to the chemoreceptor, which increases its activities.

Physiological Significance

The above results showed that EA or DPN stimulation could inhibit the defence reaction by the excitation of type II and III fibres, which could activate the ARC-vPAG-NRO pathway, release endorphin and 5-HT, and inhibit the cardiovascular sympathetic neurons in RVLM. Stimulation of the superficial nerve, e.g., SPN will have the opposite effect and is related to the release of ACh. The inputs from DPN could also modulate the baro- and chemoreceptor reflexes, which depend on the situation of the cardiovascular center. These may be the important mechanisms with which EA can inhibit arrhythmia, myocardial ischemia and hypertension, etc.

References

1. Che, M.X. and Su, Q.F. (1988) Modulatory effect of deep peroneal nerve stimulation on the carotid body chemoreceptor pressor response in rabbits. *Acta Physiol Sin*, **40**: 486–493.
2. He, S.Q. and Su, Q.F. (1983) Influence of stimulation of the deep peroneal nerve on renal nerve discharge under different levels of central sympathetic activity. *Acta Physiol Sin*, **35**: 243–249.
3. Huangfu, D.H. and Li, P. (1985) The inhibitory effect of the deep peroneal nerve inputs on defence reaction elicited by brainstem stimulation. *Chin J. Physiol Sci*, **1**: 176–184.
4. Huangfu, D.H. and Li, P. (1996) Effect of deep peroneal nerve inputs on ventral medullary defence-reaction neurons. *Chin J. Physiol Sci*, **2**: 123–131.
5. Huangfu, D.H. and Li, P. (1987a) The role of nucleus arcuatus in the inhibitory effect of deepp peroneal inputs on defence reaction. *Chin J. Physiol Sci*, **3**: 37–46.
6. Huangfu, D.H. and Li, P. (1987b) Afferent connection of the ventrolateral medulla in the rabbit—studied with HRP technique. *Chin J. Physiol Sci*, **3**: 86–95.
7. Huangfu, D.H. (1988a) The role of nucleus raphe obscurus in the inhibition of defence reaction by deep peroneal nerve stimulation. *Chin J. Physiol Sci*, **4**: 77–83.
8. Huangfu, D.H. and Li, P. (1988b) The inhibitory effect of ARC-PAG-NRO system on the ventrolateral medullary neurons in the rabbit. *Chin J. Physiol Sci*, **4**: 115–125.
9. Iriki, M. and Korner, P.I. (1979) Central nervous interaction between chemoreceptor and baroreceptor control mechanisms. In: C. McC. Brooks, K. Koizumi and A. Sato (eds.): Integrative function of the autonomic nervous system. University of Tokyo Press, 415–427.
10. Lovick, T.A., Li, P. and Schenberg, L.C. (1995) Modulation of the cardiovascular defence response by low frwquency stimulation of a deep somatic nerve in rats. *J. Auton Nerv Sys*, **50**: 147–154.

11. Su, Q.F., Che, M.X. and Cheng, G. (1991) Role of the cervical sympathetic trunk in somatic input enhancement of the carotid chemoreceptor pressor reflex in rabbit. *Acta Acad Med Shanghai*, 18: 18–21.
12. Sun, X.Y. and Yao, T. (1985) Inhibitory effect of electric needling on the defence reaction produced by hypothalamic stimulation in awake rabbits. *Acta Physiol Sci*, 37: 15–23.
13. Sun, X.Y. and Yao, T. (1986) Periaqueductal grey matter participates in the inhibitory effect of electrical needling on defence reaction. *Acta Physiol Sci*, 38: 483–490.
14. Sun, X.Y. and Yao, T. (1987) Inhibition of the defence reaction by microinjection of sodium glutamate into the arcuate nucleus in conscious rabbits. *Chin J. Physiol Sci*, 3: 259–268.
15. Wang, W. and Yao, T. (1985) Resetting of carotid sinus baroreceptor reflex during stimualtion of somatic nerve in the rabbit. *Chin J. Physiol Sci*, 1: 166–175.
16. Wang, W. and Yao, T. (1986a) Effect of somatic nerve stimualtion on the activity of the carotid sinus baroreceptor in the rabbit. *Chin J. Physiol Sci*, 2: 68–75.
17. Wang, W. and Yao, T. (1986b) Role of the cervical sympathetic nerve in the resetting of carotid sinus baroreceptor refelx during somatic nerve stimualtion in the rabbit. *Chin J. Physiol Sci*, 2: 319–326.
18. Wang, W. and Yao, T. (1987a) Effect of microinjection of sodium glutamate into the arcuate nucleus on carotid sinus baroreceptor reflex in the rabbit. *Chin J. Physiol Sci*, 3: 140–148.
19. Wang, W. and Yao, T. (1987b) Effect of somatic stimulation on baroreceptor reflex in morphine-tolerated rabbits. *Chin J. Physiol Sci*, 3: 335–340.
20. Wang, W. and Yao, T. (1987c) Role of endogenous opioid peptides in baroreflex resetting induced by deep peroneal nerve stimulation in the rabbit. *Chin J. Physiol Sci*, 3: 350–357.
21. Wang, W. and Yao, T. (1987d) Resetting of baroreceptor reflex by electroacupuncture in conscious rabbits. *Acta Physiol Sci*, 39: 300–304.
22. Wang, W. and Yao, T. (1988a) Participation of central serotonin in baroreflex resetting induced by deep peroneal nerve stimulation in the rabbit. *Chin J. Physiol Sci*, 4: 1–10.
23. Wang, W. and Yao, T. (1988b) Involvement of central acetylcholine in baroreflex resetting induced by deep peroneal nerve stimulation in the rabbit. *Chin J. Physiol Sci*, 4: 11–18.
24. Wang, W., Zhang, Z. and Yao, T. (1988) Effect of central vasopressin on the baroreflex resetting induced by deep peroneal nerve stimulation in the rabbit. *Chin J. Physiol Sci*, 4: 193–201.
25. Wang, W. and Yao, T. (1989) Autonomic efferent pattern characterizing baroreflex resetting induced by deep peroneal nerve stimulation in the rabbit. *Chin J. Physiol Sci*, 5: 128–135.

26. Yao, T. and Thoren, P. (1983) Adrenergic and pressure-induced modulation of carotid sinus baroreceptors in rabbits. *Acta Physiol Scand*, **117**: 9–17.
27. Zhang, Y.M., Li, P. and Lovick, T.A. (1994) Role of the nucleus raphe obscurus in the inhibition of rostral ventrolateral medullary neurons induced by stimulation in the ventrolateral periaqueductal grey matter of the rabbit. *Neurosci Let*, **176**: 231–234.

11 THE ROLE OF ROSTRAL VENTROLATERAL MEDULLARY NEURONS IN THE PROMOTION OF FEEDBACK MECHANISM BY ACUPUNCTURE

Peng Li

There is good evidence that neurons in the rostral ventrolateral medulla (RVLM) play an important role in maintaining blood pressure (BP) by sending direct projections to the inter-mediolateral column (IML) of the spinal cord.[1] Hilton, et al.[12] showed that the descending pathway responsible for the cardiovascular components of the defence reaction ran as a narrow strip on each side of the RVLM. This medullary area has been proved to act as a relay nucleus in the descending pathway to the sympathetic preganglionic neurons in the spinal cord.[27] Several authors[2,28,29] observed that a pressor effect could be elicited by microinjection of excitant amino acid into the RVLM in cats and rabbits. The axons of the neurons in this area project directly to the IML of the spinal cord.[26] So, the RVLM is thought to be an important cardiovascular centre that sets vasomotor tone and integrates the cardiovascular reflexes under different conditions.[34] In this chapter we will discuss the integrative function of RVLM neurons and their role in the promotion of feedback mechanisms by acupuncture.

Spinally Projecting Defence Reaction Related Neurons in the Rostral Ventrolateral Medulla

Our study[14] showed that application of glycine or electrolytic lesions of the RVLM surface led to a profound fall in BP to the level of spinal animals; moreover, the pressor response induced by hypothalamic (HYP) and midbrain (PAG) defence areas stimulation was almost abolished.

Electrophysiological evidence showed that of the units recorded in RVLM 77.5% in rats[23] and 62.5% in rabbits[14] could be excited both by HYP and PAG defence areas stimulation. Among these units 58% were activated antidromically by stimulating the lateral horn of the thoracic cord responding to PAG defence area stimulation. So, there are convergent projections from the HYP and PAG defence areas to the

RVLM neurons, which in turn project directly to the sympathetic preganglionic neurons.

For doing correlation analysis,[18] the spontaneous firing of these defence reaction-related neurones, renal sympathetic nerve discharges or variations in BP were sent to the microcomputer simultaneously. It showed that 76% of these neurons were correlated with the sympathetic nerve discharge or variations of BP. This means that most of the defence reaction-related neurons are cardiovascular neurons.

When DL-homocysteic acid (DLH 0.2M, pH 7.4, 100nL) was microinjected into the RVLM,[8] 11% of the sites injected elicited a pressor response, tachycardia and an increase in femoral vascular conductance, which was a typical characteristic pattern of defence reaction. In 68% of the sites, the pressor response was accompanied by a decrease in femoral conductance; and in the other 21%, depressor effect or no change in BP was accompanied by an increase in femoral conductance.

In another series of experiments, DLH was microinjected into the RVLM at the same site where electrical stimulation was applied. 30% of the sites stimulated electrically produced a pressor response, tachycardia and an increase in femoral vascular conductance, but the typical cardiovascular response of defence reaction could only be induced by microinjection of DLH in one site.

These results showed that different neurons in the RVLM are dedicated to the control of different particular functional components of the sympathetic outflow. The number of functionally different neurons involved are different at each injecting site, so different patterns of response can be evoked. Since the chance of muscular vasodilatation induced by micro injection of DLH is much less than that induced by electrical stimulation in the RVLM, the number of muscular vasodilator neurons in the RVLM is possibly much less than the passing vasodilator fibres.

The Integrative Function of RVLM Neurons

Several reports have described convergent inputs to the single neurons in RVLM from different sources, including HYP, dorsal and ventral PAG, NRO, chemo- and baroreceptors and splanchnic organs, and somatic inputs, etc.[3,9,21,28]. To ensure the integrative function of the RVLM neurons to different somatic inputs, unit discharges were recorded in cats.[24] Neurons in the RVLM that responded to HYP or PAG defence areas stimulation with an excitatory postsynaptic potential (EPSP) and evoked discharges, are called defence reaction-related neurons. In 19 of these defence-reaction-related neurons, 64% showed no significant response to DPN stimulation, 6% showed an excitatory response, and 11% showed inhibitory response. However, when DPN was stimulated simultaneously with HYP or PAG, in 36 units tested, 64% of the response to HYP or PAG stimulation could be inhibited by DPN stimulation, 14% showed a facilitatory response, and 22% were not significantly affected. These findings are in conformity with Huangfu and Li's report in rabbits.[15] It showed that for most of the defence reaction-related neurons, stimulation of the DPN had no significant influence on their spontaneous firing, but had an obvious inhibitory effect on their evoked response.

On the other hand, stimulation of the superficial peroneal nerve (SPN) often exerted a facilitatory effect on both the spontaneous firing (64% of the units) and evoked discharge induced by defence area stimulation (62% of the units). Gao, et al, obtained similar results in rats.[6]

The inhibitory effect of DPN stimulation and the facilitatory effect of SPN stimulation could be focused on the same neuron. Therefore, there are convergent projections from the HYP, PAG defence areas, DPN and SPN. Later we found that projections from the nucleus raphe obscurus (NRO,[9,10] ventral PAG,[31] carotid chemoreceptor,[11] baroreceptors,[5] and splanchnie nerves,[30] etc. also converged to the RVLM neuron, and some are on the same neurons. This is possibly the morphological and physiological basis in the central nervous system for the modulatory effect of acupuncture or different somatic inputs on cardiovascular function.

Promotion of the Feedback Mechanism in the Central Nervous System by Acupuncture

The biological significance of the defence reaction is possibly to mobilise and prepare the organism as a whole to cope with the changing environment and emergency. All the internal bodily changes occurring are components of the emergency reaction. On the other hand, many regulatory mechanisms act to maintain the constancy of the internal environment to restore the normal state, once it has been disturbed. It is commonly thought that the baroreceptor reflex plays an important role in the cardiovascular regulation, and has a negative feedback effect on the defence reaction. However, it was shown that the baroreflex was inhibited by stimulation of the brain stem defence centre.[32] So, it is interesting to know what is the main negative feedback mechanism during defence reaction.

In addition, there is now evidence showing that electrical stimulation of the DPN can inhibit the defence reaction or ventricular extrasystoles elicited by stimulating the HYP or PAG defence areas. The inhibitory pathway might pass through the ARC, the ventral PAG (vPAG) and the NRO, and the NRO plays an important role in the inhibition (see chapter 10).

It is not sure whether this ARC-vPAG-NRO system can only be activated by somatic nerve stimulation or whether it is also activated when the defence areas are stimulated and act as a negative feedback mechanism in the brain. This is possible, since our previous studies showed that the number of ventricular extrasystoles induced by HYP stimulation was increased by microinjection of naloxone into the ARC, vPAG, NRO or RVLM. That result suggested the release of endogenous opioids in these areas during the defence area stimulation to restrict the over-exaggerated sympathetic excitation (see chapter 7).

In this paragraph we will discuss the negative feedback mechanism of the ARC-vPAG-NRO system and how the somatic inputs induced by acupuncture promote this system.

INHIBITION OF THE DEFENSIVE PRESSOR RESPONSE BY REPETITIVE STIMULATION OF THE BRAINSTEM DEFENCE AREAS

Xia, et al.[38] found that in rabbits after defence reaction was elicited by stimulation of the HYP for several times, the leu-enkephalin in cerebrospinal fluid (CSF) increased. Gao and He[7] showed that the cardiovascular response, the characterised pattern of defence reaction, elicited by strong electric stimulation of the front paw decreased after repetitive stimulation of it, while the content of leu-enkephalin-like immunoreactive substances in CSF increased. The present study is to test whether the cardiovascular response decreases after repetitive stimulation of the defence areas, and to analyse whether the baroreceptor reflex and the endogenous opioid peptides take part in the mechanism.

In seventeen urethane-chloralose anaesthetised rabbits, after repetitive stimulation of the HYP or PAG defence area (3 sec/min) for 5 minutes, the resting BP, HR, femoral blood flow and its conductance had no obvious change. However, the magnitude of the pressor response decreased significantly, reached a minimum 15 minutes after repetitive stimulation and returned to the control level about one hour later.

When the buffer nerves were denervated (n = 6), the inhibitory effect on the pressor response still existed after repetitive stimulation of HYP or PAG, but was slightly weaker than that in the intact animals. So the baroreflex is not the direct or main cause for the inhibition of pressor response after repetitive stimulation of the defence areas.

If naloxone (0.4 mg/kg) was intravenously injected 1–2 minutes before the repetitive stimulation of HYP or PAG, the attenuation of the pressor response was mostly prevented. So, this attenuation of the defensive pressor response is not due to central fatigue, but is an inhibition related to the activation of opioids. Our previous work showed that the inhibitory effect of EA or stimulation of DPN on the defence reaction is accomplished by the release of opioid peptides.[13,15] The present work suggests that when defence reaction occurs, some antagonistic system such as opioid peptides in the central nervous system may be activated, and restrict the extent of the defence reaction via negative feedback mechanisms and could prevent the over exaggerative and pathogenic effect of the defence reaction. To make sure whether the defence reaction could activate the ARC-vPAG-NRO system, the following experiments were performed.

EXCITATORY EFFECT OF DEFENCE AREA STIMULATION ON NEURONS IN THE NRO

Gong, et al.[9] showed the direct projections from the ventral PAG and HYP to the NRO by the horseradish peroxidase technique. To study whether the neurons in NRO could be activated by stimulation of the HYP or PAG defence areas, electrophysiological recordings were carried out in twelve rabbits.[35] Of 77 neurons in the NRO observed, 53 (69%) were excited by stimulation of the PAG with double or triple pulses. Their onset latency ranged from 3–32 (10.7 ± 1.2) ms, and their effective duration varied from 1 to 55 (11.5 ± 2.0) ms.

In ten other rabbits, 55 neurons were recorded in the NRO, where 21 neurons (38%) were excited by stimulation of HYP defence area with double or triple pulses. Their onset latencies ranged from 5 to 40 (17.8 ± 2.5) ms, and their effective duration was from 1 to 55 (34.7 ± 5.2) ms. Compared with the stimulation of PAG defence area, fewer neurons in the NRO could be excited by stimulation of HYP, and their responses were of longer latency and duration. Nevertheless, there is no difference in the regional distribution of the neurons in the NRO, which responded to PAG or HYP defence areas stimulation.

In five rabbits, the HYP and PAG defence areas were stimulated simultaneously to observe whether the convergent excitatory projections from the HYP and PAG defence areas to NRO exist. Of the 24 neurons recorded in the NRO, 11 neurons (46%) received convergent excitatory projections from the HYP and PAG defence areas.

Recently, Huang, et al.[20] reported that stimulation of the dorsal PAG could induce the expression of c-fos in NRO and the nucleus paragigantocellularis lateralis (PGL) in RVLM. This means that neurons in NRO and PGL could both be excited by stimulation of the PAG defence area. Their further work showed excitatory projections from NRO to ventral PAG. So, there is a positive feedback between ventral PAG and NRO, which will reinforce this system.[19]

All these results support the suggestion that excitation of the HYP and PAG defence areas could activate some antagonistic systems to limit the defence reaction as a negative feedback mechanism, and the NRO is an important region.

Some neurons in NRO could be excited only by two or three pulses of electrical stimulation, but not by a single pulse, and some neurons in the NRO received convergent excitatory projections from HYP and PAG defence areas. So it is suggested that the excitability of some neurons in NRO is low and the neurons might generate spikes through temporal and spatial summations. This may be the reason that the pressor responses of defence reactions induced by weak stimulation are nearly constant, but those induced by strong and repetitive stimulation are attenuated.

ACTIVATION OF THE NEURONS IN NRO BY DPN STIMULATION

In our previous work[16,17] it was shown that the DPN inputs could inhibit the defence reaction elicited by stimulation of the defence areas. It was also shown that this inhibitory effect could be abolished or attenuated by microinjection of naloxone, cinanserine into or electrolytic lesions of the NRO (see chapter 7 and 10). It seems likely that activation of the ARC-vPAG-NRO system by defence area stimulation could be facilitated by the acupuncture-like somatic nerve stimulation. To examine this hypothesis, the effects of DPN and superficial peroneal nerve (SPN) stimulation on the NRO neurons were observed.[36]

Of 53 neurons in the NRO recorded, 30 units (57%) were excited by DPN stimulation (300 μA, 0.5 ms at 1 Hz with double or triple pulses) and 24 units (45%) were excited by SPN stimulation (same parameters as DPN stimulation); among them 20 units were excited by both DPN and

SPN stimulation. Six units were inhibited by DPN and SPN stimulation. The remaining units were unaffected.

In 22 NRO neurons activated by stimulation of HYP or PAG defence areas, a facilitatory effect of DPN stimulation could be observed in 17 units (77%). Meanwhile, in 12 NRO neurons activated by stimulation of HYP or PAG, a facilitatory effect of SPN stimulation could be observed in 9 units (75%). Therefore, stimulation of DPN or SPN could activate most neurons in NRO, and facilitate the excitatory effect of defence area stimulation.

These results support our suggestion that the somatic inputs induced by acupuncture could facilitate the negative feedback mechanism of the defence reaction in the brain, i.e., the ARC-vPAG-NRO system, and restrict the over excitation of the sympathetic centre.

In previous chapters, we mentioned that the effects of DPN stimulation on the defensive pressor response were inhibitory, and the effect of SPN stimulation often showed a pressor response. We also saw that most of the defence reaction-related neurons in the RVLM could be inhibited by DPN stimulation and excited by SPN stimulation. Nevertheless, in this study, the effects of both DPN and SPN stimulation on NRO neurons were mainly facilitatory. It seems that stimulation of the SPN has dual effects on the RVLM neurons, a direct excitatory effect and an indirect inhibitory effect, which passes through the NRO. The final result will depend on the functional condition of these neurons.

EXCITATION OF THE NRO INHIBITS THE DEFENCE REACTION-RELATED NEURONS IN RVLM

Gong, et al.[10] reported that the pressor response induced by stimulation of the PAG or HYP defence areas could be inhibited by continuous electrical stimulation of the NRO, or microinjection of D,L-homocysteic acid (DLH) into the NRO. In the latter case, the pressor response did not return to the control level until 20 minutes later, while the basal BP returned to the control level within 10–20 minutes. However, the pressor response induced by stimulation of the RVLM could not be inhibited by microinjection of DLH into the NRO. So, it is believed that the RVLM is the key site where the NRO neuronal excitation could inhibit the defensive pressor response induced by stimulation of PAG or HYP defence areas.

Li, et al.[22] and Zhang, et al.[39] reported that 73–78% of the defence reaction-related neurons in the RVLM could be inhibited by stimulation of the NRO. Later, Lin, et al.[25] showed a hyperpolarization of the defence reaction-related neurons during NRO stimulation. Therefore, electrophysiological studies also support the above suggestion.

THE ROLE OF GABA IN THE INHIBITION OF RVLM NEURONS BY NRO STIMULATION

Willete, et al.[37] reported that bilateral microinjection of the GABAergic agonist, muscimol, into the ventrolateral vasopressor sites of the medulla caused a marked fall in BP, and that bicuculline could block the effect of muscimol. Gong, et al.[10] observed that after microinjection of the GABAergic receptor antagonist bicuculine into the RVLM bilaterally, the inhibitory effect on defensive pressor response by the NRO stimulation was abolished or greatly attenuated within 2 minutes. This blocking effect lasted for 20–80 minutes. So it is suggested that GABA may be an inhibitory transmitter in the efferent pathway of the NRO to the RVLM. Zhang, et al.[39] recorded the neuronal firing in the RVLM, and saw that the spontaneous firing and evoked neuronal discharges induced by stimulation of the PAG defensive area diminished significantly after GABA was applied iontophoretically. On the other hand, iontophoresis of bicuculline could increase the spontaneous firing of the defence reaction-related neurons in the RVLM and block the inhibitory effect of the NRO stimulation on their evoked response induced by PAG stimulation. So GABA is possibly one of the inhibitory transmitters from the NRO to the RVLM neurons.

THE ROLE OF 5-HT IN THE INHIBITION OF RVLM NEURONS BY THE NRO STIMULATION

The RVLM is rich in 5-HT-immunoreactive nerve terminals,[33] many of which are probably derived from the serotonin containing perikarya of the medullary raphi. Lovick[28] showed that microinjection of 5-HT (10–100 nmol) into the bilateral RVLM in rats produced a significant depressor response lasting up to 69 minutes. This effect was usually accompanied by a bradycardia. It is shown that this region might be a major site of action for the central antihypertensive action of 5-HT.

Zhang, et al.[39] found that the spontaneous neuronal firing in the RVLM and the evoked discharge induced by stimulation of PAG defence area attenuated significantly when 5-HT was iontophoretically applied to the RVLM. Moreover, iontophoresis of cinaserine into the RVLM increased the spontaneous firing and blocked the inhibitory effect of the NRO stimulation on the evoked discharge induced by the PAG stimulation. These results support the view that 5-HT is also an important transmitter mediating this inhibitory effect of NRO excitation on the RVLM defence reaction-related neurons.

The relationship between GABA, 5-HT, opioids and ACh, etc. is not sure and needs further investigation.

Physiological Significance

The RVLM neurons receive convergent projections from the HYP, PAG defence areas, the baro- and chemoreceptor receptors, NRO, splanchnic afferent and various somatic afferents as well. Most of these RVLM neurons projected directly to the ILM of the spinal cord, and correlated with the sympathetic nerve discharge and BP level. So, they are important in the maintenance of haemostasis, and a key area for the modulatory effect of acupuncture. It is interesting to see that the splanchnic and somatic inputs from different parts of the body can project to the same neuron of the RVLM. This may be the physiological base that some splanchnic diseases can be treated by acupuncture applied to the acupoints that are not located on the same or nearby spinal segment of that splanchnic organ.

The above results showed that excitation of the HYP or PAG defence areas can activate the ARC-vPAG-NRO system, which acts as a negative feedback mechanism to limit the over-excitation of the sympathetic nervous system. The somatic inputs induced by acupuncture could promote this negative feedback mechanism, and inhibit the RVLM cardiovascular neurons via the release of opioids, 5-HT and GABA, etc. It is known that although psychosocial stress exists everywhere and every day in modern society, only certain people will get cardiovascular diseases. One important reason for this are the imperfect negative feedback mechanisms in the brain due to insomnia, long-term stress, etc. and lacking physical exercise and somatic inputs. Acupuncture is a good and simple way to help patients to facilitate the negative feedback mechanism and modulate the sympathetic outflow and prevent and cure some cardiovascular diseases (Fig. 11.1).

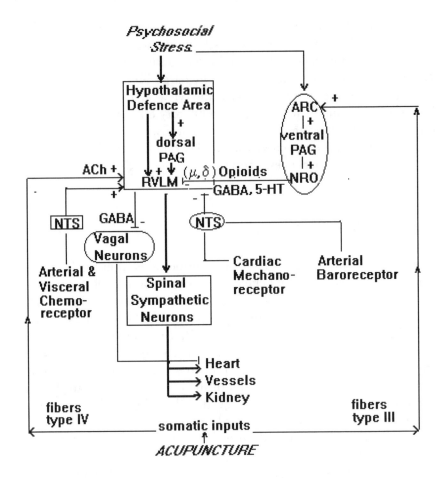

Fig. 11.1 Modulatory effect of acupuncture on cardiovascular diseases—promotion of the feedback mechanism in the brain.

References

1. Blessing, W.W., Goodchild, A.K., Dampney, R.A.L. and Chalmers, J.P. (1981) Cells groups in the lower brain stem of the rabbit projecting to the spinal cord with special reference to catecholamine-containing neurons. *Brain Res*, **221**: 35–55.
2. Dampney, R.A.L. and Giuliano, R. (1985) Cardiovascular control by cholinergic mechanism in the central nervous system. *Ann Rev Pharmacol Toxicol*, **22**: 314–381.
3. Gao, K.M. and Li, P. (1993a) Convergent inputs onto the rostral ventrolateral medullary neurons of the rat. *Chin J. Physiol Sci*, **9**: 286–296.

4. Gao, K.M. and Li, P. (1993b) Post-synaptic activity evoked in the rostral ventrolateral medullary neurons by stimulation of the defence areas of hypothalamus and midbrain in the rat. *Neuroscience Let*, **161**: 153–156.

5. Gao, K.M. and Li, P. (1994a) Effect of baroreceptor inputs on the activity of rostral ventrolateral medullary neurons evoked by stimulation of defence areas and somatic nerves. *Chin J. Physiol Sci*, **10**: 283–288.

6. Gao, K.M. and Li, P. (1994b) Responses of neurons in the nucleus paragigantocellularis lateralis to somatic nerve stimulation. *Neurosci Let*, **178**: 15–18.

7. Gao, L.Z. and He, L.F. (1988) Noxious stimulation depresses nociceptive blood pressure response-opioid peptides implicated. *Chin J. Physiol Sci*, **4**: 185–192.

8. Gong, Q.L., Huangfu, D.H. and Li, P. (1987) Exploration of cardiovascular and respiratory neuron groups in the ventrolateral medulla of the rabbit. *Chin J. Physiol Sci*, **3**: 149–156.

9. Gong, Q.L., Huangfu, D.H. and Li, P. (1988) Afferent connections of nucleus raphe obscurus in rabbits. *Chin J. Physiol. Sci*, **4**: 369–374.

10. Gong, Q.L., Lin, R.J. and Li, P. (1989) The inhibitory effect of nucleus raphe obscurus on defence pressor response. *Chin J. Physiol Sci*, **5**: 311–318.

11. Fan, W., Zhang, Z. and Lin, R.J. (1990) Effect of carotid chemoreceptor stimulation on defence reaction related units in rostral ventrolateral medulla. *Chin J. Physiol. Sci*, **6**: 129–136.

12. Hilton, S.M., Marshall, J.M. and Timms, R.J. (1983) Ventral medullary relay neurons in the pathway from the defence areas of the cat and their effect on blood pressure. *J. Physiol*, **245**: 149–166.

13. Huangfu, D.H. and Li, P. (1985) The inhibitory effect of the deep peroneal nerve inputs on defence reaction elicited by brain stem stimulation. *Chin J. Physiol Sci*, **1**: 176–184.

14. Huangfu, D.H. and Li, P. (1986a) Defence reaction-related neurons in ventral medulla of rabbits. *Acta Physiol Sin*, **38**: 383–389.

15. Huangfu, D.H. and Li, P. (1986b) Effect of deep peroneal nerve inputs on ventral medullary defence-reaction-related neurons. *Chin J. Physiol Sci*, **2**: 123–131.

16. Huangfu, D.H. and Li, P. (1987) The role of nucleus arcuatus in the inhibitory effect of deep peroneal nerve inputs on defence reaction. *Chin J. Physiol Sci*, **3**: 37–46.

17. Huangfu, D.H. and Li, P. (1988) Role of nucleus raphe obscurus in the inhibition of defence reaction by deep peroneal nerve stimulation. *Chin J. Physiol Sci*, **4**: 77–83.

18. Huangfu, D.H. and Li, P. (1988) Cross correlative analysis of ventrolateral medullary neuronal discharges and cardiovascular activity. *Acta Acad Med Shanghai*, **15**: 470–472.

19. Huang, J.H., Li, P. and Gong, Q.L. (1996) The effects of stimulation of nucleus raphe obscurus on fos-expression evoked by activating dorsal

periaqueductal gray and unit discharge in ventral periaqueductal gray in rat. *Acta Physiol Sci*, **48**: 149–156.

20. Huang, J.H., Gong, Q.L. and Li, P. (1996) The expression of c-fos in nucleus raphe obscurus and paragigantocellularis lateralis following stimulation of dorsal periaqueductal gray. *Acta Acad Med Shanghai*, **23**: 117–121

21. Li, P. (1991) Modulatory effect of somatic inputs on medullary cardiovascular neuronal function. *News in Physiol Sci*, **6**: 69–72.

22. Li, P., Gong, Q.L. and Huangfu, D.H. (1990) Excitation of the nucleus raphe obscurus inhibits the pressor-response induced by hypothalamic and midbrain defence areas stimulation. *Neurosci Let Supp.*, **37**: S18.

23. Li, P. and Lovick, T.A. (1985) Excitatory projection from hypothalamic and midbrain defence region to nucleus paragigantocellularis lateralis in the rat. *Exp Neurol*, **89**: 543–553.

24. Lin, R.J., Gong, Q.L. and Li, P. (1991) Convergent inputs to neurons in the nucleus paragiganto-cellularis leterealis in the cat. *NeuroReport*, **2**: 281–284.

25. Lin, R.J., Gong, Q.L. and Li, P. (1992) Synaptic mechanism involved in the defence-reaction-related neurons in nucleus paragigantocellularis lateralis in the cat. *Chin J. Physiol Sci*, **8**: 60–67.

26. Lovick, T.A. (1985) Descending projections from the ventrolateral medulla dn cardiovascular control. *Pflugers Arch*, **404**: 197–202.

27. Lovick, T.A. and Hilton, S.M. (1985) Vasodilator and vasoconstrictor neurons of the ventrolateral medulla in the cat. *Brain Res*, **331**: 353–357.

28. Lovick, T.A. and Li, P. (1989) Integrated function of neurons in the rostral ventrolateral medulla Progress in *Brain Res*, **81**: 223–232.

29. McAllen, R.M. and Wollard, S. (1984) Exploration of the cats medullary surface by microinjection of excitant amino acid. *J. Physiol* (London) **346**: 35.

30. Peng, Y.J., Gong, Q.L. and Li, P. (1998) Convergence of midbrain, visceral and somatic inputs onto single neurons in the nucleus paragigantocellularis lateralis in rats. (in submission).

31. Peng, Y.J., Gong, Q.L. and Li, P. (1998) Responses of neurons in the rostral ventrolateral medulla to electrical stimulation of dorsal and ventrolateral periaqueductoral gray matter. (in submission)

32. Spyer, K.M. (1984) Central control of the cardiovascular system. In Baker PF ed. Recent adv Physiol Churchill Livingstone, Edinburgh 163–199.

33. Steinbush, H.W.M. (1981) Distribution of serotonin immunoreactivity in the central nervous system of the rat cell bodies and terminals. *Neuroscience*, **6**: 557–618.

34. Sun, M.K. (1995) Central neuronal organization and control of sympathetic nervous system in mammals, *Progress in Neurology*, **47**: 157–233.

35. Wang, W.H. and Li, P. (1989) Inhibition of defensive pressor response by repetitive stimulation of brainstem defence areas. *Chin J. Physiol Sci*, **5**: 252–257.

36. Wang, W.H. and Li, P. (1991) Influence of defence area stimulation on neurons in nucleus raphe obscurus. *Chin J. Physiol Sci*, **7**: 184–189.

37. Willete, R.N., Kireger, A.J. and Barcas, H.N. (1983) Medullary γ-aminobuytric acid (GABA) receptors and the regulation of blood pressure in the rat. *J. Pharmacol Exp Thereap*, **226**: 891–899.
38. Xia, Y., Chang, A.Z. and Cao, X.D. (1989) Increased leuenkephalin immunoreactivity in cerebro-spinal fluid during stimulation of hypothalamic defence area in rabbits. *Acta Physiol Sci*, **40**: 365–367.

2 FACTORS INFLUENCING THE EFFECT OF ACUPUNCTURE

Peng Li

The above chapters discussed the effect and mechanism of acupuncture on different diseases. We can understand that the effect of acupuncture depends on many factors: the different acupoints we choose, the stimulation parameters and also the situation of the central nervous system, etc. In this chapter we will discuss these factors in more detail.

Effect of Different Acupoints

In Chapter 3, we talked about the anatomical and physiological base of acupuncture, that is to say what kind of nerve or nerve ending lies underneath the acupoints. We also described how to select acupoints, e.g., "Ah Shi" points, acupoints on the same or nearby spinal segment, and distal acupoints. Here we will show that different acupoints have different effects on blood pressure.[11] It is known that underneath Zusanli (St 36) is the deep peroneal nerve (DPN), under Xuanzhong (GB 39) is the superficial peroneal nerve (SPN), under Quchi (LI 11) is the deep radial nerve (DRN), and under Pianli (LI 6) is the superficial radial nerve. When we used a weak current of 300 μA (100 Hz, 0.5 ms duration) to stimulate these nerves, we got different effects on the mean blood pressure (MBP). Stimulation of DPN and DRN induced a depressor effect, while stimulation of SPN or SRN had a pressor effect. There are more myelinated fibres in the deep nerves and more non-myelinated fibres in the superficial nerves. Therefore, even using the same weak current, stimulation of the deep nerves will excite type II and III fibres and get a depressor effect, while stimulation of superficial nerves will excite type IV fibres and get a pressor effect. The acupoints often used to treat hypertension are Quchi (LI 11, beneath it is DRN) and Zusanli (St 36, beneath it is DPN), etc. while that used to treat hypotension is Pianli (LI 6, beneath it is SRN), etc. Xuanzhong (GB 39, beneath it is SPN) is not often used to treat hypertension or hypotension. This is an example of the anatomical and physiological basis to explain why different acupoints are used to treat different diseases.

Effect of Different Stimulation Parameters

It has long been known that stimulation of the somatic afferent causes either an increase or decrease in the arterial BP as well as the sympathetic nerve activity depending upon the stimulus parameters used.[2,10] In our experiments'[12] when we stimulate the same nerve underneath the same acupoint with a different current, we will have different results. For example, stimulating DPN or DRN with 300 μA induces a depressor response as described in the above paragraph. However, in the same experiment, stimulation of these deep nerves with a higher current (600 μA) will induce a pressor response. When the superficial nerves were stimulated with a higher current, a more marked pressor response was obtained. We know that stimulation of deep nerves with a higher current up to 600 μA will also excite type IV fibres. So, it is to similar stimulation of the superficial nerves inducing a pressor response. Doctors should remember that even are chosen the same acupoints using, different stimulation parameters can induce different results.

Effect of Acupuncture Under Different Functional States

In the previous chapters evidence has shown that stimulation of the same acupoints or the nerves underneath these acupoints produced different effects on BP and sympathetic activity according to the functional state. In chapters 5 and 6, we described that acupuncture applied on Zusanli (St 36) or stimulation of the DPN underneath it could induce a depressor effect in hypertensive animals, while it induces a pressor effect in hypotensive animals, even using the same stimulation parameters. In the experiments of the above section, we also saw that when the BP was lowered by haemorrhage, stimulation of DPN or DRN even with weak current (300 μA) will induce a pressor response rather than depressor response. The pressor response by stimulation of the superficial nerves is more significant after haemorrhage. The following experiments will show more details.

WHY DID THE DEPRESSOR EFFECT OF DPN STIMULATION DISAPPEAR AFTER HAEMORRHAGE?

In the above paragraph, we described that the DPN stimulation elicited no significant depressor effect after haemorrhage, while it was significant in hypertensive animals. In that case, what is the mechanism? We know that the MBP is determined by the tonic activity of the cardiovascular centre, which integrates many cardiovascular reflexes, i.e., the baroreflex, chemoreflex and defence reaction, etc. In this series of experiments we tried to analyse why the effect of DPN stimulation on the defensive pressor response changed after blood loss.

Effect of blood loss on the defensive pressor response

Lin, et al.[13] showed that in the urethane-chloralose anaesthetised rabbits, after moderated blood loss (10–20%), the amplitude of the pressor response induced by stimulation of the midbrain defence area (PAG) increased significantly. This is not due to the increase of inputs from the cardiac volume receptors, because the pressor response was unaltered after bilateral vagotomy.

This increase of defensive pressor response during haemorrhage is also not due to the decrease of baroreceptor inputs. Because when the MBP was reduced to the level similar to moderate blood loss by intravenous infusion of a vasodilator, nitroprusside (NP), to decrease the baroreceptor inputs, the pressor response was not increased significantly. This phenomenon was not altered after bilateral section of the aortic nerves. Only when the carotid sinus nerves were blocked by infiltration of lidocaine bilaterally was the MBP elevated and the defensive pressor response markedly decreased. So, it is suggested that the enhancement of the pressor response induced by midbrain defence area stimulation during moderate blood loss is mainly due to an increase in the chemoreceptor inputs.

Effect of DPN stimulation on the defensive pressor response after moderate bleeding

As we described in chapter 10, the pressor response induced by stimulation of the HYP or PAG could be inhibited by stimulation of DPN with low frequency and low intensity. Nevertheless, after moderate bleeding, the defensive pressor response was significantly increased and could not readily be inhibited by the DPN stimulation.[3]

It was also shown in the last section that the enhancement of defence pressor response during moderate haemorrhage was mainly due to the excitation of the cardiovascular centre and that the inputs from the chemoreceptor might play an important role. In 1989, Fan, et al.[3] showed that an increase of the carotid chemoreceptor inputs by infusion of CO_2 saturated bicarbonate solution (0.4 ml of 1 mol/Liter) into the carotid artery could induce a significant pressor response; it could also facilitate the defence pressor response induced by stimulation of the PAG. This enhanced pressor response induced by PAG stimulation during moderate haemorrhage could be abolished by bilateral infiltration of lidocaine into the sinus nerve. These results support our suggestion, i.e. that the enhancement of the pressor response was mainly due to the increase of the afferent inputs from the carotid chemoreceptor. The enhanced defence pressor response was also not inhibited by stimulation of DPN. So, it is suggested that the enhanced defensive pressor response during moderate haemorrhage could not be inhibited by DPN stimulation because the excitability of the cardiovascular centre increased with the increase of chemoreceptor inputs.

Central endogenous cholinergic mechanisms of the enhanced defence pressor response in acute moderate haemorrhage

Central cholinergic mechanisms have been shown to be involved in the regulation of cardiovascular function. In chapter 6, we described that icv administration of cholinomimetic agonists could elevate blood pressure that could be blocked by the pretreatment of an atropine injection into the RVLM. In 1990 Fan, et al.[4] showed that icv administration of the cholinergic antagonist atropine (50 μg in 100 μl) produced a significant fall in the defence pressor response, which had increased after moderate bleeding. Microinjection of atropine (5 mg in 0.5 ml) into the RVLM could also prevent the increase of defence pressor response after moderate bleeding. Therefore it is believed that after moderate bleeding the increase of the carotid chemoreceptor inputs activates the central cholinergic mechanism, especially the cholinergic receptors on the RVLM neurons that relate to the defence pressor response.

Effect of chemoreceptor and DPN stimulation on defence reaction-related neurons in the RVLM

With the aim of studying the integration of the chemoreceptor input and the defence reaction in the RVLM, neuronal discharges of 59 units were recorded in the RVLM activated by PAG defence area stimulation.[5] The carotid chemoreceptor was excited by an injection of 0.2–0.4 ml lobeline, or 1M CO_2 saturated bicarbonate solution through a cannula in the external maxillary artery, which passed into the common carotid artery near the sinus area over a period of 8–10 seconds. 90% of the units recorded received convergent excitatory projections from the PAG defence area and the chemoreceptor. When both the stimulation of the PAG and the carotid chemoreceptor were applied simultaneously, the evoked discharges of the units were much more than during stimulation of the PAG alone.

When only the PAG was stimulated, the evoked discharges of three-quartely of the defence reaction-related neurons in the RVLM were reduced by stimulation of DPN. However, if the PAG defence area and the carotid chemoreceptor were stimulated simultaneously, the evoked discharges of RVLM neurons increased enormously and could not be inhibited by the DPN stimulation. Thus the neurons in the RVLM play an important role in relaying and evidently integrating the cardiovascular components of the defence reaction, chemoreceptor pressor response and somatic inputs.

The effect of DPN stimulation depends on the excitability of the cardiovascular centre, especially the neurons in the RVLM. In normotensive and hypertensive animals, the DPN inputs could inhibit the RVLM neurons by activating the opiate, 5-HT and GABA receptors (see chapters 7, 8, 10, and 11), while after haemorrhage, the baroreceptor inputs decreased and chemoreceptor inputs increased. So the cholinergic receptors on RVLM neurons were activated, and the excitability of these neurons increased. Under such conditions, these neurons can no longer be inhibited by DPN stimulation. Moreover, the group IV fibres in the DPN, although only small in number, may also activate the cholinergic receptors in the RVLM and in turn produce a pressor effect. This is the mechanism that stimulation of the DPN underneath Zusanli (St 36) has a depressor effect upon during hypertension, but it might also have a pressor effect during haemorrhage.

Some more examples in the following paragraphs also show that under different conditions, even with no change in MBP, stimulating the same acupoint with the same parameter will have different results.

EFFECT OF DPN STIMULATION ON RENAL NERVE DISCHARGE UNDER DIFFERENT LEVELS OF BP

The renal nerve discharge (RND) is a good index of sympathetic outflows.[1] The present experiment was designed to examine the effect of DPN stimulation on RND under different levels (RND) of BP.[14] In normotensive rabbits, the BP, HR and RND, etc. were quite stable and did not change significantly over the hours. When the DPN was stimulated with a weak current (150–300 μA, 12 Hz, 0.5 ms) for 15 minutes, the RND was inhibited significantly. It even decreased further after the stimulation was stopped and then recovered slowly to the control level in just over 20 minutes. There was no change in BP and HR, and the RND did not change markedly, if the DPN was stimulated with a strong current.

When the BP was decreased from 104 ± 5 mmHg to 72 ± 16 mmHg by intravenous infusion of nitroprusside (NP, 13–27 μg/kg/min), HR increased significantly from 277 ± 11 beats/minutes to 302 ± 19 beats/minutes; the RND increased markedly and renal blood flow (RBF) decreased. Under such conditions, stimulation of DPN with a strong current (500–800 μA) had no significant effect on BP, HR, mesenteric blood flow (MBF) and FBF, but the RND increased and RBF decreased further. After the cessation of DPN stimulation, the RND and RBF slowly recovered to their control levels. If the DPN was stimulated with a low current (150–300 μA), no significant change could be observed. It is also shown that the RND is inversely related to BP. In NP-induced hypotensive animals, after the DPN was stimulated with a strong current, the RND-BP correlation curve shifted to the right. That means that at a certain level of BP, the RND increased compared with the control, suggesting a reset of the baroreflex by the DPN input.

When noradrenaline (NA) was infused at a constant rate, the BP was elevated from 107 ± 8 mmHg to 124 ± 7 mmHg, HR decreased from 277 ± 11 beats/minutes to 246 ± 8 beats/minutes; RND decreased by 50%, and RBF also decreased by 14%. Under such a situation, whether the DPN was stimulated with a weak or strong current, RND decreased further and RBF increased a little, but no significant change in BP and HR occurred. After cessation of the nerve stimulation, the RND remained at a low level for about 15 minutes and recovered slowly.

The transmitters related to the different responses were also studied. In normotensive and hypertensive (induced by NA infusion) rabbits, intravenous injection (iv) of naloxone (0.4 mg/kg) could block the inhibitory effect of DPN stimulation with a weak current, while iv scopolamine had no such effect. On the other hand, iv scopolamine could block the excitatory effect of DPN stimulation with a strong current on RND in hypotensive rabbits induced by NP infusion. Naloxone iv could not block this excitatory effect. Therefore it is shown that the inhibitory effect of DPN stimulation is attributable to the release of endogenous opioids, while the excitatory effect of DPN stimulation is related to the activation of the central cholinergic system.

EFFECT OF DPN STIMULATION ON RND DURING HYPERVOLEMIA AND HYPOVOLEMIA

This series of experiments was designed to test the effect of DPN stimulation on RND during saline loading and haemorrhage.[8,9]

Effect of DPN stimulation on hypervolemia

Two groups of rabbits were observed. (a) The controls group in which only isotonic saline (3.2 ml/minutes) was infused intravenously for 40 minutes; (b) the stimulation group in which the DPN was stimulated during the latter half of the 40 minutes period of saline loading.

In the control group, after the onset of the saline infusion, the right atrial pressure increased gradually. No significant change in mean arterial pressure (MBP) was observed during the loading period. However, as the right atrial pressure increased, the RND and HR decreased gradually, while the urinary outflow increased. At the end of the loading period, the renal nerve activity was $72 \pm 3\%$ of the control value, while the urinary outflow increased to about eight times its control value. During the recovery period, renal nerve activity gradually returned toward its pre-loading level within a few minutes, while the urinary outflow was still much greater than the control level 30 minutes after the end of saline loading. The renal blood flow (RBF) of the left kidney measured with an electromagnetic blood flow meter showed an increase during loading, and reached $112 \pm 6.9\%$ of its control value at the end of loading.

In the stimulation group, the alterations of the right atrial pressure, MBP and HR during the first of the 40 minutes loading period were similar to those in the control group. However, during the latter half of the 40 minutes period of saline loading, when electrical stimulation of the DPN was applied, a more profound inhibition of the renal nerve activity was observed which was only $56 \pm 4\%$ of its control value. After the end of the saline infusion and DPN stimulation, the recovery of both the RND and the urinary outflow progressed much more slowly than in the control group. The RBF also increased further during DPN stimulation. At the end of DPN stimulation, the RBF reached a level of $121 \pm 8.1\%$ of its preloading control value. So, there was a statistically significant difference in the level of the RND between the stimulation group and the control group during the stimulation period and the recovery period.

The effect of the opiate receptor antagonist naloxone was also investigated. In rabbits that received an intravenous naloxone (0.4 mg/kg) administration 3 minutes before the DPN stimulation, the ensuing nerve stimulation no longer elicited a further decrease in the RND as observed in the animals without naloxone treatment. Instead, it increased nearly to its pre-loading control level. On the other hand, the cholinergic receptor antagonist scopolamine (0.25 mg/kg iv) did not affect the inhibition of DPN stimulation on the RND.

Effect of DPN stimulation in nonhypotensive hemorrhagic rabbits

In this study, the rabbits were again divided into a control group and a stimulation group. Non-hypotensive hemorrhage was produced by withdrawing 10% of the total blood volume via the right femoral vein within 5 to 7 minutes. The right atrial pressure was lowered gradually during the first 10 minutes after hemorrhagic and was then maintained at a low level. The MBP was reduced slightly by no more than 5 mmHg and returned to its control level within 20 minutes. The RBF decreased to 90 ± 4.4% of its control value. There was no significant change in HR. Following haemorrhage, there was an initial rapid increase in the RND during the first 5–10 minutes, then it was maintained at a level about 20% of its control value during the rest of the experimental period.

In the stimulation group, the changes in the right atrial pressure, MBP, HR and RBF during the first 20 minutes after blood loss were similar to those in the control group. The acupuncture-like DPN stimulation was started 20 minutes after blood loss. The stimulation of the DPN caused a remarkable increase in the RND that reached a level of 150 ± 6.4% of its pre-hemorrhage control value in the first 5 minutes of nerve stimulation. The RND was then reduced gradually. The RBF decreased further to 77.6 ± 5.5% of its pre-hemorrhage control value within the first 10 minutes of nerve stimulation.

15 minutes after hemorrhage, when RND increased to 120 ± 4% of its pre-hemorrhage control value, administration of scopolamine (0.25 mg/kg, iv) caused no significant change in the RND, but abolished the further increase of RND during DPN stimulation. However, naloxone (0.4 mg/kg, iv) did not influence the excitatory effect of DPN stimulation on the RND in hemorrhagic rabbits.

Physiological significance

Saline loading and non-hypotensive hemorrhage have been often used in physiological studies for changing the blood volume and thus the atrial mechanoreceptor activity[6] without concomitant marked changes in MBP. It was shown[7] that the atrial mechanoreceptor activity was altered more markedly than that of the arterial baroreceptor during moderate change in blood volume. In our studies, the saline infusion and blood withdrawn caused only a little change in MBP but a remarkable change in the RND. These changes of RND could be greatly attenuated after bilateral vagotomy, showing the importance of the cardiac mechanoreceptor in the renal nerve response.

The present work again shows the fact that the acupuncture-like stimulation of the somatic nerve produced a modulatory effect on the renal nerve activity. It caused a decrease in RND during saline loading, but an increase after non-hypotensive blood loss. It seems likely that the blood volume determines the direction of the response of the RND. These two responses of the RND upon DPN stimulation are probably mediated by different central mechanisms. The inhibition of RND by DPN stimulation during saline loading is prevented by naloxone pretreatment, but not by scopolamine. On the other hand, the excitation of RND by DPN stimulation after non-hypertensive hemorrhage is prevented by scopolamine, but not by naloxone. These results imply that the endorphin system might play an important role in the former response while the latter response might be mainly mediated by the muscarinic cholinergic system. These results support our suggestion that the somatic inputs elicited by acupuncture exert both excitation and inhibition on the central nervous system. The RND, to be an efferent outflow, is determined by the integrative function of the central nervous system at that moment. The RND is important in the maintenance of the homeostasis of the extracellular fluids and body salts.[1] So, acupuncture can facilitate the physiological regulatory activity in response to alterations of the external or internal environment. This might be the important physiological basis of the modulatory effect of acupuncture.

Clinical Application

From the above results we can understand that the effects of acupuncture depend on three main factors: the acupoints we selected, the parameters used and the condition of the central nervous system of the patient. So, choosing the right acupoints and selection suitable stimulation parameters are important. Even using the same acupoints and the same stimulation parameters will get different effects in different patients, depending on their situation.

Therefore, evaluating the condition of the central nervous system of the patient is very important before using acupuncture to treat patients. This is why we emphasise that acupuncture is not simply a therapeutic technique; it should not be used by a nurse or technician, nor by someone who has only been trained for a few months. Even a doctor needs to understand the principles of Traditional Chinese Medicine and always have the integrative physiology and neuroscience in mind.

References

1. DiBona, G.F. (1982) The function of renal nerves. *Rev Physiol Biochem Pharmacol*, **94**: 75–181.
2. Fedina, L., Katunskill, A.Y., Khayutin, V.M. and Mitsanyi, A. (1966) Responses of renal sympathetic nerves to stimulation of afferent A and C fibers of tibial and mesenterial nerves. *Acta Physiol Acad Sci Hung*, **29**: 157–176.
3. Fan, W., Lin, R.J. and Li, P. (1989) Effect of deep peroneal nerve inputs on the cardiovascular defence reaction after acute moderate bleeding in rabbits. *Chin J. Physiol Sci*, **5**: 210–217.
4. Fan, W., Lin, R.J. and Li, P. (1990) Central endogenous cholinergic mechanism of the enhanced defence rpessor response in acute moderate gleeding rabbits. *Chin J. Physiol Sci*, **6**: 129–136.
5. Fan, W., Zhang, Z. and Lin, R.J. (1990) Effect of carotid chemoreceptor stimulation on defence reaction related units in rostral ventrolateral medulla. *Chin J. Physiol Sci*, **6**: 317–323.
6. Goetzm, K.L., Bond, G.C. and Bloxham, D.D. (1975) Atrial receptors and renal funcation. *Physiol Rev*, **55**: 157–205.
7. Gupta, P.D., Henry, J.P., Sinclair, R. and von Baumgarten, R. (1966) Responses of atrial and aortic baroreceptors to nonhypotensive hemorrhage and to transfusion. *Am J. Physiol*, **211**: 1429–1437.
8. He, S.Q. and Su, Q.F. (1983) Influence of stimulation of the deep peroneal nerve on renal nerve discharge under different levels of central sympathetic activity. *Acta Physiol Sin*, **35**: 243–249.
9. He, S.Q., Sun, X.Y. and Yao, T. (1985) Somatosympathetic responses in saline-loaded and hemorhage rabbits. *CHin J. Physiol Sci*, **1**: 1–9.
10. Johansson, B. (1962) Circulatory responses to stimulation afferents. *Acta Physiol Scand*, **57**: Suppl. 1–91.
11. Li, J., Lin, Q. and Li, P. (1993) Effect of somatic nerve stimulation on blood pressure in normotensive and hemorrhagic rats. *Acta Academic Medicine Shanghai*, **20**: 39–43.
12. Li, J. and Li, P. (1992) The influence of stimulation oof soamtic nerves under different acupoints on the blood pressure. *Shanghai J. Aup Moxib*, **11**: 39–43.

13. Lin, R.J., Shao, Y. and Gong, Q.L. (1988) Effect of blood loss on cardiovascular response induced by stimualtion of periaqueductal grey in the rabbit. *Chin J. Physiol Sci*, 5: 18–25.
14. Xiao, Y.F. and Li, P. (1983) Effect of deep peroneal nerve stimulation on renal nerve discharge under different levels of blood pressure in rabbits. *Acta Physiol Sin*, 35: 432–439.

13 SUMMARY

Peng Li

Acupuncture has been used to treat patients of various kinds of diseases for more than two and a half thousand years, and now spread to other Asian countries, Europe, North America and throughout the world. The World Health Organization lists more than 40 conditions for which acupuncture may be indicated. In this book we have described the effect and mechanism of acupuncture on pain, hypertension, hypotension, arrhythmia, myocardial ischemia and many other diseases.

Beside clinical observations, many experiments have been used to study the effect of acupuncture. It has been shown that the anatomical structure of the acupoints of different mammals and their nerve supply are similar to those of the corresponding acupoints of the human being. Stimulation of the nerves innervating the acupoints often produces the same effect as that of acupuncture or EA. The effects of acupuncture are more easily demonstrated in conscious animals, but some effects can also be shown in urethane-chloralose anesthetized animals. It is interesting to point out that acupuncture or somatic nerve stimulation has no significant effect in animals with normal cardiovascular functions, whereas it can modulate or normalize abnormal functions.

Since the late 1950s some operations have been performed under acupuncture "anesthesia". Those patients whose sympathetic activity could be inhibited by acupuncture were shown to have good analgesic effect by acupuncture. Some chemicals and herbs were used to improve the effectiveness of acupuncture analgesia. Chronic pain, such as headache, migraine, back and lumbar pain, sciatica, neuralgia, etc. could also be relieved by acupuncture or EA. The mechanism of acupuncture analgesia is complicated. It is due to the activation of type II and III fibers in the somatic nerves underneath the acupoints. These somatic inputs induce the release of endorphin, enkephaline, dynorphin and 5-HT, etc. in the brain and spinal cord and result in an analgesic effect. For clinical doctors, it is important to know how to choose patients before doing operations with acupuncture "anesthesia". For a good analgesic effect, doctors should understand how to choose the right acupoints and available stimulation parameters. Usually, low current and low frequency stimulation is effective. Sometimes, low current and high frequency stimulation is an alternative.

Clinical observations reported that acupuncture could have a depressor effect on some types of hypertension, especially for stage 1 and 2. Experimental studies showed that in SHR, NA-induced hypertensive dogs, stress-induced hypertensive rats and renal hypertension, EA (low current and low frequency) applied on Zusanli (St 36), Neiguan (Pe 6) or stimulation of the somatic nerves underneath these acupoints could inhibit the defense reaction, chemoreceptor reflex and sympathetic outflow, produce vasodilation of splanchnic arteries, and had a significant long-lasting depressor effect. This is related to the activation of type II and III fibres, and activation of the endogenous opioids system in the brain. 5-HT system might be also activated.

It is reported that acupuncture could be used to elevate low BP in hypotensive patients. In experimental studies, hypotensive animals induced by hemorrhage, intravenous infusion of NP or endotoxic shock, EA on Zusanli (St 36) or Neiguan (Pe 6) or stimulation of the somatic nerve strong enough to excite group IV fibres produced a marked pressor effect. This effect often accompanied by an increase in cardiac contractile force, cardiac output, splanchnic nerve activity and mesenteric vascular resistance, and a further decrease of renal blood flow. These effects are mainly due to the activation of the cholinergic M receptors of the sympathetic cardiovascular center of RVLM. Resetting of the baroreceptor reflex is also involved.

Clinical reports showed that some kinds of arrhythmia could be cured or improved by acupuncture. In experimental studies ventricular extrasystoles induced by hypothalamic stimulation could be inhibited by EA applied on Zusanli (St 36) or Neiguan (Pe 6), or stimulation of the DPN or MN underneath these acupoints with a low current and low frequency. This effect is due to the stimulation of type II and III fibres of the somatic nerves, which induce the release of opioids, GABA and 5-HT in the brain, inhibit the cardiac sympathetic center in RVLM and reduce the hypothalamic stimulation induced ventricular extrasystoles. In addition, the bradycardia evoked by aortic nerve stimulation could be inhibited by somatic nerve stimulation, which excited group IV fibres. The activation of which in turn activated the cholinergic M receptors in the RVLM and inhibited the neurons in the NTS and the preganglionic vagal cardiomotor neurons via a GABAergic mechanism.

Recently, it was reported that acupuncture could reduce angina attacks and improve coronary heart disease. Experimental studies showed that EA on Neiguan (Pe 6) had an inhibitory effect on reflex-induced myocardial ischemia. This is mainly due to the stimulation of Aδ fibers in the median nerve, which can activate opiate receptors in the RVLM, inhibit sympathetic outflow and have a depressor effect. It diminishes cardiac oxygen demand rather than improve blood supply, and thus has a therapeutic effect on some kinds of angina. The receptors activated in the RVLM are mainly μ and δ receptors; κ receptors may take less part in this inhibition.

Acupuncture was used to treat gastrointestinal diseases, urinary diseases, asthma, diabetes, hyperthyroidism, thyroiditis, obesity, facial nerve paralysis, paralysis after stroke, oligogalactia after labor, and also to improve uterine contractions in pregnancies past the due-date and induce ovulation etc. It even can stop smoking, alcoholism and drug abuse. In short, it was reported that acupuncture can modulate the autonomic, endocrine and immune functions and thoroughly improve nervous regeneration, etc. All these mechanism have not been studied enough. There are many topics that need further investigation.

Our work showed that the modulation of acupuncture on cardiovascular diseases is related to its influence on the defense reaction, baro- and chemoreceptor reflexes, etc. The somatic afferent impulses may reset the baroreceptor reflex via the central opioids, serotonin, vasopressin, and cholinergic mechanisms. The chemoreceptor reflex can also be modulated by the activation of somatic inputs, and be related to the opioid and cholinergic mechanisms. The RVLM neurons receive convergent projections from the HYP, PAG defense areas, the baro- and chemo-receptors, NRO, splanchnic afferent and various somatic afferent inputs. Most of these RVLM neurons projected directly to the ILM of the spinal cord, and correlated with the sympathetic nerve discharge and BP level. They are important in the maintenance of homeostasis, and a key area for the modulation of acupuncture. Excitation of the HYP or PAG defense areas can activate the ARC-vPAG-NRO system, which acts as a negative feedback mechanism to limit the over-excitation of the sympathetic nervous system. The somatic inputs induced by acupuncture could promote this negative feedback mechanism and inhibit the RVLM cardiovascular neurons via the release of endorphin, enkephaline, 5-HT and GABA, etc.

Three main factors will influence the effect of acupuncture:

(1) Different acupoints have different effect, which depend on what kind of nerve endings or fibres are beneath them, to which spinal segment they project, and which "channels" they belong to.
(2) Different stimulation parameters. Low current and low frequency

stimulation usually has an inhibitory effect, while low current and high frequency has an analgesic effect.

(3) Different functional state. Even when using the same acupoint and stimulation parameters, the effect of acupuncture depend on the integrative function of the central nervous system.

Acupuncture is a part of Traditional Chinese Medicine (TCM). It is not a simple technique. Doctors who like to use acupuncture should have studied both Western Medicine and TCM. They should also learn advanced basic medical sciences, especially integrative physiology and neuroscience. Investigation of the mechanism of acupuncture is the first step to understanding TCM scientifically. A combination of TCM and Western Medicine will not only promote the development of integrative physiology and neuroscience, but will enhance the effectiveness and reduce the cost of treating disease.

SECTION 2
INTRODUCTION

Lily Cheung

Research into Traditional Acupuncture and Moxibustion this century had shown that evidence exist for a neuro-physiological basis for acupoint stimulation.

Description of diseases or disturbances in organic functions between TCM and conventional medicine differs only because of the way Chinese medicine had developed. Thus a certain set of symptoms that had been described as chronic bronchitis can be described as "lung qi xu" in TCM.

With an increase in understanding of the mechanism of acupoint stimulation, treatment with acupuncture can only become more effective. For example, when a young man suffers with sciatica, TCM will regard this as a Bi Syndrome with interruption of the flow of qi in the Meridians. If the pain radiates down the buttock to the lower leg, we can choose from Yanglingquan (GB 34), which is a He-Sea point and specific for pain in the muscles; Huantiao (GB 30), specific for pain in the lower back, weakness of the lower extremities and for activating the meridian qi; Chengfu (UB 36), to clear and activate the meridian qi and to reduce pain in the lumbar region; local points depending on examination by palpation may be at Guanyuanshu (UB 26) and/or Dachangshu (UB 25), Xiaochangshu (UB 27), Weizhong (UB 40), a He-Sea point specific for low back pain and motor impairment, Chengshan (UB 57), specific for low back pain.

After examining the patient, we can determine which local point should be used, whether the pain is from L4 or L5 and then choose the appropriate acupuncture point. If the pain radiates to the buttock, Huantiao should be chosen as this point also overlies the sciatic nerve. If the radiation of pain spreads to the peroneal muscles, Yanglingquan will be chosen. If the pain spreads to the calf muscle instead, then Chengshan will be the point of choice. Yanglingquan will stimulate the peroneal nerve and Chengshan, the tibial nerve. Thus, the final prescription for acupuncture can be arrived at from the combined knowledge of the anatomy and the specific actions of the acupuncture points.

When there are symptoms of organic dysfunction as, for example, urinary retention, when the underlying causes of myelomeningocele, spina bifida occulta or tumours have been ruled out, the principle of treatment will be to restore normal urinary function by regulating the action of the autonomic nerves on the bladder. According to TCM, urinary bladder dysfunction will be brought on by a dysruption of kidney qi. There are specific acupoints for restoring normal function to the bladder, e.g. Shenshu (UB 23) (L1–L3); Pangguanshu (UB 28) (L5–S2); Ciliao (UB 32) (S2); Xiaoliao (UB 34) (L5–S4); Zhongji (Ren 3) (T6–T12); Qihai (Ren 6) (T6–T12).

The contraction of the bladder detrusor muscle is brought about by parasympathetic activity (S2–S3). The internal sphincter leading to the urethra is normally closed by sympathetic activity (L1–L2). When the bladder is full, nerve impulses from the cerebral cortex, increase parasympathetic activity and decrease sympathetic activity. This causes the internal sphincter to relax, and the bladder muscle to contract. At the same time, voluntary inhibition of pudendal nerve (S2–S4) activity relaxes the external sphincter.

Thus, by combining our knowledge of the specific actions of the appropriate acupoints and our understanding of the bladder physiology, we will be able to choose the combination of points that would have the most effect on that part of the autonomic nervous system. According to TCM, we should also use some distal points for a better response, e.g. Sanyingjiao (Sp 6) (L4–S3) or Taixi (K 3) (L4–S2) or Zusanli (St 36) (L4–S3), depending on the TCM diagnosis. You will note that these points are also related to the same nerves.

These are just two easy examples to illustrate the integration of scientific knowledge into a system evolved from clinical experiences over thousands of years. Acupuncture is a system we are only beginning to understand in terms of modern science. It is only our lack of a total understanding of the human physiology and a difficulty with the right models for research, that is preventing us from having scientific explanations for all the effects of acupoint stimulation and how best to use them.

RHINITIS

Male—65 years old

Complaint:

Nasal congestion and discharge for the past fifty years.

History:

The problem started with white and sticky nasal discharge especially in the cold weather and in a polluted atmosphere. This was also worse in the mornings. While still in Hong Kong, he underwent 2 rhinodysis (nasal douche) with no effect. The symptoms had been gradually getting worse. The GP had prescribed antibiotics and nasal sprays. Periodic use of these provided temporary relief. Recently, the patient had needed to blow his nose every 15 minutes in spite of the nasal sprays and antibiotics. The consultant had advised surgery which the patient had refused. As a result of his symptoms, sleep had been difficult.

On Examination:

There was copious mucous discharge and the mucous membrane appears to be very red. The tone of speech was nasal. The throat appeared to be clear and without soreness. Tongue—pale with a thin white coat. Pulse—small.

TCM Diagnosis:

Fei Qi Xu and Cold

Treatment:

Points Used	Nerves Stimulated	TCM Explanations
Yinxiang (LI 20)	CrN. V + VII	Specific point for rhinorrhoea: expels wind to reduce obstruction
Hegu (LI 4)	C6 – T1	Yuan-source point: disperses wind and heat
Shangyingxiang (Ext. Pt.)	CrN. V + VII	Specific point for problems in the nasal cavity
Quchi (LI II)	C5 – T1	Regulates qi; promotes circulation; disperses wind and clears heat; specific for allergy problems
Feishu (UB 13)	T3 – T4	Regulates Wei qi and nourishes yin

Fengchi (GB 20)   CrN. XI; C2 − C5   Crossing point; disperses wind;
                                           removes fire; nourishes yin

Electro-acupuncture and moxibustion was given on the above points. After the first treatment, the patient immediately felt able to breathe through his nose and the discharge had stopped temporarily. Daily treatment was advised. After the third day, discharge was much reduced and the sinusus needed less clearing. He was also able to sleep. All the symptoms were much reduced after 7 treatments and he was advised to only have the treatment when necessary or at least once a month. Chronic problems usually require treatment occasionally. Consequently the patient felt comfortable with just a treatment every 4 to 6 weeks.

Comments:

Stimulation of the nasopalatine nerve at Yinxiang and Shangyiangxiang can reduce nasal discharge by regulating the sympathetic and para-sympathetic activities to the upper respiratory tract. Moxibustion also enhances the action of beta-endorphins which acts as an accelerator within the immune system thus modifying allergic reactions of the body. The point, Hegu is often used in acupuncture for problems related to the area of the face. This observation was based on clinical experience.

LOCK JAW

Male—57 years old

Complaint:

Suffering with a locked jaw for the past 10 days

History:

Previous to the last ten days, opening of the mouth was accompanied by pain. He was experiencing difficulty with solid foods and finally even fluid intake was difficult. A dentist was consulted who decided that the jaw was the cause. Analgesia was prescribed but with no effect.

On Examination:

The patient was unable to open the jaw wide enough for the tongue to be seen. Pulse—fast.

TCM Diagnosis:

Rising Stomach Fire

Treatment:

Electro-acupuncture and moxibustion were used on the following points:

Points Used	Nerves Stimulated	TCM Explanations
Jiache (St 6)	CrN. VII	Clears heat and reduces fire; regulates Stomach qi; specific point for opening the jaw
Xiaguan (St 7)	CrN. V + VII	Regulates fow of Stomach qi; reduces pain; reduces motor impairment to the jaw
Hegu (LI 4)	C6 – T1	Clears heat; reduces pain

Immediately after the treatment, the jaw felt more relaxed. He was able to eat normally. Two more treatments were required before normality returned.

Comments:

The point, Hegu enhances the anti-inflammatory reaction of the body to the area of the face. Needling Xiaguan and Jiache stimulates CrN. VII to restore mobility to the jaw.

HAY FEVER

Female—43 years old

Complaint:

Spring cleaning 10 days previous triggered off asthma.

History:

Came to reside in England 20 years ago. There was no symptoms of allergy for the first 4 years. Since then she had started itching in the throat and eyes, leading to coughing and sneezing every April. Symptoms had been getting worse year by year, exacerbated by excessive dust. Sleep was disturbed. Antihistamines prescribed by the GP had only provided a reduction in some of the symptoms. The symptoms receded towards the end of spring. There was no apparent food allergy. There was a history of asthma and allergy with the mother and sister.

On Examination:

Tired looking. Tongue—swollen and pale with a thin white coat. Pulse—deep and fast.

TCM Diagnosis:

Fei Qi Xu

Treatment:

Electro-acupuncture and moxibustion were used on the following points. These were divided into two sets and used alternately.

Plan 1

Points Used	Nerves Stimulated	TCM Explanations
Yinxiang (LI 20)	CrN V + VII	Specific point for hay fever, itch, rhinorrhoea and nasal problems.
Quchi (LI 11)	C5 – T1	Regulates qi; promotes blood flow.
Lieque (Lu 7)	C5 – T1	Luo (connecting) point; ventilates lungs; expels wind; calms throat.
Zusanli (St 36)	L4 – S3	He-Sea point; strengthens body's resistance; restores normal function of body; enrich blood + qi.
Xuehai (Sp 10)	L2 – L4	Clears heat; regulates qi + blood.

Plan 2—Include Yinxiang; Quchi and Lieque and add the following:

Zhongfu (Lu 1)	C5 − T1	Clears cold; promotes qi.
Baihui (Du 20)	CrN. V	Specific for nasal obstruction; increases yang qi.
Anmian (Ext. pt.)	CrN. XI	Specific point for insomnia;
	C1 − C3	regulates lung qi.
Dingchuan (Ext.pt.)	CrN. XI	Specific point for reducing asthma; increases lung qi.

Treatment was given once a week. In addition to acupuncture and moxibustion, Chinese herbal medcine was prescribed. Enough herbs were given for a daily intake over 6 days out of 7. The following 2 prescriptions were alternated weekly.

Prescription 1		*Prescription 2*	
Xin Yi Hua	(Flos Magnoliae)	Xin Yi Hua	
Cang Er Zi	(Fructus Xanthii)	Cang Er Zi	
Sang Shen	(Fructus Mori)	Sang Shen	
Fu Ling	(Poria)	Yuan Zhi	(Radix Polygalae)
Hai Er Shen	(Radix Pseudostellariae)	Huang Qi	(Radix Astralgali Seu Hedysari)
Shu Di	(Radix Rehmanniae Praeparata)	Ye Jiao Teng	(Caulis Polygoni Multiflori)
Kuan Dong Hua	(Flox Farfarae)	Suan Zao Ren	(Semen Ziziphi Spinosae)
Zi Wan	(Radix Asteris)	Zi Wan	
Zhe Bei Mu	(Bulbus Fritillariac Thunbergil)		

In total, a course of 10 treatments were given of acupuncture, moxibustion and herbs. There were no symptoms by the end of the course. The patient was advised to come for treatment the following year before the start of the season.

A similar course of treatment was given the following year according to the above plan. Only 4 weeks of treatment was required.

On the third year, the patient felt well enough not to require treatment.

Comments:

The nasopalatine nerve and ganglion carries the sympathetic and parasympathetic supply to the mucous membrane of the nasal passages. Stimulation by acupuncture of those nerves and the regulation of the sympathetic and parasympathetic of the whole body with the help of herbs, increases the anti-allergy and anti-inflammatory function of the immune system thus moderating the antihistamine reaction more effectively than the antihistamine drugs prescribed.

HERPES ZOSTER

Male—30 years old

Complaint:

Hot and burning sensation of the left side of the chest for the past 2 days.

History:

10 days previously, sleep was restricted to 3 hours nightly due to increased work load. 2 days ago the above symptoms started to appear with the appearance of vesicles which were painful to the touch. The pain radiates towards the spine and was worse at night. He felt a bitter taste in the mouth.

On Examination:

There was a line of vesicles, one inch wide along the left dermatome of T5 to T7. He felt exhausted. Temperature—37°C. Tongue—slightly red with a thin white plus yellow coat. Pulse—wiry and small.

TCM Diagnosis:

Damp Heat Syndrome

Treatment:

Hua-Tuo points corresponding to the site of the lesion at T5 to T7 and a corresponding point further out along the intercostal nerve towards the end of the vesicle line were chosen in addition to the following:

Points Used	Nerves Stimulated	TCM Explanations
Xuchai (Sp 10)	L2 – L4	Clears blood heat; removes damp; regulates qi
Quchi (LI 11)	C5 – T1	Clears heat; removes damp; regulates qi; promotes blood flow
Taichong (Liv 3)	L4 – S2	Removes heat from the liver
Neiguan (P6)	C6 – T1	Confluent point connecting to the Yinwei Meridian; regulates qi to soothe the chest area; sedates; reduces pain

The combination of Xuehai and Quchi (these points are on the Hand and Foot Tai Yin Meridians) enhances the effect of soothing the Liver, regulating qi and reducing pain.

Taichong and Neiguan are both points on the Hand and Foot Jei Yin Meridians. This combination appears to enhance the analgesia effect on intercostal nerve pain.

In addition to the acupuncture and moxibustion, the patient was given the following prescription of herbs to be taken daily:

Long Dan Cao	Radix Gentianae
Huang Qin	Radix Scutellariae
Ze Xie	Rhizoma Alismetis
Chai Hu	Radix Bupleuri
Che Qian Zi	Semen Plantaginis
Zhi Zi	Fructus Gardeniae
Sheng Di	Radix Rehmanniae
Gan Cao	Radix Glycyrrhizae

Treatment was given every day for 3 days. The patient recovered fully.

Comments:

The herpes virus attacks specific nerve endings. In this case, needling at T5 to T7 affects the common sensory ganglion pertaining to these areas, thus enhancing the analgesia effect. At the same time the use of the other points, with the help of herbs helped to restore the body to normality. According to traditional thought, the herbs were chosen to clear liver fire and damp. The patient was advised to be cautious about overworking.

IRRITABLE BOWEL SYNDROME

Female—30 years old

Complaint:

Diarrhoea with bleeding.

History:

Periodical abdominal pain for the past 5 years, leading to diarrhoea and bleeding. Symptoms were worse before the monthly periods. Pain was relieved by bowel motions. Pain occurred 2 to 3 times daily and exacerbated when she ate bread. Other symptoms included feeling tired; poor appetite; heavy periods and frequent absence from work. Sigmoidscopy; abdominal scan; gastroscopy; stool examination and a barium meal x-ray were carried out at the hospital. Blood tests showed slight anaemia. Was given a prescription of fybrogel and colprenrin. The symptoms remained the same.

On Examination:

Complexion was pale and dull. On the left side of the abdomen, a lump was felt which was about 3 inches long and was tender on palpation. Tongue—pale with a white coat. Pulse—small and slightly deep.

TCM Diagnosis:

Weakness of the spleen and stomach

Treatment:

Electro-acupuncture and moxibustion were used to strengthen the spleen and regulate the stomach with the following:

Points Used	Nerves Stimulated	TCM Explanations
Ah Shih points on abdomen		Reduces pain
Zusanli (St 36)	L4 – S3	Lower He-sea point of the stomach Meridian; regulates digestive system
Tianshu (St 25)	T7 – T12	Front Mu Point of the large intestine; regulates qi flow to strengthen function of spleen and large intestine; stops diarrhoea.
Shangjuxu (St 37)	L4 – S1	Lower He-Sea Point of the large intestine; regulate qi flow and the

Points Used	Nerves Stimulated	TCM Explanations
		function of the stomach and spleen; stops diarrhoea.
Pishu (UB 20)	T11 – T12	Back Shu point of the spleen; regulates and strengthens function of the spleen; specific for stopping diarrhoea
Weishu (UB 21)	T12 – L1	Back Shu point of the stomach; nourishes the digestive system; improves stomach yin; specific for relieving abdominal pain
Dachangshu (UB 25)	L4	Back Shu point of the large intestine; improves large intestine function: stops abdominal pain and helps bowel movements; specific for stopping diarrhoea
Ciliao (UB 32)	S2	Regulates lower jiao; improves large intestine function; stops abdominal pain and helps bowel movements.

The combination of points Dachangshu and Zusanli is effective in regulating the digestive system, relieve abdominal spasm and pain. After 5 treatments, the diarrhoea and bleeding and the size of the lump were reduced and the bleeding during the last period was less heavy. At the end of the fifth treatment, ear studs were left in on the stomach and large intestine points. The condition remained stable for the next 6 weeks without treatment. 2 more treatments were given after the 6 week break. Her bowel movement returned to normal, the bleeding had stopped and the lump on her abdomen could no longer be felt.

After an interval of 9 weeks, there was still no abdominal pain, bowel motions remained normal, but there was some bleeding and the lump had started to make an appearance. Her period was due in a few days. At this stage, the TCM diagnosis was changed to **Spleen and Kidney Yang Xu.**

The following point were used:

Points Used	Nerves Stimulated	TCM Explanations
Sanyingjiao (Sp 6)	L4 – S3	Crossing point of the spleen, liver and kidney Meridians; strengthens spleen and kidney functions; reinforces yin qi
Daheng (Sp 15)	T8 – T12	Front Mu point; warms the middle jiao to improve digestive function
Taichong (Liv 3)	L4 – S2	Shu-stream and Yuan-source point; Gate point; soothes the

		liver; regulates qi and activates blood
Shenshu (UB 23)	L1 – L3	Back Shu point of the kidney; strengthens kidney qi
Ciliao (UB 32)	S2	Strengthens the kidney qi

Corresponding Hua-tuo points can be used instead of points on the UB Meridian. 2 treatments were given per week for the following 4 weeks. All symptoms were generally reduced. Weekly treatments were given for the next 3 months. At the end of that period, all symptoms had disappeared and no more treatments were required.

Comments:

Needling at point Zusanli balances peristalsis via the vagal nerve activity through the anterior fibialis. Some studies had shown that this point can strengthen the immune system, reduce mucous discharge and inflammation.

IRRITABLE BOWEL SYNDROME—CASE 2

Female—24 years old

Complaint:

Abdominal pain and diarrhoea

History:

For the past 8 years, the patient had been suffering with immediate abdominal pain every time she ate a salad. This was then followed by diarrhoea. Recently, extra pressure at work had initiated the diarrhoea and sometimes constipation. Certain foods, such as bananas, onions, beans and cauliflower tended to exacerbate the symptoms. Appetite was normal. Periods were also normal. Had been investigated at the hospital. Tranquillizers were prescribed. These had no effect.

On Examination:

Patient appeared to be highly strung and sensitive. Tongue—normal. Pulse—wiry.

TCM Diagnosis:

Disharmony of spleen and liver

Treatment:

Points Used	Nerves Stimulated	TCM Explanations
Tianshu (St 25)	T7 − T12	Front Mu point; regulates qi flow to strengthen function of the spleen and the large intestine; stops diarrhoea
Shangjuxu (St 37)	L4 − S1	Lower He-sea point of the large intestine; regulates qi flow and the function of the stomach and the spleen; stops diarrhoea
Taichong (Liv 3)	L4 − S2	Shu-stream and Yuan-source point and Gate point; soothes the liver; regulates qi and activates blood
Dachangshu (UB 25)	L4	Back Shu point of the large intestine; improves the large intestine function; stops abdominal pain; helps bowel movements

| Ciliao (UB 32) | S2 | Regulates lower jiao; improves the large intestine function; stops abdominal pain and helps bowel movements |

Electro-acupuncture and moxibustion were used on the above points. Studs were left on ear points, Shenmen, kidney and liver. After 2 treatments, all symptoms were reduced. After 3 further treatments all symptoms had disappeared and no more treatment was required.

Comments:

Tianshu and Shangjuxu used in combination was observed in some studies to enhance phagocytosis and at the same time increase serum globulin which in turn has a positive effect on the immune system. Using Dachangshu with Tianshu seems to be effective in regulating the large intestine function.

HYPERTENSION

Female—38 years old

History:

Started to suffer with hypertension 6 months after the birth of the second child. The blood pressure was normal during the pregnancy and before the birth. The last reading was 130/95 mmHg. Had been feeling bad tempered. Palms and soles of feet felt hot. Suffered with insomnia. Periods were irregular. Headaches had become frequent and her mouth felt dry most of the time.

On Examination:

Blood pressure was 140/100 mmHg

TCM Diagnosis:

Liver Yang Excess

Treatment:

Electro-acupuncture and moxibustion were used on the following points:

Points Used	Nerves Stimulated	TCM Explanations
Fengchi (GB 20)	CrN. XI	Refreshes the mind; specific point for reducing fire; relieves headaches; reduces hypertension
Hegu (LI 4)	C6 – C7	Yuan-source point; tranquillises the mind; specific for relieving headaches; reduces fire
Neiguan (P 6) connecting to	C6 – T1	Luo-connecting point; confluent point for Yinwei; regulates qi; relieves mental stress
Waiguan (SJ 5)	C6 – C8	Luo-connecting point; confluent point for Yangwei; regulates qi; reduces fire
Sanyingjiao (Sp 6)	L4 – S3	Clears heat; nourishes the kidney, liver and spleen
Zusanli (St 36)	L4 – S3	He-sea point; clears heat; strengthens the body's resistance; restores normal function; reduces headaches and hypertension

Immediately after the treatment, the blood pressure reading was 130/100 mmHg.

For the next treatment, the above points were used with the addition of the following:

Xinshu (UB 15)	T3 – T5	Regulates Heart qi and the functions of the heart Meridian: relieves mental stress
Jueyinshu (UB 14)	T2 – T4	Regulates heart qi; specific for treating problems of the heart and Pericardium

After the treatment, the blood pressure reading was 130/90 mmHg. A total of 10 treatments were given. The BP was stabilised and the last reading was 130/85 mmHg.

A follow up, one year later found the blood pressure reading to be 160/90 mmHg. Treatment was given using the above prescription. The BP was 140/90 mmHg afterwards. Another treatment was given the following week, after which the reading was 130/85 mmHg. The patient was discharged.

HYPERTENSION—CASE 2

Female—54 years old

History:

There was a one year history of headaches, insomnia and irregular menstruation. The last blood pressure reading was 150/100 mmHg. Antihypertensive drugs were prescribed and taken without much effect. The patient had also stopped having periods. Headaches had increased and she had started to suffer with palpitations and feeling tired all the time. She had decided not to continue with the medication.

On Examination:

Complexion was slightly red. BP—140/100 mmHg. Tongue—slightly red with a white coat. Pulse—wiry.

TCM Diagnosis:

Disharmony of Chong and Ren Meridians

Treatment:

Electro-acupuncture and moxibustion were given using the following prescription:

Points Used	Nerves Stimulated	TCM Explanations
Zusanli (St 36)	L4 − S3	He-sea point; clears heat; strengthens the body's resistance; restores normal function; reduces headaches and hypertension
Neiguan (P 6)	C6 − T1	Luo-connecting point; confluent point; regulates qi; reduces fire
Hegu (LI 4)	C6 − C7	Yuan-source point; reduces fire and headaches; tranquillise the mind
Quchi (LI 11)	C5 − T1	He-sea point; regulates qi; promotes blood flow; reduces hypertension
Jueyinshu (UB 14)	T2 − T4	Regulates the heart qi; specific for treating problems with the heart
Xinshu (UB 15)	T3 − T5	Regulates Heart qi; regulates the function of the heart Meridian; relieves mental stress

Zhongwan (Ren 12) T7 – T12   One of the eight influential points
                                         effective for hypertension

Treatment was given once weekly. After 3 weeks, the BP was
140/90 mmHg.

After a further 7 sessions, the BP was 130/80 mmHg. No more
treatment was given.

HYPERTENSION—CASE 3

Male—67 years old

History:

For the previous few days, the patient was suffering with gradually worsening headaches with affected vision and dizziness. Palpitation was also present with shortness of breath and tightness of chest. At night, the frequency of micturation was in creased. The ECG reading revealed a sinus rhythm at a rate of 60/min. The tracing indicated a left bundle branch block. Tenomin 50 mg. and Navidrex K were prescribed. A chest x-ray was also suggestive of emphysema. The heart size was normal and there was no pulmonary congestion.

On Examination:

The BP—180/110. Nails were looking purplish. He felt cold in all 4 limbs. Tongue—red. Pulse—wiry, fast and small.

TCM Diagnosis:

Liver and Kidney Yin Xu

Treatment:

Points Used	Nerves Stimulated	TCM Explanations
Zusanli (St 36)	L4 – S3	He-sea point; clears heat; strengthens the body's resistance; restores normal function; reduces headaches and hypertension
Sanyingjiao (Sp 6)	L4 – S3	Clears heat; nourishes the kidney; liver and spleen
Xinshu (UB 15)	T3 – T5	Regulates the heart qi and the function of the heart Meridian; relieves mental stress
Jueyinshu (UB 14)	T2 – T4	Regulates the heart qi; specific for treating angina or other heart problems
Shenshu (UB 23)	L1 – L3	Strengthens the function of the kidney qi; improves acuity of vision; Back Shu point of the kidney
Fengchi (GB 20)	CrN. XI	Refreshes the mind; reduces the blood pressure

| Taixi (K 3) | L4 – S2 | Nourishes the yin; tonifies kidney; restores qi |

Electro-acupuncture and moxibustion were given using the above prescription. After the treatment, the BP reading was 160/100 mmHg. The purplish tone on the nails was much reduced.

10 weekly treatments were given. At the end of the course, the BP reading had stabilised to 135/80 mmHg.

Treatment was continued once every 2 or 3 months for the following 9 years. The blood pressure reading was maintained and the patient felt better all round.

ARRHYTHMIA

Female—33 years old

Complaint:

Palpitation

History:

The patient had been suffering from palpitation for the previous 8 months. There had been a lot of stress from the family and work. She had symptoms of dizziness, fullness of the chest, tiredness and irritability. The GP had diagnosed arrhythmia. The treatment with drugs had not produced a great improvement in the symptoms.

On Examination:

Complexion—pale and tired looking. No heart murmur. Heartbeat—irregular at 80/min. Tongue—red with a thin white coat. Pulse—irregular and small.

TCM Diagnosis:

Qi Yin Xu

Treatment:

Points Used	Nerves Stimulated	TCM Explanations
Shenmen (Ht 7)	C8 – T1	Shu-stream point and Yuan-source point; regulates heart qi; nourishes the Heart; calms the mind
Neiguan (P 6)	C6 – T1	Regulates qi to soothe the chest; regulates the heart beat; relaxes the mind and relieves stress
Jueyinshu (UB 14)	T2 – T4	Back Shu point of the Pericardium; regulates the function of the heart qi
Xinshu (UB 15)	T3 – T5	Back Shu point of the heart; regulates the heart; relieves mental stress

Treatment with electro-acupuncture and moxibustion was given once a week for 10 weeks. At the end of the course, the heart rate had returned to normal with no irregularity.

SMOKING ADDICTION

Male—58 years old

History:

The patient had been smoking 20 cigarettes a day for 25 years, after which he increased his intake to 50 per day for the following 10 years. Recently, he had increased his intake further to 80–100 per day. He was suffering from a chronic cough and bringing up yellow phelgm recently. This was diagnosed as chronic bronchitis by the GP. He was advised to stop smoking. He had used nicotine gum and then hypnosis with no effect. The GP had referred him for acupuncture although the patient had no confidence in the treatment.

On Examination:

There was a strong oral odour of nicotine and fingers were stained. Tongue—deep yellow coat.

TCM Diagnosis:

Stomach & lung heat

Treatment:

Only electro-acupuncture was used on the following points:

Points Used	Nerves Stimulated	TCM Explanations
Hegu (LI 4)	C6 – T1	Yuan-source point; reduce damp heat; clears channel
Lieque (Lu 7)	C5 – T1	Luo-connecting point; one of the eight confluent points between lung and Ren channels; ventilate lung to expel wind; clears and activate channels
Zusanli (St 36)	L4 – S3	He-Sea Point; clear stomach heat & channels; strengthen spleen; reduce phelgm; reinforce qi and blood; strengthen body's resistence; restore normal function

In addition, the ear was needled at points lung; stomach; shenmen and endocrine.

Ear studs were left on points lung and stomach.

The patient was able to stop after the one treatment. He was advised to have one more treatment on the following week. His sense of smell and taste improved.

Comments:

In a chronic smoker, it had been found that the levels of adrenaline, nor-adrenaline, endorphine, dopamine and ACTH are higher than in non-smokers. The acupuncture probably helped the patient by normalising these levels. Some research had also confirmed that chronic smokers have a reduced sense of taste. In a clinical study done by Dr. Cheung on a group of 615 patients (male—263, female—352) with ages ranging from 18 years upwards, the overall success rate in stopping smoking with the help of acupuncture equals 60.47%. The number of sessions in this study ranged from 1–5.

ALCOHOLISM

Male—50 years old

Complaint:

The patient had spent most of the past 20 years in a drunken stupor.

History:

The patient was single and worked as a security guard at night. He did not have any social life or any close friends or relatives. He would drink excessively on his days off and especially during his holidays. He consumed at least one litre of whisky a day. Consequently, his appetite was poor.

On Examination:

Red complexion. Behaviour normal. Gait, unsteady. Tongue—red with thick yellow greasy coat. Pulse—fast.

TCM Diagnosis:

Liver and gall bladder damp heat

Treatment:

Acupuncture and moxibustion were given on the following points:

Points Used	Nerves Stimulated	TCM Explanations
Riyue (GB 24)	T7 – T12	Clear liver & gall bladder heat; Front Mu point of gall bladder
Qimen (Liv 14)	T6 – T12	Clear liver & gall bladder heat; Front Mu point of liver; promote blood circulation; disperse dampness
Zhongwan (Ren 12)	T7 – T12	Front Mu point of stomach; regulate function of the stomach to strengthen function of the spleen to remove dampness
Shangwan (Ren 13)	T7 – T12	Regulate function of stomach to strengthen spleen function to remove dampness
Zusanli (St 36)	L4 – S3	Resolve phelgm; clear heat; He-sea point; strengthen spleen; reduce dampness

Yanglingquan (GB 34)	L4 – S1	He-sea point; remove dampness; soothe liver and gall bladder

The ear was also needled at points Alcoholism and Liver. Ear studs were placed at these points.

After the session, the patient was able to walk more steadily. 3 more treatments were given. His tongue colour returned to normal and he was able to stop drinking.

HEROIN ADDICTION

Male—27 years old

Complaint:

3 year history of heroin inhalation.

History:

Was introduced to heroin by friends. Started with a small dose but for the past year had needed at least 1 gram a day. He needed the drug at least once every hour. He had been feeling depressed, tired, lethargic and experiencing an increase in the frequency of micturation. This was beginning to impair his efficiency at work and there was a danger of being sacked.

On Examination:

He had a weary appearance with a pale complexion and pale lips. Tongue—pale with a thick white coat. Pulse—slow.

TCM Diagnosis:

Spleen and Kidney Xu

Treatment:

Acupuncture and moxibustion was used according to the following:

Plan 1

Points Used	*Nerves Stimulated*	*TCM Explanations*
Sanyingjiao (Sp 6)	L4 − S3	Strengthen the spleen and stomach; reinforce liver and kidney; nourish yin.
Zusanli (St 36)	L4 − S3	Nourish qi + blood; reinforce liver and kidney; He-sea point
Hegu (LI 4)	C6 − T1	Yuan Source point and Gate point
Sanyangluo (SJ 8)	C6 − C8	Relief pain; increase yang qi
Taixi (K 3)	L2 − S3	Shu-stream and Yuan-source point; tonify kidney; restore qi
Shenshu (UB 23)	L1 − L3	Back Shu point of the kidney; strengthens function of kidney qi

In addition, the ear was needled at point Shenmen and Lung.

Plan 2

Sanyingjiao (Sp 6)	L4 – S3	Strengthen the spleen and stomach; reinforce liver + kidney; nourish yin
Zusanli (St 36)	L4 – S3	Nourish qi and blood; reinforce liver + kidney He-sea point
Fengchi (GB 20)	CrN XI	Refresh the mind
Neiguan (P 6)	C6 – T1	Luo-connecting point; regulate qi; specific for gastro-intestinal disturbance; relieve mental stress
Taixi (K 3)	L2 – S3	Shu-stream and Yuan-source point; tonify kidney; restore qi
Shenshu (UB 23)	L1 – L3	Back Shu point of the kidney; strengthens function of kidney qi
Shenmen (Ht 7)	C8 – T1	Shu-stream and Yuan source point; nourich and regulate heart qi; relieve anxiety

Ear points, Lung; Shenmen and Stomach was used in Plan 2

Treatment was given daily, alternating the above plans. The patient was able to gradually reduce the intake of the heroin. After 14 days, he was able to function without any heroin.

CHOCOLATE ADDICTION

Female—32 years old

Complaint:

No control over amount of chocolate eaten daily.

History:

Over the last 10 years, the patient had been consuming 1 lb. of chocolate a day. She had used hypnosis and tranquillisers without any benefit.

On Examination:

The patient appeared to be overweight. Otherwise, her general health was satisfactory. Tongue—thick yellow coat. Pulse—normal.

TCM Diagnosis:

Damp with phlegm

Treatment:

Acupuncture and moxibustion were given on the following points:

Points Used	Nerves Stimulated	TCM Explanations
Hegu (LI 4)	C6 – T1	Yuan-source point; Gate point; eliminates damp
Taiyuan (Lu 9)	C6 – C7	Resolves phlegm; Shu-stream point; Yuan-source point; one of the 8 influential points
Zusanli (St 36)	L4 – S3	He-sea point; strengthens the spleen; reduces phlegm
Fenglong (St 40)	L4 – S1	Luo-connecting point; regulates spleen to remove damp; regulates stomach to reduce phlegm

A total of 4 weekly sessions were given, after which the patient appeared to be in complete control.

5 years later, while out in New Zealand, the patient had a relapse. Treatment with acupuncture in New Zealand was unsuccessfull. On her return, she came for treatment again. That time, the patient regained control of the habit after only 2 sessions.

PSORIASIS

Single Female—18 years old

Complaint:

Peeling and scaling of skin in both knees, elbows and scalp.

History:

Had been suffering with psoriasis since the age of 14. In addition, she was also having emotional problems leading to depression and quickness of temper. Recently, the silvery scales on the anterior part of the lower leg and the lateral side of the upper arms had got worse. Her father and sister also suffer with psoriasis.

On Examination:

Lesions were bright red, with sharply outlined plaques covered with silvery scales. These were concentrated round both knees and elbows and the anterior part of the lower legs. Small papules were on the posterior part of the arms. Appetite was poor. Tongue—red with smooth coat. Pulse—wiry + fast.

TCM Diagnosis:

Blood Heat

Treatment:

Acupuncture was given on the following points:

Points Used	Nerves Stimulated	TCM Explanations
Xuehai (Sp 10)	L2 – L4	Activates blood; remove damp; clears heat
Fengchi (GB 20)	CrN. XI	Activates blood; reduce fire; relieves stagnation; calms the mind
Quichi (LI 11)	C5 – T1	He-sea point of the LI channel; activates blood; clears heat
Neiguan (P 6)	C6 – T1	Sedation; luo-connecting point; one of the 8 confluent points

The following herbs were given in addition to acupuncture. Each prescription was to be taken for 2 days.

Bai Xian Pi	(Cortex Dictamni Radicis)
Huang Qin	(Radix Scutellariae)

Bai Shao	(Radix Paeoniae Alba)
Sheng Di	(Radix Rehamanniae)
Fang feng	(Radix Ledebouriellae)
Wei Ling	(Herba Potentillae Chinensis)
Jing Jie	(Herba schizonepetae)
Gan Cao	(Radix Glycyrrhizae)

A course of 10 weekly sessions of acupuncture were given. At the end of the 6th session, normal skin had begun to appear inside the lesions, and her depression had begun to lift. There was a break for treatment for a week before the start of another course of 10 treatments. At the end of the second course, the patient was well enough for treatment to stop.

Comments:

Some research have shown that needling the above points helped to improve the circulation especially the micro-circulation to the skin. Stimulation of the points also provided an anti-inflammatory effect. Some studies have also shown that needling Neiguan would have a positive effect on the immune system by increasing brain LEK + reducing adrenal medullar LEK.

There is no permanent cure for Psoriasis. There is a possibility of recurrence. When this happens, treatment can resume.

PSORIASIS—CASE 2

Female—30 years old

Complaint:

Itchy, peeling skin

History:

Started to have symptoms of psoriasis from age 16 at both elbows, dorsum of hands, both knees and along the shin bones and dorsum of feet near the ankles. At the age of one, she developed eczema which troubled her only temporarily. The patient was vegetarian but enjoyed spicy food. Her periods were irregular with occasional constipation. There was no family history of psoriasis or eczema. Was prescribed steroids but with no results.

On Examination:

Had a reddish complexion. Skin looked red with silver scales. There were columns of darker red skin between the index and ring finger and the little finger. The skin in the area of the shin bones was light red with silver scales and a source of irritation. The skin between the lateral malleolus and medial malleolus was dark red with silver scales.

TCM Diagnosis:

Blood Heat

Treatment:

Electro-acupuncture was used on the following:

Points Used	Nerves Stimulated	TCM Explanations
Dubi (St 35)	L3	Local point of knees
Xiyan (ext. pt.)	L3	Local point of knees
Taichong (Liv 3)	L4 – S2	Remove heat from liver
Shousanli (LI 10)	C5 – C8	Local point; clears heat
Tianjing (SJ 10)	C5 – C8	Local point; clears heat

Treatment was given once weekly. On the third week, growth of normal skin was observed. The points prescription was changed to the following:

Dubi; Xiyan; Taichong; Tianjing and the following added:

Zusanli (St 36)	L4 – S3	He-sea point; enrich blood + qi; restores normal function of body

Yanglingquan (GB 34)	L4 – S1	Reduce heat
Jiaxi (St 41)	L4 – S1	Removes damp; reduce heat
Fuliu (K 7)	L4 – S2	Removes heat
Mingmen (Du 4)	L2	

Ext. Point between 2nd and 3rd metatarsal bone.

This prescription was used for the following 6 weeks. The condition of the skin gradually improved over this period. At the end of the six weeks the skin over the elbows was completely normal. Over the shin bone, normal skin was starting to appear and the area over the dorsum of hand and foot was looking much lighter. For the next 3 weeks, the following points were used: Dubi; Xiyan; Taichong; Tianjing; Yanglingquan; Jiaxi; Fuliu. The following 4 weeks, the patient was unable to come for treatment as a result of flu. During this period, the area over the shin bone, elbow and lumbar area started to have raised skin and 2 spots appeared on the face. The following points were added to the last prescription:

Fengchi (GB 20)	CrN. XI	Sedation; reduce fire and wind
Shenshu (UB 23)	L1 – L3	Back shu point of the kidney; improve function of kidney qi
Mingmen (Du 4)	L2	Local point; regulate force of qi
Ciliao (UB 32)	S2	Clear lower jiao damp-heat; improve function of LI

Treatment was then continued for 4 weeks. The spots on the face cleared, and the skin over the lumbar area improved.

URTICARIA

Female—28 years old

Complaint:

Patient had been suffering with urticaria for the past 2 years.

History:

The urticaria was triggered off by nervous tension. Her skin started to take on a reddish colour and itchy spots appearing, ranging from pin-point areas to larger ones. Tranquillisers were prescribed with good effect initially. The problem had started to worsen. Did not appear to be linked with diet but sunshine aggravated the itching. There was no family history.

On Examination:

Irritable spots were found on the front and back of the trunk and on all four limbs. Tongue—red with a yellow thin coat. Pulse—small.

TCM Diagnosis:

Wind Heat

Treatment:

Electroacupuncture was used on the following points:

Points Used	Nerves Stimulated	TCM Explanations
Neiguan (P 6)	C6–T1	Luo-connecting Point; regulates qi; relieves mental stress
Shenmen (Ht 7)	C8–T1	Shu-stream point; Yuan-souce point; reduces fire; tranquilise the mind; reduce anxiety
Xuehai (SP 10)	L2–L4	Activates blood to remove heat; clears blood heat
Fengchi (GB 20)	CrN. XI	Reduces wind; pacify fire; calms the mind
Feishu (UB 13)	T3–T4	Back shu point of the lung; regulates lung qi; reduces fire; nourishes yin

4 weekly sessions were given, after which symptoms were reduced but itchiness was still present. The following herbs were then prescribed in addition to acupuncture treatment.

Xu Zhu	(Rhizome Polygonati Adorati)
Sheng Di	(Radix Rehmanniae)
Huang Qi	(Radix Scutellariae)
Bai Xian Pi	(Cortex Dictamui Radicis)
Fang Feng	(Radix Ledehouriellae)
Tu Fu Ling	(Rhizoma Smilacix Glabrae)
Ji Li	(Fructus Tribuli)
Gan Cao	(Radix Glycyurrhizae)

The herbs were taken daily for the next 2 weeks including weekly sessions of acupuncture. Moxibustion was also used on some of the points. The urticaria stopped.

ECZEMA

Female—66 years old

History:

Suffering with eczema on both palms. Cortisone therapy had only a temporary effect.

On Examination:

Skin on both palms red and itchy. Tongue—red with a slight yellow coat.

TCM Diagnosis:

Damp Heat

Treatment:

Electro-acupuncture was used on the following points:

Points Used	Nerves Stimulated	TCM Explanations
Quchi (LI 11)	C5–T1	He-sea point; Expels wind; clears heat; regulates qi; promotes blood circulation; clears lung heat
Chize (Lu 5)	C5–C8	He-sea point; clears lung heat
Hegu (LI 4)	C6–T1	Reduces fire; tranquillises the mind
Shenmen (Ht 7)	C8–T1	Shu-stream and Yuan-source point; reduces fire; tranquillises the mind
Sanyingjiao (Sp 6)	L4–S3	Reduces heat; nourishes lung
Xuehai (Sp 10)	L2–L4	Regulates qi; activates blood; reduces wind and damp; clears heat
Fengchi (GB 20)	CrN. XI	Clears heat; disperses wind; activates channels

Ear points, Shenmen and Lung were also used.
After 5 weekly sessions, the following prescription of herbs was given in conjunction with the acupuncture.

Bai Xian Pi	(Cortex Dictamni)
Ji Li	(Fructus Tribuli)
Fang Feng	(Radix Ledebouriellae)
Jing Jie	(Herba Schizonepetae)
Dan Pi	(Cortex Moutan Radicis)
Chi Shao	(Radix Paeoniae Rubra)

Bai Zhi	(Radix Angelicae Dahuricae)
Huang Qin	(Radix Scutellariae)
Gan Cao	(Radix Glycyrrhizae)

3 prescriptions were given per week. Each prescription to be used for two days. At the same time the following herbs were used as a poultice:

Ku Shen	(Radix Sophorae Flavescentis)
Huang Bo	(Cortex Phellodendri)
Hua Jiao	(Paericarpium Zanthoxyli)
Dan Zhu Ye	(Herba Lophatheri)

After 4 weeks of acupuncture and herbs, the itching was reduced and there was less splitting of the skin.

The herbal prescription was modified.

Bai Xian Pi	(Cortex Dictamni Radicis)
Ji Li	(Fructus Tribuli)
Fang Feng	(Radix Ledebouriellae)
Jing Jie	(Herba Schizonepetae)
Gan Cao	(Radix Glycyrrhizae)
Dan Zhu Ye	(Herba Lophatheri)
Bai Shao	(Radix Paeoniae Alba)
Sheng Di	(Radix Rehmanniae)
Mu Tong	(Caulis Akebiae)

The following accompanying poultice was given:

Ku Shen	(Radix Sophorae Flavescentis)
Huang Lian	(Rhizoma Coptidis)
Fang Feng	(Radix Ledebouriellae)

Similarly, each prescription was used for 2 days, 3 prescriptions per week, together with weekly acupuncture.

After 2 weeks, the skin was still itchy, but normal in appearance. Wei Ling Cai (Herba Potentillae Chinensis) was added to the above herbal prescription. Fang Feng was removed from the poultice prescription and replaced with Deng Xin Hua (Junais Efusus).

After 2 weeks of this treatment, the skin felt normal again and treatment was stopped.

ACNE

Male—26 years old

Complaint:

Suffering with acne since 11 years old.

History:

15 years ago, papular eruptions and papulopustules started appearing on the face and the upper dorsal trunk. The discharge was white or yellow in appearance and black heads were present. Skin tended to be greasy. Tends to be worse with the intake of spicy food. He suffered the occasional bout of constipation.

On Examination:

Tongue—red with yellow greasy coat. Pulse—slippery and fast.

TCM Diagnosis:

Fei Wei Damp Heat

Treatment:

Electro-acupuncture was used on the following:

Points Used	Nerves Stimulated	TCM Explanations
Dazhui (Du 14)	C3; C4; C8; CrN. XI	Clears wind heat; nourishes yin
Xuehai (Sp 10)	L2–L4	Activates blood; removes wind and dampness; clears blood heat
Yinglingquan (Sp 9)	L3–S2	Strengthens spleen; removes dampness; clears heat; He-sea point
Zusanli (St 36)	L4–S3	He-sea point; clears stomach heat; removes wind; activates blood
Fengchi (GB 20)	CrN. XI	Clears heat; removes wind; activates blood
Hegu (LI 4)	C6–T1	Yuan-source point; removes wind and heat; specific for facial problems
Quchi (LI 11)	C5–T1	He-sea point; removes wind heat and dampness
Feishu (UB 13)	T3–T4	Back shu point of the lung; clears lung heat; regulates lung qi; nourishes yin

| Weishu (UB 21) | T12–L1 | Back shu point of the stomach; removes damp; regulates stomach function |

Yinglingquan and Zusanli together clears damp heat from spleen and stomach. Hegu and Quchi together reduces yang-ming wind-heat.

Weekly treatments were given for 4 weeks. The patient had a complete recovery.

Comments:

Hegu, Quchi and Dazhui have antibacterial and anti-inflammatory functions as well as raising immune functions.

ACNE—CASE 2

Female—25 years old

Complaint:

Had been suffering with acne for the past 8 years.

History:

Started menstruating at 11 years old. Acne appeared at age 13. Eruptions were intermittent and worse before and during menses during which time papulopastules would be present. Periods were irregular with clots. Patient had an affinity for greasy and fried food, which tended to make the skin worse. Bowel and digestive functions were normal.

On Examination:

The skin looked dull and filled with tuberculae, with papuloeruptions and papulopustules. The facial skin also looked greasy. Tongue—dull red with blood spots. Pulse—slow.

TCM Disgnosis:

Blood Stagnation

Treatment:

Electro-acupuncture was used on the following points:

Points Used	Nerves Stimulated	TCM Explanations
Sanyingjiao (Sp 6)	L4–S3	Crossing point of 3 yin channels; strengthens spleen + stomach; reinforces liver + kidney; clears heat
Hegu (LI 4)	C6–T1	Yuan-source point; removes wind and heat
Jiache (St 6)	CrN 7	Regulates qi flow
Zusanli (St 36)	L4–S3	He-sea point; clears St. heat; removes dampness; strengthens spleen
Xuehai (Sp 10)	L2–L4	Activates blood; clears blood heat
Taixi (K 3)	L4–S2	Shu-stream + yuan source point; nourishes yin
Zhongji (Ren 3)	T6–T12	Regulates Chong and Ren Mai

| Feishu (UB 13) | T3–T4 | Back shu point of the lung; activates blood; reduces stagnation; nourishes yin; moisturises facial skin |
| Pishu (UB 21) | T11–T12 | Back shu point of the spleen; activates blood; reduces stagnation; nourishes yin; moisturises facial skin |

Sanyingjiao and Zhongji in combination helps to drive qi and blood downwards.

A total of 6 weekly treatments were given and the patient had a complete recovery.

222 Mechanism of Acupuncture Therapy and Clinical Case Studies

NEURO-DERMATITIS

Female—45 years old

Complaint:

The skin of the palm on the left had been dry and rough.

History:

2 years previously, the patient was starting to suffer with anxiety as a result of stress at work. The skin of the left palm gradually become thicker, itchy and appeared redder than the right palm. Cortisone cream was prescribed, but was only effective temporarily. Sedatives were also prescribed. Again, the effect of these were only short term.

On Examination:

The skin on affected palm was dry, red, rough and thick. There was no scaling. Tongue—pale with white coat. Pulse—small.

TCM Diagnosis:

Blood Xu with Wind Dryness.

Treatment:

Electro-acupuncture was given on the following points:

Points Used	Nerves Stimulated	TCM Diagnosis
Neiguan (P 6)	C7–T1	Reduces stress
Shenmen (Ht 7)	C8–T1	Shu-stream + Yuan-source point; relieves dryness; clears Ht. fire; sedates
Xuehai (Sp 10)	L2–L4	Activates blood and clears the heat
Quchi (LI 11)	C5–T1	He-sea point; clears wind heat; regulates qi; promotes blood circulation;
Zusanli (St 36)	L4–S3	He-sea point; enriches the blood + qi; restores normal function of the body

Treatment was given on alternate days for 2 weeks and the patient was well enough for treatment to stop.

NEURO-DERMATITIS—CASE 2

Male—30 years old

Complaint:

Rough skin all over.

History:

Patient had been suffering with stress at work for a long time. One year previous, itchy patches, each the size of a 50p coin were appearing on the neck, elbows and in the popliteal fossa on both sides. These gradually increased in size especially when the level of stress increased or whenever consumption of alcohol was over a certain limit. He usually experienced dryness of the mouth. Appetite appeared to be normal.

On Examination:

The skin on the right side of the neck was rough, thick and red in an area of about 2 inches long by 1 inch wide. Similar patches about the size of a 10p coin, were also found in the inner canthus of the eyes, elbows and in the popliteal fosse. The skin looked dry throughout. Tongue—red with a thin yellow coat. Pulse—slippery and fast.

TCM Diagnosis:

Blood Heat producing Wind

Treatment:

Points for electro-acupuncture were chosen particularly according to the nerve supply.

Points Used	Nerves Stimulated	TCM Explanations
Quchi (LI 11)	C5–T1	Expels wind; clears heat; regulates qi; promotes blood flow
Xuehai (Sp 10)	L2–L4	Clears blood heat; activates blood to clear wind
Weizhong (UB 40)	L4–S2	Removes pathogenic heat from blood
Zusanli (St 36)	L4–S3	Clears heat; strengthens body resistence; He-sea point
Fengchi (GB 20)	CrN. XI	Expels wind and reduces fire
Jianjing (GB 21)	CrN. XI	Expels wind and reduces fire

A total of 15 weekly treatments were given and the patient had a complete recovery.

DYSMENORRHOEA

Female—30 years old

Complaint:

Had been suffering with dysmenorrhoea for more than 10 years.

History:

Had her first menstruation at age 13, then the next period was not until a year later. Since then her cycle tended to be 30 to 35 days. Her periods would last 7 days with heavy bleeding. From the age of 17, she would have lower abdominal pain and backache at the start of each period lasting 3 days. Analgesia was prescribed but with poor. From 18 years of age, she started on the contraceptive pill until 2 years ago. During the time relief she was on the pill, there was no pain during her cycle. Her pains had returned to trouble her at the start of each period and were now usually accompanied by vomiting. Bleeding would be dark red with clots. These symptoms would lessen by the third day.

On Examination:

The patient carried a painful expression. She had pain in the lower abdomen which was too tender for palpation. Her breasts were swollen and painful. Bleeding had been heavy, with clots. Tongue—dull red. Pulse—wiry.

TCM Diagnosis:

Qi and Blood Stagnation

Treatment:

Electro-acupuncture and moxibustion were used on the following:

Points Used	Nerves Stimulated	TCM Explanations
Zhongji (Ren 3)	T6–T12	Front mu point of the urinary bladder; regulates Chong and Ren channels
Qihai (Ren 6)	T6–T12	Tonifies kidney qi
Sanyingjiao (Sp 6)	L4–S3	Crossing point of 3 yin channels; tonifies yin; pacifies yang; reinforces liver and kidney; resoves stagnation
Xuehai (Sp 10)	L2–L4	Activates blood; resolves stagnation; regulates qi

| Shenshu (UB 23) | L1–L3 | Back shu point of the kidney; strengthens function of kidney qi |
| Ciliao (UB 2) | S2 | Strengthens kidney; regulates menstruation |

Treatment was given for 3 days consecutively before the start of the period. After 4 months, the patient had recovered.

Comments:

Stimulating the sacrum plexus of nerves probably improved the general circulation as well as the micro-circulation to the reproductive system, thus influencing the balance of hormones and reducing pain.

DYSFUNCTIONAL UTERINE BLEEDING

Female—43 years old

Complaint:

Irregular heavy periods.

History:

The patient started menstruation at age 15. The cycles vary between 21 to 45 days. Each time the bleeding lasted for about 7 days and the discharge was deep red. Her period started 6 weeks ago. It was heavy with a deep red colour and thin. She felt cold, especially in the four limbs and a soreness in the lumbar region. This was the pattern over the past year. Each time, progesterone was taken and this was effective in reducing the discomfort and duration of bleeding, until recent months when bleeding had been heavy with all the accompanying pain and progesterone had been ineffective.

On Examination:

She had a pale complexion and appeared tired. Her bleeding had been continuous. She had to use a few boxes of tampons each day and was forced to stay in doors and in bed lying on incontinent pads. Tongue—pale. Pulse—weak.

TCM Diagnosis:

Shen Xu

Treatment:

Electro-acupuncture and moxibustion were given on the following points:

Points Used	Nerves Stimulated	TCM Explanations
Guanyuan (Ren 4)	T6–T12	Front mu point; specific for irregular menstruation and gynaecological problems; tonifies kidney; reinforces source qi
Zhongji (Ren 3)	T6–T12	Front mu point; tonifies kidney function; regulates Zhong and Ren channels; specific for gynaecological problems
Zigong (ext. pt.)	T7–T12	Specific point for problems relating to the uterus

Sanyingjiao (Sp 6)	L4–S3	Reinforces liver and kidney; specific for gynaecological problems
Ciliao (UB 32)	S2	Strengthens kidney; regulates menstruation
Shenshu (UB 23)	L1–L3	Back shu poinst of the kidney; strengthens kidney qi
Taixi (K 3)	L4–S2	Shu-stream and yuan-source point; nourishes yin; tonifies kidney; restores qi
Kunlun (UB 60)	L5–S2	Jing-river point; strengthens kidney function

Point Taixi is needled through to Kunlun. Ear points were also used on Uterus and Endocrine.

After the first treatment, the bleeding reduced. The next five treatments were given at home by which time she was able to attend the surgery. Treatment was given twice a week for the next three weeks then once a week for the following four weeks. The patient recovered completely even after a follow-up 3 years later.

Comment:

The aim of the treatment was to stimulate normal ovulation and regulate the reproductive hormones. It had succeeded well in this case.

INFERTILITY

Female—36 years old

Complaint:

Unable to conceive

History:

Had been married for 3 years and unable to conceive so far. Twice in the past 2 years she had experienced abdominal pain and discomfort during intercourse while in the middle of her cycle. She had a 28–30 day cycle. Bleeding usually lasted 4–5 days, with no clots but a deep red colour and not heavy. The first day of the period is usually painful. All investigations had shown no abnormality.

On Examination:

Tongue—slight purplish with a white coat. Pulse—deep and wiry.
TCM Explanations:
Blood and Qi Stagnation

Treatment:

Electro-acupuncture and moxibustion were used on the following points:

Points Used	Nerves Stimulated	TCM Explanations
Zhongji (Ren 3)	T6–T12	Front mu point; specific for gynaecological problems; tonifies kidney; reinforces souce qi
Guanyuan (Ren 4)	T6–T12	Tonifies kidney and reinforces source qi
Sanyingjiao (Sp 6)	L4–S3	Reinforces source qi and the function of liver and kidney
Zigong (ext. pt.)	T7–T12	Tonifies the kidney and its function
Xuehai (Sp 10)	L2–L4	Regulates qi and blood circulation; regulates the function of the lower jiao
Ciliao (UB 32)	S2	Strengthens the kidney; regulates menstrual functions

Ear points were also used on Uterus and Endocrine.
Only one treatment was given. 9 months later the patient gave birth to a baby boy.

INFERTILITY—CASE 2

Female—39 years old

Complaint:

Unable to conceive.

History:

The patient fell pregnant 15 years ago but was not ready for a baby, so she had a DNC. Since then she had been unable to conceive. Investigations had shown one blocked fallopian tube and the other was oedematous. She opted for IVF and had a few unsuccessful attempts, each time the uterus was unable to retain the fertilised egg. Her cycle lasted 24–28 days with a 3 day duration of menses. She started menstruating at age 13. Menses were normal with no clots or discomfort.

On Examination:

Tongue—slightly pale with a thin white coat. Pulse—deep.

TCM Diagnosis:

Kidney Xu

Treatment:

Electro-acupuncture and moxibustion were given on the following points in the middle of her cycle on 3 consecutive days:

Points Used	Nerves Stimulated	TCM Explanations
Zhongji (Ren 3)	T6–T12	Front mu point of the urinary bladder; regulates Chong and Ren channels
Qugu (Ren 2)	T6–T12	Tonifies kidney qi; regulates menses
Zigong (ext. pt.)	T7–T12	Tonifies function of kidney qi; reinforces the liver and kidney; regulates Chong and Ren channels; nourishes the uterus
Sanyingjiao (Sp 6)	L4–S3	Reinforces source qi; reinforces the kidney
Taichong (liv 3)	L4–S2	Shu-stream and Yuan-source point of the liver; Gate point

Ciliao (UB 32)	S2	Strengthens the kidney; regulates menses
Shenshu (UB 23)	L1–L3	Back shu point of the kidney; strengthens kidney qi

The same course of treatment was given for four months. In the fourth month, follicles were found to be much larger than before during routine checks at the IVF clinic. Their sizes had not changed during hormone therapy before acupuncture was given. Thus there was a better prospect of getting good healthy eggs. The final outcome of this case was not known.

Comments:

Acupuncture probably stimulated the hypothalamus which is the link between the pituitary and the ovaries thus causing a change in FSH levels to improve follicular size.

INFERTILITY—CASE 3

Female—38 years old

Complaint:

Had not been able to conceive since 2 miscarriages.

History:

Normally enjoys good health. The first miscarriage was at 4 weeks, the second at 16 weeks. Had a 25+ days menstrual cycle, bleeding lasting 3–4 days with no dysmenorrhoea or clots. Was prescribed hormone therapy. All investigations showed no abnormality. A year had passed since her last miscarriage.

On Examination:

It had been 10 days from the end of her last period. Tongue—slightly red. Pulse—small.

TCM Diagnosis:

Shen Yin Xu

Treatment:

The following points were chosen for electro-acupuncture and moxibustion:

Points Used	Nerves Stimulated	TCM Explanations
Zhongji (Ren 3)	T6–T12	Front mu point of the urinary bladder; regulates Chong and Ren channels
Qugu (Ren 2)	T6–T12	Tonifies kidney; regulates menstruation
Zigong (ext. pt.)	T7–T12	Tonifies kidney; regulates menstruation
Sanyingjiao (Sp 6)	L4–S3	Indicated in infertility; reinforces kidney and spleen; regulates Chong and Ren channels; nourishes uterus
Yinglingquan (Sp 9)	L3–S2	He-sea point; reinforces spleen
Hiatus (ext. pt.)	S4	Tonifies function of kidney to regulate menses
Mingmen (Du 4)	L2	Regulates flow of qi; reinforces yang; strengthens life's essence

Ciliao (UB 32)	S2	Strengthens the kidney; regulates menses
Zhongliao (UB 33)	S3	Strengthens the kidney; regulates menses
Dachangshu (UB 25)	L4	Back shu point of the large intestine; regulates qi function; relieves stagnation in the abdomen

Treatment was given daily for 14 days from the middle of the period. On the third month, the following changes were made to the prescription:

Yinglingquan, Qugu and Dachangshu were omitted and the following substituted:

Taixi (K 3)	L4–S2	Shu-stream and yuan-source point; norishes yin to reduce pathogical factors; tonifies kidney to restore qi; regulates menses
Guanyuan (Ren 4)	T6–T12	Tonifies kidney; reinforces source qi; regulates menses and female fertility

After needling with the new prescription for 2 days, tests showed that the luteinising hormone levels had increased. The following month, ear points were added at Qicong, Endocrine and Uterus. Ear studs were also left in these points after needling. Tests also showed an increase in luteinising hormone levels. Treatment was stopped and the case was not followed up.

PRE MATURE EJACULATION

Male—60 years old

History:

Had a long history of premature ejaculation but had got worse recently. Had to rely on drugs to sleep. Was given injections which only had a temporary effect. Suffering with depression as a result.

On Examination:

Looking tired. Tongue—pale with white coat. Pulse—small

TCM Diagnosis:

Qi and Blood Xu

Treatment:

The following points were chosen for electro-acupuncture and moxibustion:

Points Used	Nerves Stimulated	TCM Explanations
Qugu (Ren 2)	T6–T12	Tonifies kidney; specific for premature ejaculation
Zhongji (Ren 3)	T6–T12	Regulates Chong and Ren channels; specific for premature ejaculation
Mingmen (Du 4)	L2	Regulates qi flow; strengthens essence of life; reinforces yang; specific for premature ejaculation
Hiatus (Ext. pt.)	S4	Tonifies kidney;
Sanyingjiao (Sp 6)	L4–S3	Nourishes yin; pacifies yang; reinforces spleen and liver, blood and qi; specific for problems related to the genitalia
Shenshu (UB 23)	L1–L3	Strengthens kidney function; improve sexual essence; helps sexual function
Yinglingquan (Sp 9)	L3–S2	Reinforces xu and sexual essence and helps sexual function

Ear points were used on Testes and Endocrine.

Treatment was given twice weekly. After three weeks, there was a slight improvement. Shenshu and Yinglingquan were removed from the prescription and the following added:

Ciliao (UB 32)	S2	Reinforces kidney and liver; specific for problems involving the genitals
Zhongliao (UB 33)	S3	Reinforces kidney and liver; increases seminal essence

Treatment was continued twice weekly and after 4 weeks, the patient was making good progress. Treatment was then reduced to once weekly. After a further 6 weeks the patient felt well enough for treatment to stop.

PRE-MENSTRUAL TENSION

Female—36 years old

Complaint:

Suffered with depression before periods.

History:

The PMT had been going on for a few years. Each time before the start of a period, she would feel very emotional, depressed and would ache round her temples. Her breasts would feel swollen and achey. Legs and arms would also feel swollen and she would not be able to sleep. There would also be a bitter taste in her mouth. As soon as the period started, all symptoms disappear except for some abdominal pain. Periods were irregular with clots. Appetite was poor and there was frequency of micturation especially during the night,

On Examination:

The patient was very weepy. It was about 4 days before her period was due. She felt depressed. Her breasts were tender even on slight touch. Fingers were swollen. Tongue—red with a thin white coat. Pulse—wiry.

TCM Diagnosis:

Gan Qi and Blood Stagnation

Electro-acupuncture and moxibustion were used on the following points:

Points Used	Nerves Stimulated	TCM Explanations
Neiguan (P 6)	C6–T1	Lower connecting point; regulates qi; relieves mental stress
Taiyang (ext. pt.)	CrN. V + VII	Calms the mind; reduces headache
Hegu (LI 4)	C6–T1	Yuan-source point; tranquillises the mind; reduces pain
Sanyingjiao (Sp 6)	L4–S3	Crossing point of 3 yin channels; reinforces liver and kidney qi; strengthens spleen; calms the mind
Zhongji (Ren 3)	T6–T12	Regulates Chong and Ren channels; regulates micturation;

		front mu point of the urinary bladder
Qugu (Ren 2)	T6–T12	Tonifies liver; regulates menstruation
Ciliao (UB 32)	S2	Strengthens kidney and liver; regulates menstruation
Zhongliao (UB 33)	S3	Strengthens kidney and liver; regulates menstruation
Fengchi (GB 20)	CrN. XI	Relieves stagnation; activates blood; refreshes the mind

Treatment was given for 3 consecutive days before the usual time for symptoms to occur. Another treatment was given after the end of the period. This pattern of treatment was continued for 4 months and the patient recovered fully.

Comments:

The aim of the treatment was to regulate the function of the reproductive system and thus also regulate the levels of the various hormones involved. Generally speaking, this type of condition response very well to acupuncture and moxibustion.

MENOPAUSE

Female—54 years old

Complaint:

Suffering with hot flushes.

History:

Stopped menstruating at age 41 years. Previous to that, had normal and regular periods, although heavy. Her husband passed away very suddenly, and the shock of this had triggered her periods to stop. She was getting hot flushes accompanied by sweating, feeling tired all the time, soreness in the lower back, poor appetite, mood swings, quick tempered and weepy. GP had prescribed hormone replacement. After two year on the HRT, symptoms were reduced. Whenever the patient tried to stop the HRT, symptoms would reappear. She did not want to continue with the HRT. Her mother had also suffered badly with hot flushes until she died at the age of 70.

On Examination:

She was feeling nervous. Her abdomen was swollen and felt bloated. Her chest felt too tender to be touched. Tongue—pale. Pulse—small and deep.

TCM Diagnosis:

Kidney Yang Xu

Treatment:

Electro-acupuncture and moxibustion were used on the following points:

Points Used	Nerves Stimulated	TCM Explanations
Qugu (Ren 2)	T6–T12	Tonifies kidney; reduces heat
Zhongji (Ren 3)	T6–T12	Regulates Chong and Ren channels
Neiguan (P 6)	C6–T1	Luo-connecting point; regulates qi to soothe chest; relieves mental stress
Sanyingjiao (Sp 6)	L4–S3	Crossing point of 3 yin channels; reinforces kidney and liver; clears heat; calms the mind
Zhongliao (UB 33)	S3	Strengthens the kidney; reduces heat

Ciliao (UB 32)	S2	Strengthens the kidney; reduces heat
Shenshu (UB 23)	L1–S3	Back shu point of the kidney; strengthens the functions of kidney qi

Ear points used were Zigong and Shenmen.

Weekly sessions were given. After 4 treatments, the patient was able to stop the HRT without any bad effects. 3 more sessions were given after which treatment was no longer necessary.

OVARIAN CYST

Female—25 years old

Complaint:

Ovarian cyst on the left side.

History:

Towards the end of the previous year, the patient experienced pain in her right lower abdomen, and irregular periods. She felt a lump in the area. Investigations by the gynaecologist had established the presence of a cyst and this was removed by surgery. Her periods returned to normal after the surgery. Earlier on this year, she felt a similar pain on the left side. A subsequent laproscopy showed an ovarian cyst about 4 mm. in size. A course of hormones were prescribed. The patient had felt no change in her symptoms. In fact she did not have any periods. She decided to try acupuncture two months after the diagnosis.

On Examination:

A lump could be felt in the left lower abdomen which was tender on palpation. Tongue—dull purplish with blood spots. Pulse—small.

TCM Diagnosis:

Qi and Blood Stagnation

Treatment:

Electro-acupuncture and moxibustion were given on the following:

Points Used	Nerves Stimulated	TCM Explanations
Zhongji (Ren 3)	T6–T12	Front mu point of the urinary bladder; regulates Chong and Ren Channels
Qihai (Ren 6)	T6–T12	Tonifies kidney; reinforces lower jiao qi
Sanyingjiao (Sp 6)	L4–S3	Crossing point of 3 yin channels; reinforces blood and qi; nourishes yin; pacifies yang
Yinlingquan (Sp 9)	L3–S2	He-sea point; reinforces qi
Ciliao (UB 32)	S2	Strengthens kidney; regulates menstruation
Zhongliao (UB 33)	S3	Strengthens kidney; regulates menstruation

Shenshu (UB 23)	L1–L3	Back shu point of the kidney; strengthens kidney qi
Ah Shih Point		

Weekly treatments were given. After 3 weeks, the lump was smaller and did not feel tender to palpation. A further 6 sessions were given after which the patient had a laproscopy examination and scan. All they could find was some scar tissues. There was no sign of the cyst.

Comments:

It is not usual for this problem to respond so well to acupuncture and moxibustion. More research will be needed in this area.

MORNING SICKNESS

Female—29 years old

History:

She was in the sixth week of her pregnancy. She had been suffering sickness, vomiting and nausea in the mornings and at the sight of food. She could not taste anything and felt tired and lethargic. Did not want to take any drugs.

On Examination:

She looked tired. Tongue—pale with a white coat. Pulse—slippery and slow.

Treatment:

The needles were inserted in the following points:

Points Used	Nerves Stimulated	TCM Explanations
Neiguan (P 6)	C6–T1	Luo-connecting point; regulation of qi to soothe gastro-intestinal disturbances
Zhongwan (Ren 12)	T7–T12	Front mu point of stomach; regulate stomach function; strengthens spleen function

The needles were *not* manipulated. Only moxibustion was applied to the needles. The nausea and vomiting stopped.

Neiguan and Zhongwan together act very effectively to reduce nausea and vomiting. Examination by gastroscopy had shown that needling Neiguan regulates the function of the stomach and intestines. Clinical observations had shown that stimulation of this point is good for gastric pain and abdominal disturbances.

LOW VOLUME AND POOR MOTILITY OF SPERM

Male—37 years old

History:

Had been trying to have children for many years. Investigation at the hospital showed that he suffered with a low volume and motility of his sperm in spite of having normal hormone levels.

On Examination:

Tongue—pale. Pulse—small.

TCM Diagnosis:

Kidney Xu

Treatment:

The following points were chosen for electro-acupuncture and moxibustion:

Points Used	Nerves Stimulated	TCM Explanations
Taixi (K 3)	L4–S2	Shu-stream and Yuan-source point; reinforces and nourishes kidney yin
Sanyingjiao (Sp 6)	L4–S3	Crossing point of 3 yin channels; nourishes yin; pacifies yang; strengthens spleen and stomach; reinforces liver and kidney; specific for the reproductive system
Guanyuan (Ren 4)	T6–T12	Tonifies kidney; reinforces qi; specific for the reproductive system
Qugu (Ren 2)	T6–T12	Tonifies kidney; specific for the reproductive system
Zigong (Ext. pt.)	T7–L1	Tonifies function of the kidney
Ciliao (UB 32)	S2	Strengthens kidney
Xialiao (UB 34)	S1–S4	Strengthens kidney
Shenshu (UB 23)	L1–L3	Strengthens kidney qi

Ear points were needled at Shenmen and Endocrine.

Weekly treatments were given. After 2 weeks, the following herbs were prescribed in conjunction with the acupuncture:

Yina Yang Huo	Herba Epimedii
Gou Qi Zi	Fructus Lycii
Rou Cong Rong	Herba Cistanches
Ba Ji	Radix Morindae Officinalis
Shu Di	Radix Rehmanniae Praeparata
Fu Ling	Poria
Xu Duan	Radix Dipsaci
Zhi Zi	Fructus Gardeniae
Bai Shao	Radix Paeoniae Alba

3 prescriptions were taken over a week. After a week, the tongue was looking slightly red, the pulse, small and strong. The prescription was changed to the following:

Yin Yang Huo	Herba Epimedii
Gou Qi Zi	Fructus Lycii
Ba Ji	Radix Morindae Officinalis
Shu Di	Radix Rehmanniae Praeparata
Xu Dian	Radix Dipsaci
Bai Shao	Radix Paeoniae Alba
Tu Si Zi	Semen Cuscutae
She Chuang Zi	Fructus Cnidii
Bu Gu Zi	Fructus Psorialeae
Niu Xi	Radix Achyranthis Bidentatae
Shang Shen	Fructus Mori
Shou Wu	Radix Polygoni Multiflori

The above prescription was taken for another week in conjunction with acupuncture and moxibustion. The acupuncture was continued for another 6 weeks. Treatment was stopped. Another sperm count was performed, and it was found that the immotility was reduced by 10% and the quality had improved.

HYPERPLASIA OF THE BREAST

Female—36 years old

Complaint:

Lump on the left side of the breast.

History:

4 years previously, the patient was aware of a lump on the lateral and inferior side of the left breast. There was no pain and it did not feel hard. Had used acupuncture and chinese herbs in America. There was a good response. 8 months previously, she became depressed when her husband died. She began to notice that the lump had started to appear again. Her periods had become irregular and she had begun to suffer with insomnia.

On Examination:

On palpation, the lump felt as thick as a thumb, soft, well anchored and not movable. The skin colour was normal and there was no pain. The supra- claviular lymph nodes were normal. Tongue—slightly purplish with a thin white coat. Pulse—wiry and slow.

TCM Diagnosis:

Lung Qi Stagnation

Treatment:

Electro-acupuncture and moxibustion were used on the following:

Points Used	Nerve Stimulated	TCM Explanations
Hegu (LI 4)	C6–T1	Yuan-source point of the Yang Ming Channel rich in blood and qi
Tanzhong (Ren 17)	C5–T1	Front mu point of the pericardium; one of the 8 influential points; dominates qi
Jianjing (GB 21)	Cr.N XI	Clears channels to regulate qi flow to remove mass
Ganshu (UB 18)	T9–T10	Back shu point of liver, nourishes liver and kidney yin
Tianzong (SI 11)	T3–T5	Disperses accumulation of mass; regulates qi

| Sanyingjiao (Sp 6) | L4–S3 | Strengthens stomach and spleen; reinforces liver and kidney yin qi |
| Qimen (Liv 14) | T8–T12 | Front mu point of the liver |

Weekly treatments were given and after 10 sessions the lump had completely disappeared.

Comments:

This was an unusual case. Many of the points chosen were for the suitability of the nerve connections. There were no clear explanations for the recovery of this patient and insufficient comparative studies had been performed.

CYSTITIS

Female—56 years old

Complaint:

Dysuria.

History:

2 months previously, the patient had felt uncomfortable during micturation. As time went on, she developed frequency of micturation and her urine was concentrated and smelly. There was no blood. This was her first experience of cystitis. Antibiotics were prescribed with no effect.

On Examination:

The pelvic area was tender on palpation. Tongue—normal with a thin white coat tinged with yellow. Pulse—fast.

TCM Diagnosis:

Urinary Bladder Damp Heat

Treatment:

Points Used	Nerves Stimulated	TCM Explanations
Zhongji (Ren 3)	T6–T12	Front mu point of the UB Channel; promotes urination; clears damp heat
Qihai (Ren 6)	T6–T12	Tonifies kidney qi
Sanyingjiao (Sp 6)	L4–S3	Removes dampness; reduces heat
Taixi (K 3)	L4–S2	Shu-stream and yuan-source points of the kidney channel; clears heat; reinforces kidney qi; reduces pain
Shenshu (UB 23)	L1–L3	Strengthens kidney qi; encourages diuresis
Ciliao (UB 32)	S2	Strengthens kidney; reduces heat; removes dampness
Xiaoliao (UB 34)	L5–S4	Strengthens kidney; reduces heat; removes dampness
Pangguanshu (UB 28)	L5–S1	Strengthens lower jiao; clears and regulates water dampness

Acupuncture and moxibustion were given according to the above prescription for 3 sessions on alternate days in the first week. At the same time, 3 prescriptions of the following herbs were given over 6 days:

Chai Hu	(Radix Bupleuri)
Bai Jiang Cao	(Herba Patriniae)
Yin Chen	(Herba Artemisiae Scopariae)
Che Qian Cao	(Herba Plantaginis)
Jin Qian Cao	(Herba Lysimachiae)
Pugong Ying	(Herba Taraxaci)
Huang Qin	(Radix Scutellariae)
Huang Bo	(Cortex Phellodendri)
Zhi Mu	(Rhizoma Anemarrhenae)

Frequency of micturation was reduced and the urine was less smelly. The same treatment was continued for another week. On the third week, only herbs were prescribed:

Chai Hu	(Radix Bupleuri)
Jin Qian Cao	(Herba Lysimachiae)
Pugong Ying	(Herba Taraxaci)
Zhi Mu	(Rhizoma Anemarrhenae)
Huang Bo	(Cortex Phellodendri)
Zhi Zi	(Fructus Gardeniae)
Tian Hua Fen	(Radix Trichosanthis)

After a week of the above herbal prescription, micturation was normal, and she did not feel any discomfort. She was advised to continue the herbs for one more week.

Comments:

The process of micturation depends on the co-ordination of the sympathetic and parasympathetic activities. The external sphincter of the bladder is controlled by the pudendal nerve (S2–S4). Sympathetic supply to the bladder arises from L1–L2 spinal segments. When choosing points for the treatment, these were taken into consideration in conjunction with the traditional functions of those points. Stimulation of these areas certainly helped to normalise the function of the bladder and the kidney.

CYSTITIS—CASE 2

Female—38 years old

Complaint:

Dysuria.

History:

General health had been good. About 4 years ago she had experienced intermittent dysuria which got better with increased fluid intake. About 2 years ago, she had the same discomfort again but that time micturation was accompanied by a burning sensation. Increased fluid intake did not have any effect that time. At the same time she experienced low back pain, increased thirst and dryness of the mouth.

On Examination:

She had a pained expression. There was slight pressure pain in the area of the lower abdomen. There was also palpation tenderness in the lumbar region of L2–L3. Flexion of the spine was painful. Tongue—red. Pulse—fast and small.

TCM Diagnosis:

Kidney Yin Xu

Treatment:

Electro-acupuncture and moxibustion were used on the following:

Points Used	Nerves Stimulated	TCM Explanations
Zhongji (Ren 3)	T6–T12	Front mu point of the urinary bladder; promotes urination
Guanyuan (Ren 4)	T6–T12	Tonifies function of the kidney; reinforces kidney qi; reduces heat; removes dampness
Sanyingjiao (Sp 6)	L4–S3	Crossing point of 3 yin channels; reinforces kidney; nourishes yin
Taixi (K 3) through	L4–S2	Pacifies yang; reinforces kidney; nourishes yin; specific for problems involving micturation.
Kunlun (UB 60)	L5–S2	Jing-river point; strengthens function of kidney and restores qi

Shenshu (UB 23)	L1–L3	Back shu point of the kidney; strengthens kidney; reinforces kidney qi; strengthens lower back
Pangguanshu (UB 28)	L5–S2	Back shu point of the urinary bladder; regulates water pathways; reduces stiffness of the back

Stimulating Guanyuan and Sanyingjiao in combination is effective for restoring urinary bladder function and improve micturation. Needling Taixi through to Kunlun improves function of the kidney and effective for reducing low back pain.

In addition to the above treatment once a week, 6 prescriptions of Jin Qian Cao (Herba Lysimachiae) were to be taken over 2 weeks.

By the third week no more treatment was necessary.

URINARY RETENTION

Male—65 years old

Complaint:

Had been suffering from retention for the past 10 hours.

History:

Had surgery to remove bladder stones 2 years ago. 10 days previous to consultation, he had difficulty in passing urine. Was catheterised in hospital. 2 days later, he had retention again, and was relieved by catheterisation. He had to be catheterised for a third time during this period. When he came for consultation, he had been unable to pass urine for 10 hours.

On Examination:

His bladder was painful and swollen and too sensitive for palpation. Tongue—normal with a thin white coat. Pulse—fast.

TCM Diagnosis:

Shen Yang Xu

Treatment:

Points chosen for electro-acupuncture and moxibustion were:

Points Used	Nerves Stimulated	TCM Explanations
Shenshu (UB 23)	L1–L3	Back shu point of the kidney; strengthens kidney qi; encourages diuresis
Pangguanshu (UB28)	L5–S2	Back shu point of the urinary bladder; strengthens lower jiao; clears and regulates water pathways
Ciliao (UB 32)	S2	Strengthens the kidney
Sanyingjiao (Sp 6)	L4–S3	Crossing point of 3 yin channels; strengthens the kidney
Zusanli (St 36)	L4–S3	Reinforces liver and kidney blood and qi

The abdomen was too distended for needles to be inserted. After stimulating the above points for 20 minutes, they were removed, and the patient was asked to stand. Digital pressure was applied to points Qugu (Ren 2) and Zhongji (Ren 3) and patient was asked to flex his spine. The patient had to pass urine immediately and he was able to empty his bladder satisfactorily. He was taught how to apply the pressure on those two points to help him empty his bladder. He did not need any more treatment.

URINARY BLADDER STONE

Male—31 years old

Complaint:

Suffered with painful and blood-stained micturation. He could also feel a hardness in one area of the urethra.

History:

Since the age of 18 years, he had been passing a stone every other day. It had become less during the last year. 10 days previously, he passed one. The size of the stones ranged from 2 mm. to 5 mm. They were tubular and transparent.

On Examination:

He had a painful expression. In the lower $\frac{1}{3}$ of the urethra, a hard lump could be felt. It left him in pain all the time. Tongue—red with a yellow coat. Pulse—wiry and fast.

TCM Diagnosis:

Urinary Bladder Damp Heat.

Treatment:

Point used for electro-acupuncture and moxibustion were:

Points Used	Nerves Stimulated	TCM Explanations
Sanyingjiao (Sp 6)	L4–S3	Crossing point of 3 yin channels; nourishes yin; pacifies yang; removes dampness and heat
Zhongji (Ren 3)	T6–T12	Front mu point of the urinary bladder; regulates Chong and Ren Channels
Qihai (Ren 6)	T6–T12	Tonifies heat; reinforces lower jiao heat
Pangguanshu (UB 28)	L5; S1–S2	Back shu point of the urinary bladder; strengthens lower jiao; clears and regulates water pathways
Ciliao (UB 32)	S2	Strengthens kidney; reduces heat; removes damp
Xiaoliao (UB 34)	L5; S1; S2; S4	Strengthens kidney; reduces heat; removes damp

Shenshu (UB 23)	L1–L3	Back shu point of the kidney; strengthens function of kidney qi

After the needles had been stimulated for 45 minutes, the patient requested to be allowed to empty his bladder. During micturation, he felt pain and the urine was blood stained and a 3 mm. tubular stone was passed. The following prescription of herbs was prescribed, one prescription to be taken daily for 3 days.

Jin Qian Cao	(Herba Lysimachiae)
Che Qian Cao	(Herba Plantaginis)
Huang Bo	(Cortex Phellodendri)
Zhu Ling	(Polyporus Umbellatus)
Ze Xie	(Rhizoma Alismatis)
Fu Ling	(Poria)
Niu Xi	(Radix Achyranthis Bidentatae)

After 3 days of the above prescription, Jin Qian Cao and Che Qian Cao were prescribed for drinking as a tea. No more acupuncture or moxibustion was required. The patient had no more problems.

ENURESIS

Female—9 years old

Complaint:

Suffered with urinary incontinence twice nightly.

History:

Had been wetting the bed since she was 3 years old. Each time, she was only aware of the event afterwards. Various methods have been used including alarms and no drinks nearing bedtime. Nothing had worked so far.

On Examination:

She looked pale and tired. Tongue—pale with a thin white coat. Pulse—deep.

TCM Diagnosis:

Urinary Bladder Xu and Cold

Treatment:

Electro-acupuncture and moxibustion were used on the following points:

Points Used	Nerves Stimulated	TCM Explanations
Guanyuan (Ren 4)	T6–T12	Tonifies kidney; reinforces qi
Zhongji (Ren 3)	T6–T12	Regulates Chong and Ren Channels; promotes regular micturation
Sanyingjiao (Sp 6)	L4–S3	Crossing point of 3 yin channels; nourishes yin; pacifies yang
Pangguanshu (UB 28)	L5–S2	Back shu point of the urinary bladder; strengthens lower jiao; clears and regulates water passage;
Ciliao (UB 32)	S2	Strengthens kidney
Xiaoliao (UB 34)	L5; S1; S2; S4	Strengthens kidney qi
Shenshu (UB 23)	L1–L3	Strengthens function of kidney qi

Using Guanyuan, Zhongji and Sanyingjiao together is particularly effective for treating enuresis.

TRANSVERSE PRESENTATION OF THE FOETUS
Female—34 years old

Complaint:

At 33 weeks the foetus was in a transverse position.

On Examination:

This is the patient's first child (Primugravida). When she was examined on the 28th week of her pregnancy at the hospital, the foetus was found to be in transverse presentation. After several attempts, they were unable to rectify the situation.

Treatment:

Only one acupuncture point Zhiyin (UB 67), was used bilaterally. Neutral manual manipulation and moxa were applied.

During the treatment, the patient felt the foetus move. After the treatment which lasted 45 minutes, an examination showed that the head of the baby had moved down to the pelvis. The patient was taught how to apply moxa to the same points at home. She came back the third day for an examination, and the head of the baby was at 45°. The same treatment was given for 45 minutes after which another examination showed that the baby was in the normal position. The patient was advised to apply moxibustion to point Zhiyin 3 times a day. She had a normal delivery.

Comments:

According to traditional chinese medicine, stimulation of the above points helps to regulate qi to reverse the position of the foetus.

BREECH PRESENTATION OF THE FOETUS
Female—35 years old

History:

At 28 weeks, regular examination at the hospital showed the foetus in a breeched position. The doctors were unable to rectify this.

Treatment:

Only moxibustion was used on point Zhiyin (UB 67). After 40 minutes of treatment, the foetus had moved to the normal position. She was taught to continue the treatment 3 times a day. A regular check was kept at the hospital. She was able to give birth normally.

HYPERTROPHY OF THE PROSTATE

Male—72 years old

Complaint:

Increased frequency of micturation especially at night. Cannot empty bladder fully each time.

History:

For the past 5 years, the patient had been suffering with frequency of micturation. In the night, he had to get up as much as 5 times. He experienced a delayed start and did not seem to be able to empty the bladder fully. The stream was also weak. His lower abdomen felt distended.

On Examination:

He had been put on the waiting list for surgery on his prostate which was found to be enlarged. Digital examination of the prostate confirmed enlargement and tenderness of the prostate. All this had made him feel exhausted. Tongue—pale with a white and greasy coat. Pulse—weak.

TCM Diagnosis:

Kidney Yang Xu

Treatment:

The following points were chosen for acupuncture and moxibustion:

Points Used	Nerves Stimulated	TCM Explanations
Guanyuan (Ren 4)	T6–T12	Front mu point of the small intestine; tonifies kidney; increases yang qi
Qugu (Ren 2)	T6–T12	Tonifies kidney
Yinlingquan (Sp 9)	L3–S2	Strengthens spleen; reinforces blood and qi; nourishes congenital kidney qi
Taixi (K 3)	L4–S2	Nourishes yin; tonifies kidney; restores qi
Shenshu (UB 23)	L1–L3	Tonifies kidney qi
Ciliao (UB 32)	S2	Strengthens kidney qi
Xialiao (UB 34)	L5–S4	Strengthens kidney qi
Mingmen (Du 4)	L2	Reinforces yang qi and kidney qi
Hiatus of sacrum	(Ext. Pt)	

Treatment was given twice a week. After the third week, the patient was only disturbed a maximum of 3 times in the night. Starting each time was also less effort. The combination of points were changed to the following:

Guanyuan
Yinlingquan
Mingmen
Hiatus of sacrum
Sanyingjiao (Sp 6)   L4–S3   Crossing point of 3 yin channels;
                                               reinforces kidney
Qihai (Ren6)   T6–T12   Tonifies kidney qi

The combination of Sanyingjiao and Qihai is effective for reinforcing kidney yang qi. The second formula of points was alternated with the first. After a further 5 weeks, the treatment was stopped and to await the results of a follow-up appointment at the hospital in 4 weeks time. At the check up, the doctors suggested that no surgery was necessary if the patient continued to be able to pass urine at the improved rate. He was only waking up twice in the night. The starting was normal although the stream was still weak. The patient had further treatments, once fortnightly for a total of 4 treatments.

Comments:

Stimulation of the parasympathetic nerves, probably improved the circulation to the prostate gland increasing SIgA levels, at the same time reducing inflammation and pain. The prostate gland is supplied by the pelvic splanchnic nerves (S2, 3, 4). Stimulating this system reduces endocrine dysfunction, and therefore has an effect on the prostatic hyperplasia.

ACUTE DISSEMINATED ENCEPHALO-RADICULOPATHY

Male—30 years old

Complaint:

Paralysed in all 4 limbs for the past year.

History:

Just over a year ago, the patient had flu. One week after recovery, there was a sudden numbness in the legs, and he experienced difficulty with walking. Electromyography confirmed a diagnosis of encephalomyelitis with nerve root involvement. Cortisone therapy was prescribed and there was an initial dramatic improvement for 2 weeks, after which the upper limbs were showing signs of nerve involvement. Cortisone therapy was continued, but lacked the desired effect. Gradually, his arms and legs became paralysed. Acute disseminated encephalo-radiculopathy was the final diagnosis.

On Examination:

He had dropped feet. Unable to lift arms. The most he could achieve was pick up a teaspoon. No reflexes. Complexion—pale. Tongue—pale with a thick white coat. Pulse—small.

TCM Diagnosis:

Qi Xu with Phlegm Obstruction

Treatment:

Electro-acupuncture and moxibustion were used on the following points:

Points Used	Nerves Stimulated	TCM Explanations
Yanglingquan (GB 34)	L4–S1	He-sea point; specific for muscles and tendons
Huantiao (GB 30)	L2–S3	Activates nerves and relieves rigidity of muscles
Fengshi (GB 31)	L2–L4	Clears channels; improves blood circulation; disperses wind and cold
Chengshan (UB 57)	L4–S2	Activates channels; relaxes muscles and tendons
Shenshu (UB 23)	L1–L3	Back shu point; increases kidney qi; strengthens lower back and leg

Qihaishu (UB 24)	L3	Regulates qi; improves circulation; activates channels
Dachangshu (UB 25)	L4	Regulates functions of large intestine and small intestine channels; regulates qi flow
Ganshu (UB 18)	CrN. XI; T9−T10	Regulates functions of liver channel; nourishes liver and kidney yin; back shu point of the liver
Sanyingjiao (Sp 6)	L4−S3	Crossing point of 3 yin channels
Xuehai (Sp 10)	L2−L4	Activates blood and regulates qi; removes wind
Zusanli (St 36)	L4−S3	He-sea point; restores body functions to normality; enriches blood and qi; strengthens spleen and reduces phelgm; reinforces liver and kidney
Hegu (LI 4)	C6−T1	Yuan-source point; eliminates phlegm
Quchi (LI 11)	C5−T1	Regulates qi; promotes circulation; promotes blood flow

Treatment was given daily, 6 days a week. After 1½ months, he was able to walk with one walking stick and some support.

The combination of points was changed to the following:

Points Used	Nerves Stimulated	TCM Explanations
Yanglingquan		
Huantiao		
Fengshi		
Sanyingjiao		
Xuehai		
Shenshu		
Qihaishu		
Dachangshu		
Hegu		
Shousanli (LI 10)	C5−C8	Specific for motor impairment of the upper limb
Weizhong (UB 40)	L4−S2	He-sea point; specific for the motor impairment of the lower limb; relaxes muscles
Taichong (Liv 3)	L4−S2	Shu-stream and yuan source point; regulates qi and activates blood

The above combination was alternated with the following:

Yanglingquan		
Zusanli		
Quchi		
Futu (St 32)	L2–L4	Promotes circulation; regulates qi
Fenglong (St 40)	L4–S1	Luo-connecting point; strengthens spleen to resolve phlegm
Zhongzhu (SJ 3)	C8–T1	Shu-streampoint; specific for impairment of elbow and arm
Deltoid point (Ext. Pt)	Axillary nerve	Specific for impairment of arm
Chinglo (Ext. Pt.)	L4–S1	Clears the mind

After 2 months of treatment, the patient was able to walk on his own with just the help of 2 sticks. The patient then had a rest from treatment for 4 weeks. Treatment was continued for another 3 months, during which the patient was encouraged to walk regularly for exercise. At the end of the 3 months, the patient was able to walk without aids, and the treatment was stopped.

PARALYSIS

Female—21 years old

Complaint:

Bilateral paralysis of the lower limbs.

History:

For the past 2 years, the patient had been unable to walk without the aid of underarm crutches. It started with abnormal feelings in both legs. There was a history of being hit by a football in the lumbo-sacral area prior to the appearance of symptoms. Doctors at the hospital had diagnosis a bilateral medial tibial syndrome. Physiotherapy was prescribed but to no effect. She had undergone some exploratory surgery but it was inconclusive. When her symptoms persisted, further surgery was advised.

On Examination:

There was no atrophy of the leg muscles. Reflexes were weak. Responses to pin-prick tests were reduced. She could not stand without support. Tongue and pulse appeared normal.

TCM Diagnosis:

Blood and Qi Xu

Treatment:

Points Used	Nervers Stimulated	TCM Explanations
Shenshu (UB 23)	L1–L3	Back shu point of the kidney; reinforces kidney qi; strengthens the lower back and legs
Pangguanshu (UB 28)	L5–S1	Back shu point of the urinary bladder; strengthens the lower jiao and clears UB pathways.
Zhongliao (UB 33)	L5–S3	Strengthens kidney
Weizhong (UB 40)	L4–S2	He-sea point; specific for motor impairment of the legs
Chengshan (UB 57)	L4–S2	Activates channels; effective for problems associated with muscles and tendons
Yinmen (UB 37)	L5–S2	Specific for motor impairment of the legs

Fengshi (GB 31)	L2–L4	Clears channels; improves circulation
Yanglingquan (GB 34)	L4–S1	He-sea point; specific for problems with muscles and tendons
Kunlun (UB 60)	L5–S2	Jing-river point; strengthens kidney function
Xuehai (Sp 10)	L2–L4	Activates blood; regulates qi
Yinlingquan (Sp 9)	L3–S2	He-sea point; reinforces spleen
Sanyingjiao (SP 6)	L4–S3	Crossing point of 3 yin channels; reinforces kidney
Taixi (K 3)	L4–S2	Shu-stream and yuan-source point; restores qi; tonifies kidney

Daily treatment was given. Each time only 8 points were chosen from the above for electro-acupuncture and moxibustion.

In the 2nd week, the patient could stand without the crutches and was able to take 2 steps with encouragement. By the third week, she was able to walk without crutches. She had a complete recovery after 6 weeks and treatment was stopped.

RESTLESS LEG SYNDROME

Female—52 years old

Complaint:

Soreness, pain and a feeling of distension in the deeper part of the calf muscles of both legs.

History:

Sleep was usually disturbed more than once by a feeling of soreness, distension and pain in the calf muscles. This was relieved by massage and movement. Investigations at the hospital had not revealed any abnormalities. This had been going on for just over 6 months.

On Examination:

Tongue—dull red with a thin white coat. Pulse—small and wiry.

TCM Diagnosis:

Liver and Kidney Yin Xu with blood stagnation

Treatment:

Points Used	Nerves Stimulated	TCM Explanations
Yanglingquan (GB 34)	L4–S1	One of the 8 influential points for muscles and tendons
Taixi (K 3) needled through to	L4–S2	Yuan-source point; improves kidney qi; earth point dominating muscles
Kunlun (UB 60)	L5–S2	Together with taixi, raises kidney qi
Weizhong (UB 40)	L4–S2	Reduces rigidity and contracture of tendons
Chengshan (UB 57)	L4–S2	Reduces rigidity of muscles and tendons
Shenshu (UB 23)	L1–L3	Back shu point of the kidey; raises kidney qi
Pangguanshu (UB 28)	L5–S2	Back shu point of the urinary bladder

Shenshu and Pangguanshu have a superficial and deep relationship. The combination of Shenshu and Pangguanshu, enhances the effect of raising kidney qi.

Electro-acupuncture and moxibustion were used once a week on the above points. In the meantime, the following herbs were prescribed:

Chi Shao   (Radix Paenoniae Rubra)
Gan Cao   (Radix Glycyrrhizae)
Dan Shen   (Radix Salviae Miltorrhizae)
Han Lian Cao   (Herba Ecliptae)
Dang Gui   (Radix Angelicae Sincnsis)
Ye Jiao Teng   (Caulis Polygoni Multiflori)

The patient was treated for 4 weeks with acupuncture, moxibustion and herbs. At the end of this period she had recovered well enough for treatment to stop.

Comments:

The cause for this syndrome is unknown. Acupuncture and moxibustion can treat this condition quite successfully.

PARALYSIS DUE TO TRAUMA TO THE SCIATIC NERVE

Female—2 years old

Complaint:

Paralysis of the right leg.

History:

She was suffering with a fever just over 4 months ago and was hospitalised. 2 injections were given to help reduce the fever. The fever subsided within the week and when she was about to be discharged, they discovered that she had a dropped left foot and she had difficulty walking. She was retained for treatment with physiotherapy and after 3 months there was no visible improvement and she was transferred to the Great Ormond Street Hospital. After investigations the doctors concluded that the paralysis was due to trauma to the sciatic nerve from an injection. More physiotherapy did not result in any improvement.

On Examination:

No muscle tone on the right leg below the knee. Knee and ankle jerk reflexes were absent. Responses to light touch and pin-prick tests to the affected leg were also absent. There was no voluntary movement of the affected limb. She could not stand on one leg. The tongue and pulses appear normal.

TCM Diagnosis:

Wei Syndrome

Treatment:

Acupuncture and moxibustion were used and the neutral manipulation was applied to the needles. Points were chosen only for their relationship to the nerves.

Points Used	Nerves Stimulated
Shenshu (UB 23)	L1–L3
Pangguanshu (UB 28)	L5–S2
Ciliao (UB 32)	S2

Treatment on the above points were given 3 times a week for 4 weeks. Cotton wool test at this stage showed a slight response from the toes.

From the 5th week, 5 to 6 points were chosen each time from the following:

Points Used	Nerves Stimulated
Zusanli (St 36)	L4–S3
Jiaxi (St 41)	L4–S1
St.Futu (St 32)	L2–L4
Biguan (St 31)	L2–S1
Tiaokou (St 38)	L4–S1
Sanyingjiao (Sp 6)	L4–S3
Yinlingquan (Sp 9)	L3–S2
Weizhong (UB 40)	L4–S2
Chengshan (UB 57)	L4–S2
Shenmai (UB 62)	S1–S2
Kunlun (UB 60)	L5–S2
Taixi (K 3)	L4–S2
Zhaohai (K 6)	L4–S1
Fuliu (K 7)	L4–S2
Yanglingquan (GB 34)	L4–S1
Xuanzhong (GB 39)	L4–S1
Qiuxu (GB 40)	L4–S1
Taichong (Liv 3)	L4–S2
Xingjian (Liv 2)	L4–S1

Mid-point of the space between 4th and 5th metatarsals.

After a further 3 weeks of treatment, she could stand on her own. After another 2 weeks, she could rotate the foot internally although the foot tended to evert. She was also able to take 2 steps with some help. 2 more weeks of treatment followed and she took more steps. At this stage the treatment was reduced to twice a week for another 14 weeks, after which she had a break from treatment for 4 weeks.

Treatment was resumed twice weekly. At this stage she was able to run and jump although the right foot was one size smaller than the left foot. After a further 10 weeks of treatment, the circumference of the leg 4 inches below the knee was only less than the corresponding point on the left by 1 inch. At the level of 2 inches below the knee, the circumference was the same on the right as on the left. She had begun to experience normal sensations to needle stimulation and was thus less cooperative. Treatment was thus reduced to once a week. Throughout the treatment, the patient had kept up her appointments with the consultant at the hospital who was also monitoring her progress.

After another 36 weekly treatments, she was able to run and play with no difficulty, although a discrepancy in shoe size remained. Treatment was stopped. Her progress was monitored once yearly. So far all was satisfactory.

BELL'S PALSY

Male—10 years old

Complaint:

Left sided facial palsy.

History:

Was obvious to his mother on seeing him one morning 4 days ago. He experienced a numbness of the left side of his face and could not help dribbling. He was unable to close the left eye completely.

On Examination:

There were no forehead lines on the left and there was a loss of the nasolabial fold. He could not close the left eye and the effort was accompanied by the upward rolling of the eyeball. There was a track of saliva from the left angle of the mouth. He was unable whistle or blow out his cheeks. There was also a loss of taste over the anterior $\frac{2}{3}$ of the tongue. Tongue—pale with a thin white coat. Pulse—small and wiry.

TCM Diagnosis:

Wind Cold Damage to the Channels

Treatment:

Points Used	Nerves Stimulated	TCM Explanations
Jiache (St 6)	CrN. V–VII	Removes wind; regulates qi
Xiaguan (St 7)	CrN. V–VII	Disperses wind; regulates qi
Dicang (St 4)	CrN. V–VII	Disperses wind; activates channels
Taiyang (Ext. pt.)	CrN. V–VII	Expels wind

Electro-acupuncture and moxibustion were given daily. After 3 treatments the face had returned to normal. A further 2 treatments were given and no more treatment was required.

BELL'S PALSY—CASE 2

Female—30 years old

Complaint:

Left-sided facial palsy.

History:

She started having symptoms of pain in the left ear and a slight fever about 6 months ago. She noticed the palsy and numbness one week after the start of the symptoms. She lost control of the muscles of the mouth on the left and the angle was lowered. Taste was also reduced. The GP prescribed drugs and she took them for 3 months without effect.

On Examination:

She had the typical symptoms. Tongue—slightly red with a yellow coat. Pulse—wiry.

TCM Diagnosis:

Wind Heat
   Treatment with electro-acupuncture and moxibustion were used on the following:

Points Used	Nerves Stimulated	TCM Explanations
Jiache (St 6)	CrN. V–VII	
Xiaguan (St 7)	CrN. V–VII	
Dicang (St 4)	CrN. V–VII	
Taiyang (Ext. pt.)	CrN. V–VII	
Hegu (LI 4)	C6–T1	Clears heat; disperses wind; specific for problems with the mouth and face
Jingming (UB 1)	CrN. V–VII	Reduces wind and heat

Weekly treatments were given. After 10 treatments she had recovered fully.

BELL'S PALSY—CASE 3

Female—49 years old

Complaint:

Left-sided facial palsy.

History:

4 months previously, she suffered a basal skull fracture on falling from a bus. She had contusional brain injuries (temporal and frontal lobes) with blood in the mastoid air cells and a widening of the Laribdad Suture. After 2–3 days, she developed a left-sided facial nerve palsy, trigeminal neuralgia on the same side, accompanied by deafness and tinnitus in the left ear. Investigations included routine blood tests which were normal; a CT brain scan which confirmed the above injuries; skull x-rays which showed no fractures. The facial nerve EM6 revealed a possibility of recovery; an audiogram confirmed left-sided deafness with poor prognosis of recovery. She was referred to the consultants at ENT and Neurosurgery. She had been given advanced neurophysiotherapy but with no effect.

On Examination:

Tongue—dull with a thin white + a hint of yellow coat. Pulse—normal

TCM Diagnosis:

Stagnation Blood and Qi.

Treatment:

Points Used	Nerves Stimulated	TCM Explanations
Jiache (St 6)	CrN. V–VII	
Xiaguan (St 7)	CrN. V–VII	
Dicang (St 4)	CrN. V–VII	
Hegu (LI 4)	C6–T1	Yuan-source point of Yang-ming channel
Yinxiang (LI 20)	CrN. V–VII	Expels wind
Yifeng (SJ 17)	CrN. V–VII; C1–C8	Activates qi and clears channels; disperses wind
Fengchi (GB 20)	CrN. V–VII + XI	Activates blood to remove stagnation; disperses fire and wind

Electro-acupuncture and moxibustion were given in the above combination twice weekly. 3 months later she could close her eye; the angle of her mouth returned to normal; the naso-labial fold was visible and she formed muscles to whistle and blow out her cheeks. Treatment was then reduced to once weekly. 3 months on, there was only a slightly abnormality when she smiled. Treatment was stopped. A follow-up one year later confirmed that her facial muscles had recovered completely.

MIGRAINE

Female—33 years old

Complaint:

Weekly attacks of migraine.

History:

Seemed to be triggered off by pressure of work. It could affect either side of the head. Painkillers had helped but for the past 5 or 6 years it had been gradually getting worse especially just before a period. Recently the headaches had been frontal extending down to the neck with blurred vision and vomiting. There was a pulsating feeling at the temples with diarrhoea and facial numbness which could last 3 days. Painkillers had been ineffective recently. There was no history of food allergy and no other members of the family suffered with migraine.

On Examination:

The occiput felt tender on palpation with radiation of the pain down the neck and across top of shoulders. The temples also felt tender. Tongue—slightly red with a thin white coat. Pulse—small and fast.

TCM Diagnosis:

Shao Yang Type headache

Treatment:

Electro-acupuncture was used on two combinations of points.

Plan 1

Points Used	Nerves Stimulated	TCM Explanations
Fengchi (GB 20)	CrN. XI	Removes liver and gall bladder wind; relieves stagnation; activates blood and qi; calms the mind and relieves spasm of the blood vessels; reduces pain
Jianjing (GB 21)	CrN. XI	Clears channels to regulate flow of qi
Neiguan (P 6)	C6–T1	Luo-connecting point; regulates qi and reduces vomitting
Touwei (St 8)	CrN. V	Expels wind; reduces headaches
Taiyang (Ext. Pt.)	CrN. V + VII	Expels wind; reduces headaches

| Zusanli (St 36) | L4–S3 | Regulates functions of body; reduces wind |

Plan 2
Fengchi (GB 20)
Jianjing (GB 21)
Touwei (St 8)

| Taichong (Liv 3) | L4–S2 | Regulates liver qi; activates blood; reduces headaches; Gate point |
| Hegu (LI 4) | C6–T1 | Removes wind; reduces pain; Gate point |

Treatment was given once a week, alternating Plan 1 and 2. She had a total of 20 treatments with a break in between. She had a good recovery.

MIGRAINE—CASE 2

Female—39 years old

Complaint:

Migraine at the top of the head and between the eyebrows for over 10 years.

History:

The pain also radiates down the neck. There was nausea and vomiting each time, and the eyes became sensitive to light. The pain was like pin pricks. It occurred at least once a month and usually lasted two days. Recently, she had been having the migraine at least once a week each of one day duration. Seemed to be linked to stress at work. There was a family history of sensitive skin and hay fever. She seemed to suffer more during the hay fever season.

On Examination:

It was the hay fever season, so she was having symptoms of nasal congestion. The top of the head was aching, her eyes were red. Tongue—yellow white coat. Pulse—small and wiry.

TCM Diagnosis:

Jie Yang Type Headache.

Treatment:

Two combination of points were chosen for electro-acupuncture and moxibustion:

Plan 1

Points Used	Nerves Stimulated	TCM Explanations
Baihui (Du 20)	CrN. V; C2	Regulates yang qi; specific for headaches and nasal obstruction
Yintang (Ext. pt.)	CrN. V + VII	Specific for headaches and nasal obstruction
Hegu (LI 4)	C6–T1	Reduces pain; specific for problems on the face
Fengchi (GB 20)	CrN. XI	Nourishes yang; refreshes the mind; removes liver and gallbladder wind; activates circulation; removes stagnation

Xuehai (Sp 10)	L2–L4	Regulates qi and blood circulation; disperses wind; activates blood; specific for allergy
Neiguan (P 6)	C6–T1	Luo-connecting point; regulates qi; reduces vomitting
Dazhui (Du 14)	C3; C4; C8; CrN. XI	Regulates qi flow; nourishes blood; reduces fever; relieves mental stress

Plan 2
Fengchi (GB 20)

Quchi (LI 11)	C5–T1	He-sea point of the large intestine; dispel wind; clears heat; promotes blood flow; specific for allergy
Yinxiang (LI 20)	CrN. V + VII	Specific for hay fever and nasal disorders
Zusanli (St 36)	L4–S3	Reduces wind; specific for nasal disorders and hay fever
Waiguan (SJ 5)	C6–C8	Luo-connecting point; dispels wind; regulates qi; promotes blood circulation

Treatment was given once weekly alternating the two plans. The patient recovered after 20 treatments.

Stimulation by acupuncture appears to help the immune system, and endorphine release would reduce the pain of the headache. The right combination of points is important for this case.

FACIAL PARALYSIS

Male—28 years old

Complaint:

Left facial paralysis with reduced hearing in the left ear.

History:

Suffered with flu one month previously. Pain started in the ear about a week after recovery from the flu accompanied by dizziness. Was advised by the doctor to rest and a viral infection was suspected. A few days later, he began to notice that the left side of the face was paralysed and there was a loss of hearing in the left ear. He could not help dribbling as a result. A course of steroids was prescribed to last a week. There was no change to the symptoms.

On Examination:

The naso-facial groove on the left side was less pronounced. The left eye would not close properly. He could not purse his lips or blow out his cheeks. Tongue—pale with a thin white coat. Pulse—weak.

TCM Diagnosis:

Kidney Blood Qi Xu

Treatment:

Electro-acupuncture and moxibustion were used on the following:

Points Used	Nerves Stimulated	TCM Explanations
Ermen (SJ 21)	CrN. V	Promotes and regulates functions of the ear; activates qi to improve hearing
Tinghui (GB 2)	CrN. V + VII	Improves hearing
Sizhukong (SJ 23)	CrN. V + VII	Specific for eye problems; regulates qi; activates blood
Yifeng (SJ 17)	CrN. V: VII + XI	Specific fot facial paralysis; clears channels to improve hearing
Hegu (LI 4)	C6–T1	Yuan-source point; disperses wind and heat
Waiguan (SJ 5)	C6–C8	Clears and activates channels; specific for facial paralysis and ear problems; regulates qi and promotes blood circulation

Treatment was given twice weekly. After 15 sessions, there was still a slight drooping of the mouth and there was no improvement in the hearing. The combination of points was changed to the following:

Ermen (SJ 21)
Tinghui (GB 2)
Yifeng (SJ 17)
Taixi (K 3)   L4–S2   Shu-stream and yuan-source
                                               point; nourishes yin; tonifies
                                               kidney; restores qi
Zhongzhu (SJ 3)   C8–T1   Regulates qi; improves vision and
                                               hearing

After a further 5 weekly treatments, the patient's face and hearing had returned to normal.

MÉNIÈRE'S SYNDROME

Male—39 years old

Complaint:

Tinnitus, dizziness and nausea.

History:

The first episode was during a bout of flu about 10 years ago. A similar episode followed about 2 years later. Since then each bout of flu had been accompanied by tinnitus, dizziness and nausea about 2 or 3 times a year. Each episode would last about a week. Drugs had helped so far. The symptoms of tinnitus and dizziness have become more frequent, about once every 2 or 3 weeks. The symptoms were worse if there was more stress or pressure at work. The tinnitus had a high pitch and drugs had not reduced the symptoms. After a consultation at the ENT Department, it was diagnosed as Ménièr's Syndrome.

On Examination:

Dizziness was exacerbated when his eyes were closed. Complexion and lips were pale. BP—130/80. Tongue—pale with a thin coat. Pulse—small.

TCM Diagnosis:

Heart and Spleen Qi Xu

Treatment:

Points Used	Nerves Stimulated	TCM Explanations
Yifeng (SJ 17)	C1–C8; CrN.V + VII	Activates blood; unblocks channels; improves hearing; reduces tinnitus
Tinghui (GB 2)	C2–C3; CrN.V + IX	Improves hearing and reduces tinnitus
Neiguan (P 6)	C6–T1	Stops nausea and vomiting; regulates heart qi; relieves mental stress
Baihui (Du 20)	CrN.V	Increases yang qi; reinforces blood and qi; refreshes and restores the mind
Taichong (Liv 3)	L4–S1	Calms the liver and dispels wind to regulate heat qi; activates blood and regulates qi

Zusanli (St 36)   L4–S3   Reinforces spleen; dissolves
                                         phlegm; reinforces blood and qi;
                                         reinforces kidney

Treatment with electro-acupuncture and moxibustion were given using
the above combination twice weekly. After 2 months, treatment was
reduced to once a week for the next 4 months, then reduced to once a
fortnight for the following 3 months and finally once a month for the
next 4 months. The patient recovered well enough for treatment to
stop. 10 years later he wrote to say that he was in good health.

Comments:

The stimulation of the above points helped to regulate the autonomic
nervous system to improve blood circulation in the inner ear and to
relieve hydrops (water retention in the inner ear). Acupuncture and
moxibustion are very effective for this type of condition.

MÉNIÈRE'S DISEASE—CASE 2

Female—48 years old

Complaint:

Vertigo.

History:

Patient was very busy at work and developed flu symptoms. Very soon after, the symptoms of vertigo started to appear, accompanied by nausea, vomiting and tinnitus. A consultant at the ENT department 3 days previously concluded that the patient was suffering with Ménière's disease. The standard medication was prescribed. The intensity of the vertigo was reduced but there was no effect on the intensity of tinnitus. This had left the patient with a very poor appetite. There had been a similar episode in the previous year, when the GP had prescribed the same medication which did alleviate the symptoms temporarily. The flare-ups occur every time work became intense.

On Examination:

The patient was suffering with dizziness and had to be accompanied by her husband. This feeling was worse on rotation of the neck. Complexion—pale. Lips—pale. She felt lethargic. BP—130/80 mmHg. Tongue—pale with teeth marks and a white coat. Pulse—deep and small.

TCM Diagnosis:

Qi and Blood Xu

Treatment:

Electro-acupuncture and moxibustion were used on the following points:

Points Used	Nerves Stimulated	TCM Explanations
Yifeng (SJ 17)	CrN.XI; C2–C3	Promotes and regulates the functional activities of the ear qi; improves hearing
Ermen (SJ 21)	CrN.VII	Also promotes the functional activities of the ear qi; improves hearing
Zhongzhu (SJ 3)	C8–T1	Improves hearing
Tinghui (GB 2)	CrN.VII; C2–C3	Same function as Yifeng and Ermen

Tinggong (SI 19)   CrN.VII   Specific point for eliminating
                                     tinnitus; improves hearing

Weekly treatments were given. After 10 sessions, the patient was symptom free.

Comments:

The points around the ear are related to the great auricular nerve and the auricular temporal nerve. Stimulation of these nerves helps to regulate the function of the autonomic nervous system to improve the circulation to the inner ear and to reduce the hydropa.

TRIGEMINAL NEURALGIA

Female—40 years old

Complaint:

Pain and spasm on both sides of the face, left worse than the right.

History:

One year ago, she was experiencing a lot of stress at home, resulting in insomnia. She also had pain in her teeth, the left worse than the right. The last 6 months she had been having headaches which radiates to the shoulders. Insomnia had increased and the pain was worse. She was given an injection which did not have any effect. The occurrence of pain occurred at irregular intervals each lasting 3 or 4 minutes.

On Examination:

She had a pained expression and looked tired. Tests with cotton wool and pin pricks brought a painful response. Pain was worse with finger pressure. The sensation travelled along the lower mandible and in the front of the ear, then close to the nose, following the 2nd and 3rd branch of the trigeminal nerve. Tongue—slight purplish with a white coat. Pulse—tight.

TCM Diagnosis:

Stagnation of Blood and Qi

Treatment:

Treatment was given with electro-acupuncture and moxibustion on the following:

Points Used	Nerves Stimulated	TCM Explanations
Sibai (St 2)	CrN.V + VII	Disperses wind; reduces pain; activates blood
Xiaguan (St 7)	CrN.V + VII	Disperses wind; regulates qi
Jiache (St 6)	CrN.V + VII	Disperses wind; regulates qi
Yifeng (SJ 17)	CrN.V + VII; C1–C8	Activates qi; clears channels; disperses wind
Taiyang (Ext. pt.)	CrN.V + VII	Clears wind; activates blood
Jianjing (GB 21)	CrN.XI	Clears heat; regulates qi; reduces pain in the shoulders and neck

Weekly treatments were given. A total of 20 treatments were given with a break in between.

Comments:

The points were chosen for their relationship to the nerve supply as well as for their specific traditional functions.

TRIGEMINAL NEURALGIA—CASE 2

Female—47 years old

Complaint:

Pain in the left upper and lower jaw.

History:

She had a similar episode 3 years ago which resolved with some drugs. This episode started 4 months ago and was much worse. Pain was exacerbated by drinking and brushing her teeth. Each bout of pain lasted from several seconds to several minutes and caused her to salivate excessively. Drugs had not helped and surgery was the only other option.

On Examination:

She had a painful expression. The left side of the face was painful with the cotton and pin prick tests and with finger pressure. Tongue—red with a yellow coat. Pulse—wiry.

TCM Diagnosis:

Yang Ming Stomach Heat

Treatment:

Points Used	Nerves Stimulated	TCM Explanations
Sibai (St 2)	CrN.V + VII	Disperses wind; reduces pain
Jiache (St 6)	CrN.V + VII	Disperses wind; regulates qi
Xiaguan (St 7)	CrN.V + VII	Disperses wind; regulates qi
Yinxiang (LI 20)	CrN.V + VII	Disperses wind; clears heat and channels
Yifeng (SJ 17)	CrN.V + VII; C1–C8	Disperses wind; clears channels; activates qi

Treatment with electro-acupuncture and moxibustion were given once weekly. Pain was relieved after 2 sessions. She felt well enough to stop treatment after another 2 sessions, and she was advised to come when necessary.

2 months later, it started with a bout of drinking and she only needed 1 treatment.

TINNITUS

Female—60 years old

Complaint:

A low whistling noise in the right ear.

History:

Had been suffering with the tinnitus for 10 years. Recently, she had been experiencing a dry mouth, bitter taste, a sore lumbar region, constipation and occasionally, insomnia. As a result, the whistling seemed to have got more pronounced.

On Examination:

Tongue—slightly red with a white coat. Pulse—small

TCM Diagnosis:

Shen Yin Xu

Treatment:

Points Used	Nerves Stimulated	TCM Explanations
Yifeng (SJ 17)	CrN.V + VII; C1–C8	Activates blood; clears channels; improves hearing
Fengchi (GB 20)	CrN.XI	Pacifies fire; calms the mind; specifically for insomnia
Tinghui (GB 2)	CrN.V	Removes heat from the liver and gall bladder to reduce tinnitus
Ermen (SJ 21)	CrN.V	Improves and regulates functional qi of the ear thus suitable for problems associated with the hear
Tinggong (SI 19)	CrN.V	Improves and regulates functional qi of the ear
Shenshu (UB 23)	L1–L3	Back shu point of the kidney; strengthens function of kidney qi; improves ear function
Taixi (K 3)	L4–S2	Shu-stream and yuan-source point; tonifies kidney qi; disperses pathogenic xu heat; moisturise yin
Sanyingjiao (Sp 6)	L4–S3	Strengthens spleen and stomach; reinforces kidney and liver; clears heat; calms the mind

Electro-acupuncture and moxibustion were used, twice weekly. Each of the points, Tinghui, Ermen and Tinggong were used in rotation. After 20 sessions, the patient recovered completely.

Comments:

Using point Shenshu and Taixi particularly seemed to have a good effect on this type of condition. According to traditional thought, the kidney opens out into the ear, so improving kidney qi has a better chance of helping conditions associated with the ear. As far as tinnitus is concerned, acupuncture and moxibustion is effective for some and not others. Sometimes it can only reduce the level of noise that the patient hears.

CHRONIC LARYNGITIS

Male—35 years old

Complaint:

Suffering with a sore throat for more than a year.

History:

His throat had felt dry and painful intermittently. It had felt worse recently, with a burning sensation, dry mouth and frequent liquids were required. He tended to eat spicy foods which usually exacerbated the symptoms. Tended to have dry stools but not constipation. Sleep had been disturbed recently with the soreness and dryness of the throat.

On Examination:

The throat appeared red. Tongue—dull red with a thin white coat. Pulse—small and wiry.

TCM Diagnosis:

Xu Huo Shang Yang (Flaring-up of Xu Fire)

Treatment:

Points Used	Nerves Stimulated	TCM Explanations
Sanyingjiao (Sp 6)	L4–S3	Crossing point of 3 yin channels; nourishes yin
Yuyi (Lu 10)	C6–C7	Reduces fire to relieve sore throat
Kongzui (Lu 6)	C5–C7	Reduces fire; regulates lung qi to relieve sore throat
Zusali (St 36)	L4–S3	He-sea point; clears heat; strengthens body's resistence

Electro-acupuncture and moxibustion were given on the above points once a week for six weeks. In the seventh week, acupuncture were given in addition to the following herbs which were to be taken daily:

Sheng Di	(Radix Rehmanniae)
Mai Dong	(Radix Ophiopogonis)
Bai Shao	(Radix Paconiac Alba)
Dan Pi	(Cortex Moutan Radicis)
Bei Mu	(Bulbus Fritillariac Cirrhosae)
Xuan Shen	(Radix Scropholariae)

Bo He   (Herba Menthae) (To be added to the brew only in the last
                 5 minutes)
Gan Cao   (Radix Glycyrrhizae)

After 2 more weeks of herbs and acupuncture, the patient was
discharged.

Comments:

The symptoms here are also due to abnormal activity of the vagus nerve
which can be regulated by acupuncture. Herbs are generally effective for
this type of problem.

ASTHMA

Female—69 years old

Complaint:

Asthmatic for 25 years.

History:

It was triggered of 25 years ago by a flu and cough. Since then, each time there is a change in the weather, or excessive dust or when she was near a cat, she would suffer an attack. Her chest would feel tight and she would feel breathless. She would need to be in an upright position. Subsequent coughing spells would bring up bubbly white phlegm which was not too thick. She disliked the wind and her arms and legs always felt cold. She felt tired and had been experiencing frequency of urine. Laxatives were required on alternate days to clear her bowels. There was a family history of allergy and from a child, she had been sensitive to yeast, dust, pollen and cat fur.

On Examination:

Pale complexion. All 4 limbs felt cold. Her chest was barrel-shaped. Lips were slightly white. There was a wheezing sound in her airways. Tongue—pale and slightly swollen with a thin white coat. Pulse—deep and small.

TCM Diagnosis:

Shen Yang Xu

Treatment:

Points Used	Nerves Stimulated	TCM Explanations
Dingchuan (Ext. pt.)	C3–C8	Specific for asthma
Feishu (UB 13)	T3–T4	Back shu point of the lung; regulates lung qi
Tanzhong (Ren 17)	C5–T1	Soothes the chest; relieves cold and asthma
Fenglong (St 40)	L4–S1	Strengthens the spleen and resolves phlegm
Zusanli (St 36)	L4–S3	He-sea point; strengthens spleen; removes phlegm; reinforces blood and qi of liver and kidney; restores functions of the body

Dazhui (Du 14)	C3; C4; C8	Crossing point of the Yang Channels of the Hand + Leg; improves yang qi; removes wind and cold; relieves asthma
Zhongfu (Lu 1)	C5–T1	Front mu point of the lung; promotes lung qi; relieves asthma; reduces fullness of chest
Shenshu (UB 23)	L1–L3	Back shu point of the kidney; strengthens the kidney function to increase yang qi

Electro-acupuncture and moxibustion were used on the above combination of points. Treatment was given twice a week for the first 2 weeks then once weekly. A total of 20 treatments were given with a rest in between. Her condition was stabilised and she was advised to have treatment either once monthly or when necessary.

Comments:

The combination of points, Zhongfu and Feishu is effective for relieving asthma. The combination of Dazhui and Zhongfu, is traditionally used for improving lung function.

Acupuncture and moxibustion are generally effective in helping to manage asthma rather than affecting a cure.

HAY FEVER

Male—62 years old

Complaint:

Chronic sinus congestion.

History:

Had a 20 year history of allergy especially in the summer which also caused a general itching in addition to sinusitis. 4 years ago he started having additional symptoms of earaches although there was no hearing loss. In addition there were also symptoms of constipation, a burning sensation in his stomach and his digestive system always felt gaseous. 15 years ago he had an operation on his prostate to reduce urethral blockage. Consequently, his urine passage was not as smooth as it should be and the doctors had advised a second operation.

On Examination:

He looked pale and tired. It was not the hay fever season, but his sinuses were still blocked. His lower abdomen felt distended with a heavy sensation on palpation. Tongue—pale with a white coat. Pulse—slow.

TCM Diagnosis:

Lung and Kidney Xu

Treatment:

Electro-acupuncture and moxibustion were used on the following points:

Points Used	Nerves Stimulated	TCM Explanations
Yinxiang (LI 20)	CrN.V + VII	Specific for nasal obstruction, rhinorrhoea and hay fever
Zusanli (St 36)	L4–S3	Reinforces blood and qi and kidney; strengthens spleen and stomach
Qugu (Ren 2)	T6–T12	Tonifies the kidney
Zhongji (Ren 3)	T6–T12	Front mu point of the urinary bladder; regulates the Ren channel; promotes urination
Shenshu (UB 23)	L1–L3	Back shu point of the kidney; strengthens the kidney and reinforces kidney qi

Ciliao (UB 32)	S2	Strengthens the kidney; specific for urinary problems

In addition, ear points on Prostate Gland and Kidney were also punctured. Treatment was given weekly with ear studs left in. After the third week there was less nasal congestion and there was a definite improvement with his micturation. After another 3 weeks of treatment, there was no more nasal congestion and micturation was normal. The patient then complained about pain in his left knee joint and the MCP joints of his right hand. Treatment was thus concentrated on these areas using the following:

Xiyan (St 35) and corresponding point on the medial side of the patella	L3	For relief of pain in the knee joint
Qugu (Ren 2)		
Zhongji (Ren 3)		
Point between 2nd + 3rd right metacarpals	C7–T1	Local Ah Shih points
Point between 3rd + 4th right metacarpals	C7–T1	Local Ah Shih points

The patient had 3 more treatments and had recovered well enough for treatment to stop.

EPILEPSY

Female—14 years old

Complaint:

Epileptic since puberty.

History:

Started menstruating at age 12. Six months later, she started having symptoms before, during or after her periods. They usually occur in the morning or during the night. She would fall suddenly, her eyes rolling upwards and would start to convulse for a few seconds. There were no warning signs. She had been treated with drugs while she was in Hong Kong without any improvement. In fact, the attacks had increased to a few times weekly. Her memory was poor and her sleep disturbed. There was no family history of epilepsy.

On Examination:

She looked pale and tired. Tongue—slight red and dry with a little coating. Pulse—small.

TCM Diagnosis:

Liver and Kidney Yin Xu

Treatment:

Points Used	Nerves Stimulated	TCM Explanations
Neiguan (P 6)	C6–T1	Luo-connecting point; regulates qi flow; relieves mental stress; reduces epileptic fits.
Shenmen (Ht 7)	C8–T1	Shu-stream point and yuan-source point; tranquillises and reduces anxiety; helps to reduce insomnia
Sanyingjiao (Sp 6)	L4–S3	Nourishes yin and balances yang; reinforces liver and kidney
Yintang (Ext. pt.)	CrN.V–VII	Calms the mind; specific for insomnia and convulsions
Baihui (Du 20)	CrN.V + C2	Refreshes the brain to restore the mind; nourishes yin to alleviate convulsions and insomnia
Fengchi (GB 20)	CrN.XI	Refreshes the mind; reduces insomnia and convulsions

| Anmian (Ext. pt.) | CrN.XI; C1–C3 | Reduces insomnia |
| Shenshu (UB 23) | L1–L3 | Strengthens function of kidney qi; reinforces yang; back shu point of kidney |

Treatment with electro-acupuncture and moxibustion were given on the above points once a week. After two sessions her convulsions had ceased. Treatment was then given before the start of each period and in between periods, for another 3 months. She recovered completely.

DIZZINESS

Male—66 years old

Complaint:

Started having dizzy spells 3 years ago.

History:

The dizzy spells were controlled to a certain extent by stemetil. 3 months ago, he was prescribed prochlorperazin 5 mg. There was some improvement. He had been complaining of tightness of the neck muscles and his hearing is reduced. He was also taking β-blockers to reduce high blood pressure.

On Examination:

He felt as if he was walking on the deck of a boat in rough seas all the time. Tongue—slight red with a slight yellow coat. Pulse—wiry.

TCM Diagnosis:

Gan Yang Rising

Treatment:

Electro-acupuncture and moxibustion were used on the following:

Points Used	Nerves Stimulated	TCM Explanations
Neiguan (P 6)	C6–T1	Calms the mind; reduces dizziness
Quchi (LI 11)	C5–T1	He-sea point; regulates yang qi; promotes blood flow
Zusanli (St 36)	L4–S3	He-sea point; strengthens body's resistence; restores normal function; reinforces liver and kidney
Taixi (K 3)	L4–S2	Shu-stream and yuan-source point; tonifies kidney qi
Ermen (SJ 21)	CrN.V	Improves and regulates functional qi of the ear; improves hearing
Yifeng (SJ 17)	CrN.XI; C7	Activates blood and clears channels to improve hearing
Shenshu (UB 23)	L1–L3	Back shu point of the kidney; increases kidney qi function; improves hearing

Jueyinshu (UB 14)	T2–T4	Back shu point of the pericardium; regulates flow of liver & heart qi; regulates stomach function to reduce nausea
Fengchi (GB 20)	CrN.XI	Reduces wind; calms the mind
Xinshu (UB 15)	T3–T5	Back shu point of the heart; relieves mental stress

After the first treatment, the dizziness had disappeared. Two more treatments were given to reinforce the first treatment and the patient was well enough for treatment to stop.

SLEEP WALKING (SOMNAMBULISM)

Female—32 years old

Complaint:

She had been suffering with the problem for the past year.

History:

It all started with the shock of her mother's death and having to leave her home country. She realised the extent of her problem when she was woken up one morning in the nearby park on a bench. When she was escorted back to her home, all her doors had been left ajar. Since then she had tried blocking all her doors and windows up before retiring to bed, although she would find herself waking up in various parts of the house. She dreamt a lot and even appeared to move furniture during her sleep. The GP had prescribed tranquillisers which made her worse.

On Examination:

She had a pale complexion. She felt tired and had lost her appetite. Tongue—normal. Pulse—deep and small.

TCM Diagnosis:

Heart Blood Xu

Treatment:

Points Used	Nerves Stimulated	TCM Explanations
Shenmen (Ht 7)	C8–T1	Shu-stream and yuan-source point; regulates qi; tranquillises the mind and reduces anxiety
Neiguan (P 6)	C6–T1	Luo-connecting point; nourishes heart; regulates qi; calms the mind to relieve mental stress
Zusanli (St 36)	L4–S3	He-sea point; reinforces blood and qi; restores normal function
Baihui (Du 20)	CrN.V; C2	Strengthens the brain; tranquillises the mind
Yintang (Ext.pt.)	CrN.V + VII	Unblocks the channels; calms the mind
Xinshu (UB 15)	T3–T5	Back shu point of the heart; regulates heart qi; relieves mental stress

Pishu (UB 20)	T11–T12	Back shu point of the spleen; reinforces blood
Dazhui (Du 14)	CrN.XI; C3; C4; C8	Regulates flow of qi; nourishes blood; relieves mental stress

Electro-acupuncture and moxibustion were used on the above points and an ear stud was retained at point Shenmen.

A total of 6 weekly treatments were given. Each time, a stud was retained at ear point Shenmen. She completely recovered after the 6 treatments.

NAIL BITING

Female—45 years old

Complaint:

Had not been able to stop biting her nails since childhood.

History:

She would be biting the nails of all 10 fingers, if she was not busy and especially when watching television or travelling. The appearance of her nails had made her very self conscious. She had seen a psychiatrist and a hypnotist but without success.

On Examination:

There were no tips to her fingernails. Tongue—slightly red with a thin yellow coat. Pulse—wiry and small on the left side, slippery and strong on the right.

TCM Diagnosis:

Gan Yin Xu with Stomach Fire Excess

Treatment:

Points Used	Nerves Stimulated	TCM Explanations
Ququan (Liv 8)	L2−S2	He-sea point; reinforces liver; tonifies kidney; reduces fire
Taichong (Liv 3)	L4−S2	Shu-stream and yuan-source point; reinforces liver xu
Fuliu (K 7)	L4−S2	Jing-river point; reduces fire; tonifies kidney; moisturises to reduces dryness; nourishes yin; reinforces kidney and liver; warms yang qi
Zusanli (St 36)	L4−S3	He-sea point; pacifies stomach fire; reinforces liver and kidney
Fenglong (St 40)	L4−S1	Luo-connecting point; regulates stomach and spleen
Taibai (Sp 3)	L4−S1	Shu-stream and yuan source point; reduces fire; relieves mental stress; regulates stomach and spleen
Yintang (Ext. pt.)	CrN.V + VII	Unblocks the channels and calms the mind

Anmian (Ext. pt.)   CrN.XI; C1–C3   Inhibits excess activity of the
                                             brain

Points Fenglong, Taibai and Zusanli in combination are effective in clearing stomach damp and stomach heat and in reducing stomach fire.

Electro-acupuncture and moxibustion were used on the above points once a week. After 10 weeks she felt confident that she did not need to bite her nails anymore and treatment was stopped.

INSOMNIA

Male—36 years old

Complaint:

Had been suffering from insomnia for several months.

History:

Even from a child he had reacted to stress by not sleeping. It was accompanied by palpitation and anxiety, with trembling hands, dry mouth, and at the moment a sore lower back.

On Examination:

He looked exhausted. Tongue—slightly red. Pulse—fast and small.

TCM Diagnosis:

Yin Xu with Fire Excess and Kidney Xu

Treatment:

Electro-acupuncture and moxibustion were given on the following points:

Points Used	Nerves Stimulated	TCM Explanations
Shenmen (Ht 7)	C8–T1	Yuan-source point; calms the mind
Neiguan (P 6)	C6–T1	Luo-connecting point; nourishes the heart; calms the mind to relieve mental stress
Sanyingjiao (Sp 6)	L4–S3	Crossing point of 3 yin channels; nourishes yin; pacifies yang
Taixi (K 3)	L4–S2	Shu-stream and yuan-source point
Baihui (Du 20)	CrN.V	Crossing point of 3 yang channels of the hand and leg and the Du channel; regulates brain function;
Yintang (Ext. pt.)	CrN.V + VII	Calms the mind

The combination of Neiguan and Sanyingjiao is effective in clearing heat in the upper part of the body. A total of 10 weekly treatments was required.

INSOMNIA—CASE 2

Male—37 years old

Complaint:

Had been sleeping very badly for the past month.

History:

He worked mainly on computers and had been very busy recently. The intensity of work he had caused him to sleep badly and in the past 2 months he had been having headaches as well. Recently, his shoulders and lower back had also been aching and a week ago his left ear had felt swollen.

On Examination:

He was a thin man, and he was looking tired. Tongue—red. Pulse—small and fast.

TCM Diagnosis:

Disharmony of Heart and Kidney

Treatment:

Electro-acupuncture and moxibustion were used on the following combination of points:

Points Used	Nerves Stimulated	TCM Explanations
Shenmen (Ht 7)	C8–T1	Yuan-source point; calms the mind
Neiguan (P 6)	C6–T1	Luo-connecting point; nourishes the heart; calms the mind to relieve mental stress
Baihui (Du 20)	CrN.V	Regulates brain function; crossing point of the yang channels of the 3 hand and leg and the Du channels
Yintang (Ext. pt.)	CrN.V + VII	Calms the mind
Anmian (Ext. pt.)	CrN.XI; C1–C3	Calms the mind and specific for sleeping
Fengchi (GB 20)	CrN.XI	Calms the mind; in combination with Shenmen is good for insomnia

| Shenshu (UB 23) | L1–L3 | Back shu point of the kidney; improves kidney qi |
| Taixi (K 3) | L4–S2 | Shu-stream and yuan-source point; nourishes kidney yin and improves kidney qi |

Weekly treatments were given. After 10 sessions the patient was sleeping normally.

Comments:

Shenmen and Neiguan together are effective for reducing Ht Fire. Electro-stimulation to Baihui and Yintang helps to raise the levels of 5HT. Insomniacs are found to have a low level of 5HT. Perhaps, if stimulation is successful in raising 5HT levels, the patient will be able to sleep better.

DEPRESSION

Male—32 years old

Complaint:

Recent onset of depression

History:

He had been having symptoms of feeling low, tired, fragile, having a poor appetite and no interest in sex. His sleep was disturbed and he suffered with constipation. Blood tests were normal.

On Examination:

Tongue—normal with a white coat. Pulse—wiry.

TCM Diagnosis:

Liver Qi Stagnation

Treatment:

Electro-acupuncture and moxibustion were used on the following points:

Points Used	Nerves Stimulated	TCM Explanations
Baihui (Du 20)	CrN.V	Regulates brain functions and the yang channels
Yintang (Ext. pt.)	CrN.V + VII	Calms the mind
Shenmen (Ht 7)	C8–T1	Yuan-source point; calms the mind
Neiguan (P 6)	C6–T1	Luo-connecting point; nourishes the heart; calms the mind to relieve mental stress
Zusanli (St 36)	L4–S3	Reinforces qi and blood
Dazhui (Du 14)	CrN.XI; C3; C4; C8	Regulates qi flow; relieves mental stress
Mingmen (Du 4)	L2	Regulates qi flow; strengthens essence of life; improves yang qi
Hiatus (Ext. pt.)	S4	Improves function of the reproductive system

Ear points, Shenmen and Liver were also needled. Treatment was given once a week. Only 10 treatments were required.

Comments:

The combination of Baihui and Yintang helps to improves yang qi and restore normal function. Points Zusanli and Dazhui together are also effective in improving yang qi.

OBESITY

Female—21 years old

Complaint:

Had been obese since childhood.

History:

Felt insecure and did not relate well to people including colleagues at work. Did not communicate well even with the rest of the family at home. She had long hair to cover her face and would only go out if accompanied by someone she trusted. She had tried various methods to loose weight and was even under hospital supervision for a period of time. None of the methods had worked.

On Examination:

She weighed 228 lbs. She was very shy.

TCM Diagnosis:

Damp with phlegm

Treatment:

2 combination of points were used for electro-acupuncture and moxibustion:

Plan 1

Points Used	Nerves Stimulated	TCM Explanations
Hegu (LI4)	C6–T1	Yuan-source point; eliminates damp
Quchi (LI 11)	C5–T1	He-sea point; regulates qi; promotes blood flow; relieves dampness
Zusanli (St 36)	L4–S3	He-sea point; clears channels; strengthens spleen to disperse phlegm and damp; restores normal function of the body
Xuehai (Sp 10)	L2–L4	Activates blood; clears channels; disperses damp
Zhongwan (Ren 12)	T7–T12	Front mu point of the stomach; one of the 8 influential points; regulates functions of the stomach

		to strengthen spleen function and to warm middle jiao to remove damp
Tianshu (St 25)	T7–T12	Front mu point of the large intestine; regulates function of the middle jiao and stomach and the flow of qi to strengthen the functions of the spleen and the large intestine; specific for reducing weight

At the same time, ear points Hunger and Stomach were needled and studs were retained after each session.

Plan 2
Hegu (L14); Quchi (LI 11); Zusanli (St 36); Tianshu (St 25) and:

Sanyingjiao (Sp 6)	L4–S3	Strengthens the spleen to remove dampness; promotes diuresis
Fengshi (GB 31)	L2–L4	Promotes blood circulation; activates channels; disperses dampness
Shuidao (St 28)	T 7–T12	Removes dampness; promotes diuresis

Ear points Hunger, Stomach and Endocrine were used and studs retained.
   Treatment was given once a week alternating Plan 1 with Plan 2.
   After the first treatment, her weight was 219 lbs. After 25 sessions, the patient's weight was down to 126 pounds. She was satisfied with that weight. She gained in confidence during this time, became more sociable and was able to start a relationship with a boy she met.

Comments:

After stimulation with electro-acupuncture and moxibustion, levels of plasma cortisol are raised with a corresponding fall in aldehyde ketones. There also appears to be a corresponding rise of triglycerides and total cholestoral contents. A clinical study over a period between 1979 and 1983 by Dr Lily Cheung involving 30 males and 154 females revealed that the effective rate of the treatment was 50.54%.

GALL STONES

Male—44 years old

Complaint:

Pain in the upper abdomen.

History:

Pain was worse after eating and radiates to the right scapula accompanied by nausea and a bitter taste in the mouth. It had got worse recently and after the evening meals, the pain was like a nagging toothache. Investigations at the hospital had revealed presence of gall stones. He decided not to have surgery.

On Examination:

The patient was obese. There was slight pressure pain on the right lower ribs and obvious pain in the area T9 to T11 on the right side. Tongue— normal with a thin yellow coat. Pulse—wiry and small.

TCM Diagnosis:

Liver Qi Stagnation

Treatment:

Points Used	Nerves Stimulated	TCM Explanations
Zusanli (St 36)	L4–S3	He-sea point; strengthens body's resistence and restore normal function; reduces nausea and vomiting
Zhongwan (Ren 12)	T7–T12	Front mu point of the stomach; one of the 8 influential points; stops vomiting
Zhangmen (Liv 13)	Intercostal nerves 8 to 12	Front mu point of the spleen; controls rising qi; one of the 8 influential points
Qimen (Liv 14)	Intercostal nerves 8 to 12	Front mu point of the liver; promotes blood circulation to remove blood stagnation
Ganshu (UB 18)	T8–T10	Back shu point of the liver; regulates function of liver qi; relieves pain in the hypochondria region

| Danshu (UB 19) | T9–T11 | Back shu point of the gall bladder; regulates function of the gall bladder |
| Yanglingquan (GB 34) | L4–S1 | He-sea point; one of the 8 influential points; relieves liver and gall bladder, reduces pain |

Electro-acupuncture and moxibustion were used on the above points once a week. At the same time, herbs were prescribed to be taken once daily:

Jin Qian Cao	(Herba Lysimachiae)
Yu Jin	(Radix Curcumae)
Huang Qin	(Radix Scutellariae)
Zhi Shi	(Fructus Aurantii Immaturus)
Yin Chen	(Herba Artemisiae Scopariae)
Ji Gu Cao	(Abrus)

After 2 weeks of treatment and herbs, there was only one episode of pain.10 more treatments were given during which there was no pain or discomfort. A further check-up at the hospital revealed that surgery was not necessary. He was advised to continue with acupuncture and herbal medicine once a month. Over a period of 12 months, there were no symptoms.

Comment:

The autonomic nervous system which supplies the gall bladder can be stimulated through T5–T9. Points Zhongwan, Zhangmen Qimen and Ganshu relate to the same nerve segments. The herbs prescribed promote choleresis and these herbs are commonly used for treatment of jaundice and cholycystitis.

PEPTIC ULCER

Male—25 years old

Complaint:

Upper abdominal pain and heartburn.

History:

A few years ago, stress of work and having to sit an examination caused anxiety and headaches. 2 years ago, he started having symptoms of heartburn, indigestion and loss of appetite. The heartburn was usually relieved by food. In the mornings he would have a bitter taste in his mouth which would also feel dry. After some investigations, a peptic ulcer was diagnosed. So far medication has had no effect.

On Examination:

He had a pale complexion. He was still suffering with anxiety. On palpation of the upper abdomen, it felt tender. Palpation in the area of the spine T7–T12 showed it was tender along both sides of the spine. Tongue—normal with a slight yellow coat. Pulse—wiry.

TCM Diagnosis:

Disharmony of Liver and Stomach

Treatment:

Electro-acupuncture and moxibustion were given on the following points:

Points Used	Nerves Stimulated	TCM Explanations
Zhongwan (Ren 12)	T7–T12	Front mu point of the stomach; regulates function of the stomach; relieves gastric pain and vomiting
Zusanli (St 36)	L4–S3	He-sea point; strengthens and regulates the spleen and stomach; strengthens body's resistence and restores normal functions
Taichong (Liv 3)	L4–S2	Shu-stream and yuan-source point; soothes the liver; regulates qi; activates blood
Neiguan (P 6)	C6–T1	Luo-connecting point; regulates qi; soothes the chest; reduces gastrointestinal disturbance;

		relieves mental stress; reduces gastric pain and vomiting
Ah Shih points at	T7–T12	Local points to help reduce pain
Pishu (UB 20)	T11–T12	Back shu point of the spleen; regulates function of the spleen
Weishu (UB 21)	T12–L1	Back shu point of the stomach; nourishes stomach yang

A total of 6 weekly treatments were required.

Comment:

Experiments have shown that stimulation of Zusanli can stimulate the body to raise the levels of endorphins, thus raising the pain threshold. Gastroscopy had shown that stimulating Zusanli can regulate the movements of the stomach.

CONSTIPATION

Female—37 years old.

Complaint:

Unable to have bowel motions for the last 4 days.

History:

Normal pattern for bowel motion was once every 2 to 3 days and usually with the help of laxatives. Stools were usually dry accompanied by some bleeding due to the presence of haemorrhoids. There was a time a few years previously when it seemed to be worse before her periods. Her periods had been irregular recently, and her constipation had gradually got worse. In the mornings, she would have a bitter taste in her mouth, which would tend to be dry. The use of laxatives recently did not help to clear her bowels. Her abdomen felt swollen and her appetite was lost.

On Examination:

The abdomen felt distended but there was no palpation pain. External haemorrhoids were observed. Tongue—red with a dry and yellow coat. Pulse—slippery.

TCM Diagnosis:

Yang Ming Stagnation Heat

Treatment:

Points Used	Nerves Stimulated	TCM Explanations
Zusanli (St 36)	L4–S3	He-sea point; clears heat; strengthens the spleen and nourishes the stomach; clears the channels
Shangjuxu (St 37)	L4–S1	Lower He-sea point of the large intestine; regulates stomach qi; pacifies yang ming heat
Tianshu (St 25)	T7–T12	Regulates qi flow to strengthen function of the spleen and the large intestine; specific for constipation
Dachangshu (UB 25)	L4	Back shu point of the large intestine; regulates function of the

		large intestine and the small intestine; regulates flow of qi to relieve stagnation in the abdomen
Ciliao (UB 32)	S2	Strengthens the kidney; regulates menstruation; reduces heat; improves the function of the large intestine

Electro-acupuncture only was used on the above points. Immediately after the treatment the patient felt the need to have a bowel motion and some very dry stools were passed. Only one more treatment was given the following week, after which the patient appeared to have no more problems.

One year later, the patient returned for treatment to her knee joint. She confirmed that there were no more problems with her bowel motions.

LOCK JAW—CASE 2

Male—23 years old

Complaint:

Suffered with locked jaw and pain on both sides for several years.

History:

The problem started with a bout of flu. The pain radiates to the neck and across the shoulders. She was prescribed physiotherapy which had variable temporary effects. No drugs had been prescribed. Movement of the jaw was very limited with the result that she had difficulty eating solid foods. She had also been suffering with intermittent headaches. Her urine appeared concentrated.

On Examination:

Tongue—slightly pale with a thin white coat. Pulse—slow.

TCM Diagnosis:

Blood Qi Xu with Pathological Wind Dampness in the Channels

Treatment:

Electro-acupuncture and moxibustion were used on the following points:

Points Used	Nerves Stimulated	TCM Explanations
Xiaguan (St 7)	CrN.V + VII	Crossing point of Foot Yang-ming Channel + Xiaoyang Channel; regulates qi; disperses wind
Jiache (St 6)	CrN.VII	Clears Yang-ming channel; specific point for problems with the jaw; regulates qi; disperses wind
Jianjing (GB 21)	CrN.XI	Clears channels and regulates qi; reduces heat; reduces pain along shoulder and neck
Fengchi (GB 20)	CrN.XI; C2–C5	Removes wind and fights external syndromes; activates blood; effective for pain in the neck and across shoulders
Tinggong (SI 19)	CrN.V	Crossing point for the Hand Tai-yang and the Foot + Hand Xiao-yang Channels

Treatment was given once a week. Points, Xiaguan, Jiache and Tinggong together help to activate qi and blood to remove wind and clear the channels.

After 2 sessions, pain was reduced and there was more movement in the jaw.

After 10 sessions, the patient had a complete recovery.

APHTLOUS STOMATITIS

Female—52 years old

Complaint:

Recurring ulcers in the mucous membranes of the mouth

History:

For the past 3 years, she had been having frequent ulcerations of the mouth and tongue. They gave her considerable pain especially when drinking hot or cold fluids. As a result the mouth felt dry and bitter. She suffered with some tinnitus and dizziness as well. There were also symptoms of indigestion, poor appetite, bad temper and restlessness. The sores were worse whenever she slept badly. Her periods had stopped for 2 years. She had tried many methods but without any success.

On Examination:

She had halitosis. The oral mucous membranes had small and big ulcers which were red rimmed and yellow white centers. The mandibular lymph nodes were swollen but movable and without pain. Tongue—pale with a little coat. Pulse—small and rapid.

TCM Diagnosis:

Pi Shen Xu and Xu Fire Excess

Treatment:

Electro-acupuncture and moxibustion were applied to the following points:

Points Used	Nerves Stimulated	TCM Explanations
Hegu (LI 4)	C6–T1	Yuan-source point; reduces fire; specific for problems associated with the face and mouth
Sanyingjiao (Sp 6)	L4–S3	Crossing point of the 3 yin channels; regulates the spleen and the stomach; reinforces the kidney and liver; nourishes yin and reduces fire
Zusanli (St 36)	L4–S3	He-sea point of the stomach; clears heat; strengthens the spleen and the stomach and regulates qi

Yongquan (K 1)	L5–S2	Nourishes yin to reduce pathological qi fire; relieves mental stress; brings down rising fire
Xiaguan (St 7)	CrN.V + VII	Local point to activate channel; regulates qi flow and relieves pain

The patient recovered after 20 weekly treatments.

STROKE

Female—63 years old

Complaint:

Had a stroke 4 days ago with a right sided weakness in the limbs, numbness and slow speech.

History:

Generally a weak constitution. She had a raised blood pressure but was not on medication. The symptoms appeared during a stressful holiday when she got very tired and had a quarrel with her son. Her hand and feet felt cold and her appetite was poor. She had no control over micturation.

On Examination:

BP–180/80. She looked pale and tired looking. The lips were pale, speech and responses was slow. There did not appear to be any facial weakness. Knee jerk response was reduced. There was numbness in the right arm and the right leg was weak. Tongue—pale with a purplish tinge with a white coat and blood spots. Pulse—wiry and small.

TCM Diagnosis:

Qi Xu and Blood Stagnation

Treatment:

Electro-acupuncture and moxibustion were used on 2 combinations of points:

Plan 1

Points Used	Nerves Stimulated	TCM Explanations
Hegu (LI 4)	C6–T1	Gate point and yuan-source points; expels wind
Taichong (Liv 3)	L4–S2	Gate point; reduces wind; activates blood; regulates qi
Quchi (LI 11)	C5–T1	Regulates qi; promotes blood flow; specific for reducing BP
Fengchi (GB 20)	CrN.XI	Reduces wind; regulates liver; activates blood and resolves phlegm

Zusanli (St 36)	L4–S3	He-sea point; strengthens spleen; resolves phlegm; reinforces qi and blood of the liver and kidney; restores normal functions
Sanyingjiao (Sp 6)	L4–S3	Reinforces qi and blood of the liver and kidney
Pangguanshu (UB 28)	L5–S2	Back shu point of the urinary bladder; strengthens the lower jiao to clear the water channels
Ciliao (UB 32)	S2	Strengthens the kidney and the lower extremity
Qihai (Ren 6)	T6–T12	Tonifies kidney qi
Jinjinyuye (Ext. pt.)	CrN. 12	Stimulates qi

The combination of points Quchi and Fengchi lowers BP more effectively. Point Jinjinyuye is stimulated only by pricking with the needle.

Ear points used in addition were "Lower Blood Pressure" and Kidney.

Plan 2

Points Used	Nerves Stimulated	TCM Explanations
Hegu (LI 4)		
Waiguan (SJ 5) needled through to Neiguan (P 6)	C6–T1	Regulates qi and promotes circulation
Taixi (K 3) needled through to Kunlun (UB 60)	L4–S2	Taixi is a shu-stream point and yuan-source point; reinforces kidney; nourishes yin; clears channels; strengthens functions of the kidney
Huantiao (GB 30)	L2–S3	Unblocks channels; removes wind; relieves rigidity of muscles, tendons and joints of the legs
Weizhong (UB 40)	L4–S2	Relaxes rigidity of the lumbar region and the knee
Yanglingquan (GB 34)	L4–S1	Shu-stream and one of the 8 influential points for tendons and weakness of the joints; activates channels
Lianquan (Ren 23)	CrN.V + VII; C1–C3	Regulates flow of qi; specific for aphasia and stiffness of tongue
Shenshu (UB 23)	L1–L3	Back shu point of the kidney; strengthens the function of kidney qi; strengthens the lower back and legs

Treatment was given daily, alternating Plan 1 and 2. After 4 weeks, she was able to control micturation, BP was down to 150/80 and there were improved movements in the affected limbs.

After another 6 weeks, she had improved sufficiently for treatment to stop. The patient was advised to take up Tai Chi and some running.

Six months later, she went to Indonesia. During that time, her speech and movements were normal but there was some problem with her walking. She had acupuncture there for 2 weeks.

11 years later, she wrote to say that she had completely recovered.

SJOGREN'S SYNDROME

Female—30 years old

Complaint:

The patient was suffering with parotitis and symptoms of dry mouth, eyes and vagina.

History:

About 4 years ago, the patient had a swelling of the parotid gland and severe conjunctivitis a few months later. Since then her eyes had been dry, sore and itchy with a white discharge. Last year, her saliva gland was blocked. She was hospitalised and Sjogren's Syndrome was diagnosed. In the mornings, she would feel dizzy. She had also been constipated.

On Examination:

She was looking tired. Her mouth, eyes and tongue was very dry and she had to use artificial tears. Tongue—red. Pulse—deep and small.

TCM Diagnosis:

Liver and Kidney Yin Xu

Treatment:

Points Used	Nerves Stimulated	TCM Explanations
Xiaguan (St 7)	CrN.V + VII	Activates channels and flow of qi to help stop pain; specific for problems of the parotid gland
Jiache (St 6)	CrN.VII	Regulates flow of qi; specific for problems of the parotid gland
Yifeng (SJ 17)	CrN.V; VII; XI	Clears channels; specific for problems of the parotid gland
Quchi (LI 11)	C5–T1	He-sea point; clears heat; regulates qi; promotes blood flow
Xuehai (Sp 10)	L2–L4	Regulates qi; clears blood heat
Sanyingjiao (Sp 6)	L4–S3	Regulates funciton of lower jiao; crossing point of 3 yin channels so reinforces kidney and liver qi and clears heat
Shenshu (UB 23)	L1–L3	Back shu point of the kidney; strengthens kidney qi

Ciliao (UB 32)   S2   Strengthens kidney qi; reduces
                                           heat

Electro-acupuncture and moxibustion were given on the above points once a week. After 3 weeks, there was more mucous discharge in the mouth and vagina and the parotid gland was less swollen.

After a further 3 weeks of treatment, the right parotid gland and the right eye began to feel normal and the secretions the vagina were normal. The eye and gland on the left side was still problematic.

After another 2 weeks, the left eye and gland started to improve.

4 weeks later, all symptoms had disappeared. A follow-up check one year later found the patient well. There was one episode of swelling in the parotid gland which subsided with some antibiotics.

Comments:

The symptoms experienced by the patient were due to a depressed auto-immune system. This usually responds well to acupuncture and moxibustion.

TIEGE'S DISEASE

Male—36 years old

Complaint:

Pain in the areas between the ribs and the left side of the sternum.

History:

Just over a year ago, he had a bout of flu and a cough, after which the pains started. Deep breathing and coughing would aggravate the pain. There was no redness or heat in the area, just a slight swelling. Analgesia was prescribed and only temporary relief was obtained.

On Examination:

The 3rd cartilage on the left side was painful on palpation and the area was slightly swollen. There was no redness. The pain was aggravated by coughing and deep intake of breaths, but the pain was localised. The liver and spleen felt normal on palpation. Tongue—pale with a thin white coat. Pulse—tight.

TCM Diagnosis:

Wind Cold, Blood and Qi Stagnation

Treatment:

Points Used	Nerves Stimulated	TCM Explanations
Ah Shih point at the 3rd cartilage	3rd intercostal nerve	
Tanzhong (Ren 17)	C5–T1	Front mu point of the pericardium; reinforces qi and soothes the chest
Neiguan (P 6)	C6–T1	Luo-connecting point; regulates qi; soothes chest
Waiguan (SJ 5)	C6–C8	Regulates qi; promotes blood circulation; dispels wind

Electro-acupuncture and moxibustion were given weekly for 6 weeks. The pain was gradually reduced and by the end of the 6 treatments, there was no more pain or swelling.

Comments:

Ah shih points are effective as they are pathological reaction areas of pain. Stimulating these points helps to increase circulation to the area, thus reducing inflammation and helping to increase levels of endorphins to relieve the pain.

RHEUMATOID ARTHRITIS

Female—29 years old

Complaint:

Pain in practically all her joints, especially on the right side.

History:

She had been having pain in her joints for at least 6 years. Rheumatoid arthritis was diagnosed 3 years ago when interphalangeal and metacarpophalangeal joints became red and swollen. The pain had gradually got worse in the knee, wrists and lumbar joints. Movements were limited. Analgesia had very little or no effect. Steroid therapy had more effect but she had been unable to stop it without the pain returning. She had decided to gradually come off her steroids.

On Examination:

The hands, knees and wrists on both sides were red and swollen. There was bilateral ulnar deviation. When the lumbar region was palpated, it was painful. Tongue—slightly red with a thin coat and purplish spots on both sides. Pulse—fast and slippery.

TCM Diagnosis:

Wind and Damp Bi Syndrome

Treatment:

Electro-acupuncture and moxibustion were applied to the following points:

Points Used	Nerves Stimulated	TCM Explanations
Dazhui (Du 14)	CrN.XI; C3; C4; C8	Reduces heat; regulates flow of qi; moisturises the tissues
Hegu (LI 4)	C6–T1	Clears heat; reduces wind; warms channels
Waiguan (SJ 5)	C6–C8	Luo-connecting point; regulates qi; moisturises blood; reduces fire
Xiyan (Ext. pt.) & Dubi (St 35)	L2–L4	Activates channels; relieves pain
Zusanli (St 36)	L4–S3	Clears heat; resolves dampness; reinforces blood and qi; reinforces the kidney and liver; regulates blood flow; he-sea point

Yanglingquan (GB 34)	L4–S1	He-sea point and shu-stream point; one of the 8 influential points for tendons and joints; clears heat; regulates qi
Shenshu (UB 23)	L1–L3	Strengthens the lower back and leg and the function of kidney qi
Sanyingjiao (Sp6)	L4–S3	Crossing point of the 3 yin channels; clears heat; dispels dampness; reinforces the kidney and liver

Treatment was given once weekly. She had a total of 30 treatments. A check-up 2 years later revealed that the patient was still feeling well enough not to require analgesia.

Comments:

The combination of points Hegu and Yinlingquan is effective in clearing heat and nourishing yin. Some studies had shown that this combination can modify the ESR and increase the levels of interleukin 2 to enhance the immune system.

RHEUMATOID ARTHRITIS—CASE 2

Male—60 years old

Complaint:

Pain in both knee joints.

History:

Had been diagnosed as rheumatoid arthritis. The pain was affected by weather change especially in the winter. It felt worse at night and when walking up the stairs, squatting and with flexion and extension of the joints. Application of a warm compress would help to soothe the discomfort but the pain is getting out of control.

On Examination:

He had a pale complexion. There was slight swelling on both knees but no redness. Crepitus was present on both knees. There was acute pain on palpation. Tongue—pale with a white coat. Pulse—tight.

TCM Diagnosis:

Cold Bi Syndrome

Treatment:

Points Used	Nerves Stimulated	TCM Explanations
Xiyan (Ext. pt.) & Dubi (St 35)	L3	Ah-shih points; activates channels; relieves pain
Zusanli (St 36)	L4–S3	He-sea point; disperses damp; reduces cold; activates qi and blood; strengthens the body; restores normal function
Yanglingquan (GB 34)	L4–S1	He-sea point; disperses wind; removes damp; strengthens bone; reinforces muscles and tendons; reduces pain

Treatment with electro-acupuncture and moxibustion was given once a week. A total of 20 treatments were given and the patient felt much better.

BI SYNDROME

Male—52 years old

Complaint:

Pain in the lower back and on the right side of the neck.

History:

About 2 months ago, the patient was involved in a car accident during which he was propelled forward causing pain in his neck and radiation of the pain to the occiput. The right side of the lumbar also became very painful with radiation to the cheek of the buttock. X-ray examinations had not revealed any abnormality. A corset was made for him and he went through a course of physiotherapy. There had been no change.

On Examination:

The right side of the neck felt swollen. Movements were restricted by pain with pressure pain in the occipital area and between C4 and C5, C5 and C6. In the lumbar region, the muscles on the right side of L4, L5 and S1 were tense and painful on palpation.

TCM Diagnosis:

Post Trauma Bi Syndrome

Treatment:

Electro-acupuncture and moxibustion were given on the following points:

Points Used	Nerves Stimulated	TCM Explanations
Fengchi (GB 20)	CrN.XI; C2–C5	Unblocks the channels
Jianjing (GB 21)	CrN.XI	Unblocks the channels

Ah-shih points between C4 and C5; C5 and C6 were also needled.

Treatment was given twice weekly. After 4 sessions, the neck was freer and the pain much reduced.

After a further 6 sessions, the pain had gone and the neck was moving normally. Treatment was stopped.

BI SYNDROME—CASE 2

Male—40 years old

Complaint:

Pain in the lumbar region.

History:

About one month ago, he had been sunbathing all weekend and on Monday he had difficulty getting out of bed. It gradually got worse, and the GP advised him to rest and prescribed a course of analgesia and physiotherapy. The pain had not gone away. Recently, the pain had been triggered off every time he got up from a sitting position.

On Examination:

Spinal flexion was painful and restricted. There was pressure pain between L4 and L5 and the muscles in the region were tensed. He only managed SLR to 45°. He cannot straighten his leg in the recumbent position. Tongue—pale with a thin white coat. Pulse—small.

TCM Diagnosis:

Bi Due to Cold and Damp Stagnation

Treatment:

Electro-acupuncture and moxibustion were used on the following points:

Points Used	Nerves Stimulated	TCM Explanations
Ah-Shih between L4 and L5	L3–L5	Specific point for pain in this area
Renchong (Du 26)	CrN.V + VII	Regulates the flow of qi; promotes blood circulation; using the principle of needling upper part of the body to treat the lower part
Weizhong (UB 40)	L4–S2	He-sea point; specific for relaxing rigidity and pain in the lumbar region
Yanglingquan (GB 34)	L4–S1	One of the 8 influential points to reinforce tendons and muscles; dispels cold; removes damp

After 6 weekly sessions, he was better.

BI SYNDROME—CASE 3

Male—78 years old

Complaint:

Pain in the lumbar region.

History:

He had a bad fall at 11 years old. From 1960 he had not been able to sit for long periods. In 1979, after 3 sessions of physiotherapy, he felt more pain. Investigations showed that the disc material was causing pressure on the nerves. A laminectomy was performed in 1979, but it made no difference to the pain he was experiencing. He started using the TENS machine and was having acupuncture at the hospital. 4 years after the laminectomy, he came for consultation.

On Examination:

There was pressure pain in the region of L2–S1. Flexion of the spine and coughing was painful. SLR was 60°. Tongue—pale with a thin white coat and teeth marks. Pulse—weak.

TCM Diagnosis:

Kidney Qi Xu; Qi and Blood Stagnation from Trauma

Treatment:

Electro-acupuncture and moxibustion were used on the following combination of points:

Points Used	Nerves Stimulated	TCM Diagnosis
Ah-shih point in the region L2–S1		Relaxes muscles and reduces pain
Shenshu (UB 23)	L1–L3	Strengthens kidney qi; back shu point of the kidney
Weizhong (UB 40)	L4–S2	He-sea point; relaxes rigidity; reduces pain in the lumbar region
Taixi (K 3) needled through to Kunlun (UB 60)	L4–S2	Taixi is a shu-stream and yuan-source point; reinforces kidney; restores qi and reduces pain. Kunlun clears qi stagnation; strengthens the lumbar region and improves the function of the kidney

Treatment was given weekly for 10 weeks. After this period he had no more pain and was advised to come for treatment once a month. After 4 months he was well enough to stop treatment.

Comments:

The aim of the treatment was to relax the muscle spasm, reduce tension on the nerve and to improve blood circulation.

BI SYNDROME—CASE 4

Male—55 years old

Complaint:

Pain in the lumbar region.

History:

20 years ago, he had a laminectomy which was successful. 10 years later, the pains started again. Originally, he had a slipped disc at L3–L4. 6 years after the laminectomy, he had one episode of pain as a result of increased work, when the pain radiated to both legs and he was unable to walk or flex his spine. He did recover from that episode.

On Examination:

He had to rest in bed. He had a painful expression and was unable to turn onto either side. On palpation of the spine, there was pain at the levels of L3 – L4 and L2 – L3 and the pain was worse on the right side of L3 – L4. Knee jerk and ankle jerk reflexes were reduced. SLR test was not possible due to pain. Tongue—red. Pulse—wiry and fast.

TCM Diagnosis:

Shen Yin Xu

Treatment:

Electro-acupuncture and moxibustion were given on the following points:

Points Used	Nerves Stimulated	TCM Explanations
Ah-shih points at the level of L2–L3		Reduces pain and relaxes the muscles
Guanyuanshu (UB 26)	L4–L5	Tonifies the kidney and regulates the channels
Shenshu (UB 23)	L1–L3	Back shu point of the kidney; strengthens the functionn of kidney qi
Taixi (K 3)	L4–S2	Shu-stream and yuan-source point; nourishes yin; tonifies the kidney
Mingmen (Du 4)	L2	Drains the channels; regulates the function of qi; reinforces yang

Weizhong (UB 40)   L4–S2   He-sea point; regulates rigidity
                                          and pain in the lumbar region

Treatment was given daily for 6 days. 2 weeks later, he was able to walk. Only one more treatment was required after that.

Comments:

Needle stimulation of the above points would have helped the micro-circulation in the area, restore nerve function and reduce pain and inflammation.

BI SYNDROME—CASE 5

Female—64 years old.

Complaint:

Post-operative pain.

History:

Long years of smoking had caused gangrene in the right leg, and in 1982, an amputation was performed below the knee. 5 months since, she was still suffering with pain from the medial side of the right knee and the popliteal fossa to the tip of the stump. The pain was especially bad at the tip of the stump. Analgesia prescribed had no effect on the pain.

Treatment:

Points Used	Nerves Stimulated
Yinlingquan (Sp 9)	L4–S1
Yanglingquan (GB 34)	L4–S1
Zusanli (St 36)	L4–S3
Shangjuxu (St 37)	L4–S1
Weizhong (UB 40)	L4–S2

The points were chosen according to the nerve supply. Only light penetration with the needles were used and stimulation provided with electricity. Moxibustion was used at the same time. The pain was reduced. A total of 10 treatments, twice weekly were required.

BI SYNDROME—CASE 6

Female—54 years old

Complaint:

Suffering with headaches and pain in the neck and across the shoulders.

History:

Started having recurrent headaches about 6 or 7 years ago. Came under the care of a rheumatologist in Australia without any results. Investigations had shown hyperosteogeny and osteosclerosis of the cervical spine especially at the levels of C2 and C3. Since about a year ago, the headaches had been between the eyebrows with radiation down to the neck and across the shoulders. The symptoms had caused pressure at work and with family relationships. Back in this country, she was treated with manipulation, traction, auto- suspension, lignocaine and triamcinolone injections. Benefits had been temporary, but she had never really been free from pain. In the meantime, the left leg had been gradually been beginning to trouble her but with only modest physical signs. Headaches had always been accompanied by clear signs at C2.

On Examination:

She had a painful expression. Palpation on the forehead did not produce any pressure pain. Palpation on the left side of the neck was not tender. There was definite pressure pain at C2. The muscles across the shoulders were tense and painful on palpation. Tongue—red with a yellow coat. Pulse—small.

TCM Diagnosis:

Qi and Blood Stagnation

Treatment:

Electro-acupuncture and moxibustion were given on the following points:

Points Used	Nerves Stimulated	TCM Explanations
Ah-shih points between C2 and C3		Reduces pain
Fengchi (GB 20)	CrN.XI; C2–C5	Activates qi and blood; removes stasis
Jianjing (GB 21)	CrN.XI	Regulates qi flow; specific for pain in the cervical region

| Taiyang (Ext. pt.) | CrN. II + VI | Specific for headaches |
| Houxi (SI 3) | C8–T1 | Shu-stream; confluence point connecting to Du channel for back and shoulder problems and osteosclerosis |

Treatment was given once a week. A course of 10 treatments was given. After a week's rest a further course of 10 was required before the patient was well enough.

SPONDYLOSIS

Male—69 years old

Complaint:

Pain in the neck and across the shoulders.

History:

Had been suffering for 15 years. The pain had gradually got worse in the last 6 months. On the right side the upper extremity was feeling numb and the pain was radiating to the ring finger, middle finger and the little finger. The patient was a builder and 25 years ago had injured his neck in a fall down a flight of stairs. He had to recover in a hospital but was left with a recurrent frozen shoulder. The neck was painful on rotation to the right with pain along the right arm and accompanied by a slight dizziness. Symptoms were relieved by rest. In the past 6 months, the pain had got worse and sleep had been disturbed. Movement of the neck had been limited by pain. Cold weather would make the symptoms worse. A recent x-ray revealed degeneration and nerve compression at the level of C5–C6. A course of physiotherapy and analgesia only slightly reduced the symptoms.

On Examination:

The neck movement was still restricted. Palpation of the neck caused pain at C5 and C6 especially on the right side, with radiation down the arm to the lateral 3 digits on the right side. Bicep and tricep reflexes on the right was reduced. Tongue—purplish. Pulse—wiry and small.

TCM Diagnosis:

Stagnation of Qi and Blood

Treatment:

Points Used	Nerves Stimulated	TCM Explanations
Hua-tuo at C5 + C6	C6–C7	Reduces pain
Shaohai (H 3)	C7–T1	He-sea point; improves blood circulation to reduce blood stagnation
Houxi (SI 3)	C8–T1	Expels wind to reduce neck stiffness
Fengchi (GB 20)	CrN.XI; C2–C5	Dispels wind; activates channels, qi and blood; relieves stagnation

Jianjing (GB 21)	CrN.XI	Clears channels to regulate flow of qi, stiff neck and pain in the shoulder
Jianzhen (SI 9)	C5–T2	Promotes blood circulation to remove blood stagnation
Quchi (LI 11)	C5–T1	Expels wind; regulates qi; promotes blood flow

Electro-acupuncture and moxibustion were given once a week. After 10 treatments, the amount of pain was reduced, but not completely gone.

NECK PAIN

Female—50 years old

Complaint:

Sudden onset of pain in the neck.

History:

4 weeks ago, pain started in the neck on waking , with radiation down the right side of the arm to the hand. There was numbness in the fingers on the right and movement of the neck was restricted. It was giving her a headache and sleep had not been possible. X-rays had shown mid-scoliosis with a concave to the left, and early spondylitic changes were present at C5/C6 and C6/C7 levels.

On Examination:

She had a painful expression. Her neck was stiff. On palpation, there was pain at C5 and C6 and a painful spot medial to the right scapula. Tongue—dull and purplish. Pulse—wiry and small.

TCM Diagnosis:

Blood and Qi Stagnation

Treatment:

Points Used	Nerves Stimulated	TCM Explanations
Ah-shih Points at the levels of C5/C6; C6/C7; T3; T4; T6	Corresponding cervical nerves	Reduces pain
Quchi (LI 11)	C5–T1	He-sea point; regulates qi; promotes blood flow
Tianzong (SI 11)	CrN. 11; T3–T5	Regulates qi
Ext. Pt. on Deltoid	C6	Reduces muscle spasm; promotes flow of qi
Fengchi (GB 20)	CrN.XI	Regulates blood; activates qi
Jianjing (GB 21)	CrN.XI	Regulates flow of qi

Electro-acupuncture and moxibustion were given once weekly. After 3 sessions, the patient could move the neck freely and there was no more pain. Treatment was stopped. A follow-up check many years later revealed that she had no more trouble with her neck.

ARTHRITIS

Male—35 years old

Complaint:

Aches in various joints since coming to England 2 years ago.

History:

His joints had started to ache especially in the Spring and damp weather. The worst pain was in the left knee joint and the middle finger on the left hand was red and swollen. He was unable to walk properly. Tablets prescribed had not brought him much relief.

On Examination:

He had a pained expression and was walking badly. The left knee joint looked swollen and was painful on palpation. The middle finger particularly on left hand was swollen. Tongue—red with a dry yellow coat. Pulse—fast.

TCM Diagnosis:

Hot Bi Syndrome

Treatment:

Points Used	Nerves Stimulated	TCM Explanations
Dubi (St 35)	L3	Reduces pain and swelling
Xiyan (Ext. pt.)	L3	Ah-shih point to reduce pain
Yinlingquan (Sp 9)	L3–S2	He-sea point and Ah-shih point; reduces heat; removes damp;
Sifeng (Ext. pts.)	C7–T1	Specific for painful joints in the fingers
Daling (P 7)	C7–T1	Clears heat

Electro-acupuncture and moxibustion were given on the above points. At the same time the following herbs were prescribed to be taken daily:

Qin Jiao	(Radix Gentianae Macrophyllae)
Fang Feng	(Radix Ledebouriellae)
Gui Zhi	(Ramulus Cinnamomi)
Du Huo	(Radix Angelicae Pubescentis)
Wei Ling Xian	(Radix Clematidis)
Sang Ji Sheng	(Ramulus Taxilli)

Bai Zhu   (Rhizoma Atractylodis Macrocephalae)
Shudi   (Radix Rehmanniae Praeparata)
Gan Cao   (Radix Glycyrrhizae)

After 2 daily sessions of acupuncture and moxibustion and herbal therapy the pain was reduced. He was advised to continue treatment with just herbs. After a further 8 doses of herbal therapy, he was free from pain.

SCIATICA

Male—53 years old

Complaint:

Pain in the lumbar region radiating to the left leg.

History:

Started about 2 years ago suddenly, for no apparent reason. The pain radiated to the left buttock and down the left thigh to the leg. It had made walking difficult. Sneezing and coughing would exacerbate the pain. He could only lie down in one position. Analgesia had little or no effect. Was given 12 injections of cortisone but relief was only for a short period.

On Examination:

He was limping, and was in obvious pain. Standing up from a sitting position also triggered off more pain. SLR was 45°. Knee jerk reflex was reduced on the left side. Flexion of spine was not possible. Palpation of the lumbar region revealed pain at L5 and S1. Sensation was reduced in the posterior thigh and leg. Tongue—pale with a white coat. Pulse—deep.

TCM Diagnosis:

Kidney Xu

Treatment:

Electro-acupuncture and moxibustion were given on the following points:

Points Used	Nerves Stimulated	TCM Explanations
Ah-shih points at Hua-Tuo L5/S1	L4–S2	Reduces pain
Shenshu (UB 23)	L1–L3	Strengthens function of kidney qi; strengthens the lower back and leg
Weizhong (UB 40)	L4–S2	Relaxes rigidity and pain of the lumbar region and knee
Chengshan (UB 57)	L4–S2	Relieves rigidity fo the muscles and tendons; reduces pain
Guanyuanshu (UB 26)	L4–L5	Tonifies the kidney; regulates the channels
Pangguanshu (UB 28)	L5–S2	Specific for pain and stiffness of the lower back

Huantiao (GB 30)   L2–S3   Luo-connecting point; relieves
                                            rigidity of the muscles, tendons,
                                            joints and leg

Treatment was given twice weekly. The points chosen had a close relationship to the sciatic nerve. The aim was to reduce inflammation and relieve the pressure on the nerve in addition to reducing pain.

After 4 sessions, the pain was reduced and he could walk better. After one more session he was well enough for treatment to stop.

TENDON ACHILLES PAIN

Male—40 years old

Complaint:

A painful area in the right Achilles tendon.

History:

He was training frequently for a marathon. When the pain started, he continued training in spite of the pain. It became swollen. He was prescribed analgesia and advised to rest for a week. The swelling was reduced but the pain remained.

On Examination:

He was walking with a limp. There was one particularly painful spot on palpation. There was still a slight swelling but no redness. It felt comparatively warmer than the left side. There was no problem with plantar flexion. Dorsal flexion was painful.

Treatment:

Points Used	Nerves Stimulated	TCM Explanations
Taixi (K 3) needled through to Kunlun (UB 60)	L4–S2	Reduces pain and inflammation
Sanyingjiao (Sp 6)	L4–S3	Reduces pain and inflammation

Treatment was given once a week. After two sessions, he felt completely better. Since then he had continued running and entering marathons but with only the occasional treatment.

ANKLE PAIN

Male—40 years old

Complaint:

Pain in the left ankle for the past 2 days.

History:

Sprained the left ankle. It was still swollen and painful. He had to walk with the help of a stick. Analgesia was giving temporary relief.

On Examination:

The ankle was red and swollen, obscuring the lateral swollen.

TCM Diagnosis:

Bi Syndrome

Treatment:

Points Used	Nerves Stimulated	TCM Explanations
Daling (P 7)	C7–T1	Shu-stream and yuan source point; part of Jie Yin Channel of the Hand and Foot
Kunlun (UB 60) needling through to	L4–S2	Jing-river point point; reduces stagnation and pain
Taixi (K 3)		Shu-stream and yuan-source point; reduces stagnation and pain
Xuanzhong (GB 39)	L4–S1	One of the 8 influential points; clears channels; strengthens the muscles, tendons and reinforces bones
Qiuxu (GB 40)	L4–S1	Yuan-source point; relieves rigidity of joints; reduces pain and swelling
Shenmai (UB 62)	S1–S2	Improves circulation; reduces pain

Daling is chosen in these conditions because it is the reflection of the ankle joint on the upper limb. This point is effective for acute ankle strain. This was the only point used on the first session with just neutral manipulation. The patient was advised to move the ankle when the needle was manipulated. Immediately after the treatment, the patient was able walk without his stick and the pain was less.

2 days later, the swelling was very much reduced and the lateral malleolus was visible. The pain was also reduced. The rest of the above points were then used for electro-acupuncture and moxibustion. Treatment was given on alternate days, and after 2 further sessions, the ankle was completely better.

Comments:

The use of Daling for acute ankle strain is from experience over the centuries. It seemed to reduce pain and inflammation very effectively in these circumstances.

TENNIS ELBOW

Male—39 years old

Complaint:

Pain in the right lateral epicondyle for the past 5 months.

History:

Had been playing tennis for many years. Started playing on a more regular basis recently. The pain was worse in the cold weather. Gripping would trigger the pain along the arm. Had a cortisone injection which gave relief for two days. Was given a second injection which had no effect.

On Examination:

The right lateral epicondyle was painful on palpation and extended to the medial and lateral forearm. There was a slight swelling visible and the pain was made worse by gripping. Tongue—pale and dull with a thin white coat. Pulse—normal.

Diagnosis:

Bi syndrome

Treatment:

Electro-acupuncture and moxibustion were used on the following points:

Points Used	Nerves Stimulated	TCM Explanations
Ah Shih		
Quchi (LI. 11)	C5–T1	He-Sea point; promotes blood flow
Shousanli (LI. 10)	C5–C8	Clears channel.

Treatment was given on alternate days, and the pain was gone after 3 treatments. A follow-up 6 years later, revealed that the patient no longer suffered with the same problem in spite of continued tennis.

Comment:

This is a common complaint and not just among tennis players. The effectiveness of acupuncture is probably partly due to the anti-inflammatory reaction resulting from the needle stimulation.

DE QUERVAIN'S TENOSYNOVITIS

Female—44 years old

Complaint:

Pain extending from the right shoulder to the right wrist.

History:

The patient had been suffering for the past few years. It was diagnosed as De Quervain's Tenosynovitis of the right wrist and thumb and capsulitis of the right shoulder joint. Pain was present around the rotator cuff muscles and in the neck. Movement was limited in the affected shoulder. She was not able to lift up a cup of tea and requires assistance for many daily tasks. The first consultation with the GP was in 1995 and painkillers were prescribed. The condition worsened over the following year and finally the patient was unable to continue working. She was given multiple steroid injections at the wrist. Acupuncture was tried at one stage. She attended the local pain clinic but so far all attempts had failed to reduce the pain. Consequently, she felt tearful and depressed. A report from the Rheumatology Department in 1996 revealed that she had been suffering from intermittent pain in the neck and right hand for 5 years. The report also states that, she had additional symptoms of parasthesia in the 4th and 5th fingers of the right hand and weakness when gripping. There was pain on later flexion of the affected arm. There was a reasonable range of movement otherwise. She was taking Voltoral 50 mg. three times a day as well as Coproxamol and Codidramol without reduction of the pain. A course of physiotherapy was tried without any success. There were no neurological findings in the arms. There was a presence of tenderness over the acromio-clavicular joint. Range of movement of the shoulder was normal and pain free. The area over the anatomical snuffbox on the right was tender. Cervical x-rays were normal. NSA creams, the TENS machine and ultrasound treatment had been used. An MRI scan of the wrists was normal.

On Examination:

The patient's symptoms had not altered from the above.

Treatment:

Points Used	Nerves Stimulated	TCM Explanations
Jianjing (GB 21)	CrN.XI	Reduces pain in the shoulder and neck; clears the channels

Jianqian (Ext. Pt.)	C4; C5; C6	Reduces pain in the shoulder and neck; clears the channels
Jianzhen (SI 9)	C5–T2	Promotes blood circulation
Ext. Pt. on Deltoid Muscle	C5–C6	Local point to reduce pain
Dorsum of wrist	C5–C6	Ah Shih point to reduce pain
Yangxi (LI 11)	C6–C7	Jing-river pt. of the Large Intestine; expels wind, relaxes muscles and ten- dons; relaxes the rigidity of local joints

Acupuncture and moxibustion were given on the above points. The patient came for treatment irregularly. After 7 sessions, the pain was reduced. She decided to return to work, but the pain soon returned as a result.

GOLFER'S ELBOW

Female—25 years old

Complaint:

Pain in the medial epicondyle on the right side.

History:

The patient has been a computer keyboard operator for more than 4 years. About one year ago, she felt pain on flexion and external rotation of the forearm with radiation of the pain along the ulnar side of the arm. Lifting any object with the arm became impossible and was starting to affect her work. Sleep was disturbed.

On Examination:

The medial epicondyle was painful on palpation. Gripping was painful. Extension and internal rotation of the lower arm caused pain to radiate to the little finger. Tongue—red with a slight yellow coat. Pulse—small.

Diagnosis:

Bi syndrome due to Qi and Blood Stagnation

Treatment:

Electro-acupuncture and moxibustion were used on the following:

Points Used	Nerves Stimulated	TCM Diagnosis
Shaohai (Ht 3)	C5–T1	He-sea point; regulates qi to promote blood circulation
Xiaohai (SI 8)	C7–T1	He-sea point; reduces fire; removes stasis
Shenmen (Ht 7)	C8–T1	Shu-stream and Yuan-source point

After four weekly treatments, there was a significant reduction in pain. The following point was added:

Yinlingquan (Sp 9)	L3–S2	He-sea point of the Spleen; removes damp and reduces heat

Only two further treatments were needed. The pain had completely gone.

Comments:

Yinlingquan and Xiaohai are both He-sea points. According to TCM, problems in the upper limb can be treated by corresponding points in the lower limbs.

FROZEN SHOULDER

Female—68 years old

Complaint:

Pain in the left shoulder for the past 3 months.

History:

She had a similar pain about 1 year ago in the right shoulder which was relieved by a cortisone injection. The present pain was radiating along the trapezius and up the neck with difficulty in lateral rotation and abduction of the shoulder. There was no history of trauma. Sleep was disturbed. 2 injections had been given with no effect. Analgesia prescribed was also ineffective.

On Examination:

On palpation, pain was present over the anterior border of the acromio-clavicular joint, the anterior and posterior end of the axillary fold and over the middle deltoid. There was pain on lateral rotation of the shoulder. Tongue—slightly red with a thin white coat and teethmarks. Pulse—deep and small.

TCM Diagnosis:

Bi syndrome from Qi Stagnation

Treatment:

Electro-acupuncture and moxibustion were given on the following:

Points Used	Nerves Stimulated	TCM Explanations
Jianqian (Ext. Pt.)	C4–C6	Ah-Shih point; reduces pain and increase mobility of the joint
Jianyu (LI 15)	C4–C6	Clears and activates the channel to ease joint movement and reduces pain
Jianzhen (SI 9)	C5–T2	Relieves pain
Tiaokou (St. 38) needle through to Chengshan (UB 57)	L4–S2	Improves circulation and reduces pain; relieves rigidity of the muscles and tendons

First, Tiaokou was needled through to Chengshan. While manipulating the needle, the patient was asked to move the shoulder at the same time until movement became freer. Then the rest of the points were needled with electrical stimulation.

FROZEN SHOULDER—CASE 2

Male—31 years old

Complaint:

Frozen shoulder for the past 2 days.

History:

Slept with a window open 2 days ago. On waking, the patient felt a stiffness radiating from the upper part of the spine to the right shoulder. He was unable to move the shoulder and was unable to dress himself. He had taken some analgesia but without effect.

On Examination:

The area over the right side of the neck, scapula and shoulder was tense and painful on palpation. Movement of the right shoulder was negligible. Tongue—pale. Pulse—wiry and slow.

TCM Diagnosis:

Wind Cold affecting Meridians

Treatment:

Points Used	Nerves Stimulated	TCM Explanations
Fengchi (GB 20)	CrN.XI	Dispels wind to remove external syndromes; reduces pain and stiffness in the neck
Jianjing (GB 21)	CrN.XI	Clears the channels to regulate the flow of qi; reduces stiffness and pain in the neck
Lieque (Lu 7)	C5–T1	Expels wind and reduces neck rigidity; luo-connecting point

Electro-acupuncture and moxibustion were given on the above points. After the treatment the patient felt much better. Only one more treatment was required in the following week.

CARPAL TUNNEL SYNDROME

Male—63 years old

Complaint:

Numbness in the thumb, index and middle fingers on the right

History:

Symptoms appeared 2 months ago. Had been working in a kitchen for the past 40 years. Duties generally involve cutting up food. The pain in the past 3 weeks had been in the wrist, radiating up to the elbow. Was not able to sleep.

On Examination:

The tourniquet test had a similar effect with a delay in motor conduction at the wrist on the affected side.

TCM Diagnosis:

Blood and Qi Stagnation

Treatment:

Points Used	Nerves Stimulated	TCM Explanations
Daling (P 7)	C7–T1	Regulates qi and blood; specific for contractive pain in the lower arm
Neiguan (P 6)	C6–T1	Regulates the flow of qi; reduces pain
Quchi (LI 11)	C5–T1	Regulates qi and promotes blood flow; reduces motor impairment
Shousanli (LI 10)	C5–C8	Regulates qi; reduces motor impairment

Electro-acupuncture and moxibustion were given on the above points. The points chosen affect the radial and median nerves thus improving blood circulation and reducing water retention to help relieve the symptoms.

PAIN IN THE GUMS

Female—34 years old

Complaint:

Had been suffering for 2 years with painful gums.

History:

The patient had difficulty biting because of the pain. Cold food or liquids also made the pain worse. A check by the dentist did not reveal any obvious abnormalities except for some slight swelling. After a course of antibiotics, the problem remained.

On Examination:

The gums were slightly red. There was no halitosis. The teeth were slightly loose. Tongue—slightly red. Pulse—small and fast.

TCM Diagnosis:

Xu Fire causing pain in the gums

Treatment:

Points Used	Nerves Stimulated	TCM Explanations
Jiache (St 6)	CrN.VII	Clears heat; reduces pain
Xiaguan (St 7)	CrN.V; CrN.VII	Regulates flow of qi; reduces pain
Hegu (LI 4)	C6–T1	Yuan-source point; removes heat; specific for problems in the mouth
Taixi (K 3)	L4–S2	Yuan-source and shu-stream point; nourishes yin to reduce pathogenic heat; tonifies kidney qi

Only electro-acupuncture was used on the above points. Weekly treatments were given. After 3 weeks, the patient was better.

Index